NUTRITION COUNSELING & COMMUNICATION SKILLS

NUTRITION COUNSELING & COMMUNICATION SKILLS

Katharine R. Curry, PhD, RD

Professor Emeritus
Dietetics and Nutrition Department
Florida International University
Miami, Florida

Amy Jaffe, MS, RD, LD

Director, Dietetic Internship Program
Dietetics and Nutrition Department
Florida International University
Miami, Florida

W.B. SAUNDERS COMPANY

A Division of Harcourt Brace & Company
Philadelphia London Toronto Montreal Sydney Tokyo

W.B. SAUNDERS COMPANY

A Division of Harcourt Brace & Company

The Curtis Center
Independence Square West
Philadelphia, Pennsylvania 19106

Library of Congress Cataloging-in-Publication Data

Curry, Katharine.
  Nutrition counseling and communication skills/Katharine Curry,
Amy Jaffe.—1st ed.

  p.   cm.

  ISBN 0–7216–7298-1

  1. Nutrition counseling.   I. Jaffe, Amy, MS, RD, LD.   II. Title.

RM218.7.C87   1998

362.1'76—dc21   97-34828

NUTRITION COUNSELING AND COMMUNICATION SKILLS   ISBN 0–7216–7298–1

Printed in the United States of America.

Last digit is the print number: 9   8   7   6   5   4   3   2   1

This book is

dedicated to

My daughter, Sally,

and the memory of

my son, Mark

KRC

Evan, Adam, Jesse,

and Dylan

AJ

REVIEWERS

Barbara Eldridge, RD, LD
Good Samaritan & St. Mary's Cancer
  Institute
West Palm Beach, FL

Carol Springer Fishbein, PhD
Licensed Psychologist
Anorexia and Bulimia Resource Center
Coral Gables, FL

Cynthia Hamilton, MS, RD, LD, CNSD
Cleveland Clinic Foundation
Cleveland, OH

Mary Jacob, PhD, RD
California State University
Long Beach, CA

Joan Jarcik, MS, RD
Eating Disorder Specialist
Western Psychiatric Institute and Clinic
University of Pittsburgh Medical Center
Pittsburgh, PA

Diane Juskelis, MS, RD, LD, CNSD
Mercy Hospital Medical Center
Des Moines, IA

Idamarie Laquatra, PhD, RD
Nutrition Consultant
Pittsburgh, PA

Chrysa Mahoney, MS, RD, CD
Fletcher Allen Health Care
Burlington, VT

Marilyn Y. Sampley, PhD, RD, LD
Morehead State University
Morehead, KY

Frances J. Tyus, RD, LD
Cleveland Clinic Foundation
Cleveland, OH

Mary Vaughn, RD, MA, LD
Ingalls Memorial Hospital
Harvey, IL

Sharon Weston, MS, RD
Geisinger Medical Center
Danville, PA

PREFACE

The seeds for this book were sown in the 1960s when a young dietitian climbed out of an ambulance after giving "diet instructions" to a patient on his way home. "What is wrong with this picture?" she said to herself, realizing the patient had not heard a word she had said. He was thinking about going home. "Discharge diets" tended to be like that. Patients eager to resume life at home were not at a teachable moment. Her hospital practice began to change, and readiness of patients began to be recognized.

When the opportunity to join a university faculty presented itself, so did the opportunity to nurture her growing ideas about effective nutrition education and counseling. Her professional interests lay in the development of interpersonal skills that would enhance the translation of nutrition knowledge into healthy food habits. Courses in nutrition education and counseling ensued at both the undergraduate and graduate levels. As the dietetics and nutrition program grew, so did the need for another person to assume the responsibilities of preparing students in counseling skills. A former student with private counseling experience became a colleague and together they began to enhance and expand their expertise in nutrition counseling. Projects that began as classroom instructional materials evolved into a booklet which served as the basis for this book.

The purpose of this book is to help students, dietitians, and nutrition professionals learn and apply interpersonal skills. Employing a problem-solving model, the various chapters cover counseling strategies and techniques, psychological theories, life span considerations for counseling, cross-cultural counseling, emotional factors of nutrition, eating disorders, ethics, and professional aspects of practice. Each chapter opens with goals, learning objectives, and key terms. Numerous case examples and sample dialogues are used throughout the book to illustrate the techniques and theories. At the end of each chapter, students will find Suggestions for Further Learning that challenge them to think critically about different counseling techniques and situations.

Developing this book as it is now presented has been not only a significant professional development for us, but also a very personal experience in the growth of friendship and mutual respect. We had a great deal of fun, a smattering of pain and suffering, and magnificent discussions as we brought to fruition what we have to say to dietetics and nutrition professionals, present and future.

It is of good fortune that other professionals have developed in the overall understanding of the broad scope of dietetics and nutrition practice over the last few

years. There is a burgeoning of interest in counseling and communication skills. In
health care, effectiveness is mandatory for the professional who wishes to excel as
a part of the health-care team.

KATHARINE R. CURRY, PhD, RD

AMY JAFFE, MS, RD, LD

ACKNOWLEDGMENTS

No one can undertake writing a textbook without generous help from a myriad of people. We have been fortunate to be blessed with an excellent group of professionals, friends, and relatives. We wish to express our appreciation and thanks to each of the following:

Our Editor, Maura Connor, who trusted us, nurtured us, and never failed us throughout the entire project; and the staff at W.B. Saunders Company who were uniformly professional and supportive: Victoria Legnini, Editorial Assistant; Shelley Hampton, Production Manager; and Annette Ferran, Copy Editor.

Professionals in the field of psychology who read parts of the manuscript and provided significant guidance: Roslyn Pass, PhD; Eileen Lowe, LCSW; and Scott Brinkmeier, PhD.

Those who read parts of the manuscript and offered medical and/or technical guidance: A. Thom Reece, MD; Bridgett Wilson, RD; Rod Wilson; Katherine Kemling, PhD; Colleen Babcock, RD; Tammy Beasley, RD.

Reviewers, known and unknown, whether we liked the comments or not, were extremely helpful. They made this book much better than it might have been.

People in Colorado Springs who provided access to their library service: Yvonne Steinhauer, RD, Dietetic Internship Director, and Dick Maxwell, RN, librarian, at Penrose Hospital; Dolly Spinuzzi, interlibrary loan, and Lorenzo Guerreri, resource specialist, Pike's Peak Community College; and typist Edna Huston.

Friends and colleagues in Miami, Florida, who helped smooth the road many a time: Judy Blucker, PhD, Acting Dean, and Evelyn Enrione, Associate Dean, at the College of Health, Florida International University, and their staff, Heather Salt, Candace Reese, Tina Coffelt, Kathy Hartnett-Moor, and Susan Yellin; and typists Becky Rodriguez, Zaida Agramonte, Lupe Noboa, and Abbe Breiter; she who also provided technical support and was there for the last marathon; Ezekiel Perez, for leg work in the library; and Linda Hron, MSW, RN, and Beverly Worsdale, for being there emotionally when needed.

Last, and first, and always, our family members both near and far, not already mentioned, and especially Evan, Adam, Jesse, and Dylan Jaffe, Cheryl Reece, and Sally and David Woody.

KATHARINE R. CURRY, PhD, RD

AMY JAFFE, MS, RD, LD

CONTENTS

CHAPTER 5

CHAPTER 6

CHAPTER 7

CHAPTER 8

CHAPTER 9

CHAPTER 1

An Overview of Nutrition Counseling

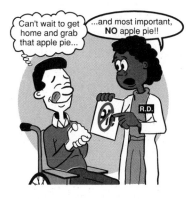

Can't wait to get home and grab that apple pie...

...and most important, NO apple pie!!

R.D.

GOALS

The major goals of this chapter are (1) to provide the rationale behind the development of the book, (2) to briefly present the historical background from which medical nutrition therapy and nutrition counseling in the field of dietetics and nutrition have grown, and (3) to discuss the ways in which this book can be used.

Learning Objectives

At the end of this chapter the reader will be able to:

1. Define key terms that are used throughout the book.

2. Explain medical nutrition therapy and counseling and their place in dietetics and nutrition practice.

3. Use the remainder of the book to enhance interpersonal communication and nutrition counseling skills to facilitate healthy nutrition lifestyles for specific clients.

The ultimate goal is that, by the end of this book, the reader will know more about human beings, will be more creative, sensitive, and flexible, and will have improved skills in counseling people about nutrition.

Key Terms

▶ Nutrition Lifestyle: the way in which people nourish themselves, affected by environmental factors such as socioeconomic status as well as internal factors such as biological needs, personality, values, and beliefs.

▶ Dietitian/Nutritionist/Dietetic Practitioner: a registered dietitian or other professional with a comprehensive scientific background in dietetics and nutrition.

▶ Medical Nutrition Therapy: the process of guiding a client toward a desirable nutrition lifestyle as needed for the treatment and/or prevention of certain disease states and for solving problems that are barriers to change.

▶ Nutrition Counseling: the process of guiding a client toward a healthy nutrition lifestyle by meeting normal nutritional needs and solving problems that are barriers to change. *Medical nutrition therapy* and *nutrition counseling* are essentially interchangeable; but in general, the term *medical nutrition therapy* is

1

used in this text in situations in which medical treatment of disease is involved, and the term *nutrition counseling* is used when counseling is an approach to disease prevention and general good health.

▸ **Medical Nutrition Therapist or Nutrition Counselor:** professional dietitian or nutritionist who engages in nutrition counseling.

▸ **Medical Model:** a prescriptive style of health care in which the professional instructs the client/patient what to do and expects passive compliance.

▸ **Guidance Model:** a participative style of health care in which the professional and client/patient work together to plan a nutrition lifestyle that will meet the goals of the client/patient's overall lifestyle.

▸ **Client/Patient:** the recipient of medical nutrition therapy, nutrition counseling, and/or other nutrition health care. The preferred term is *client,* although there are certain settings (hospitals, long-term care, doctors' offices) in which people receiving health care are called *patients.*

This book is about people—clients, patients, and interested individuals—who must or want to make nutrition choices that will enhance and lengthen a healthy life; in other words, to develop a healthy nutrition lifestyle. It is directed toward those professionals who advance the science of nutrition and translate that knowledge into human food choices. This is a major function of dietitians and nutrition professionals (Payne-Palacio & Canter, 1996; Derelian & Gilbride, 1995). The purpose of the book is to help preprofessional students and professionals to better understand clients and to increase counseling skills.

Traditionally, the professional nutrition community has been more focused on biological aspects of nutrition, but it is clear that physiological biochemistry provides only partial answers to problems in human nutrition. The natural tendency of this still-young profession is to move toward a comprehensive approach to human nutrition—to recognize its central role in every aspect of human life. Formal instruction in social and psychological aspects of nutrition have been added to preprofessional education as an essential component of professional competence. In addition, practicing professionals have become acutely aware that the marketplace requires skill in interpersonal relations and counseling. There is a surge of activity in continuing education to upgrade interpersonal skills of all types, including counseling skills.

The rapid growth of scientific information and an understanding of the inextricable nature of biological, sociological, and psychological factors in human life have made an encompassing approach to human nutrition inevitable. The inter-relationships are circular: "you eat what you are" and "you are what you eat" (Barer-Stein, 1979). The body has the opportunity to make use of nutrients only after an individual has made the choice to put something into the mouth (except in cases of young children or individuals so ill that they cannot feed themselves). In the past, this created a dichotomy of focus among students of nutrition—the nutrition phenomena that occur before the lips (BL) and the nutrition phenomena that occur after the lips (AL). People studied these phenomena from one point of view or the other, sometimes disregarding the data, facts, concepts, and theories of other points of view. Sociologists, anthropologists, and psychologists have focused on BL phenomena. Dietitians, nutritionists, and health researchers have tended to focus on AL phenomena. There is a trend toward interdisciplinary research; hopefully, it will continue and result in a much more comprehensive understanding of how to ensure optimal human nutrition. The field of dietetics and nutrition is unique in the endeavor to comprehend both. Practice is in the arena of applying scientific knowledge to facilitating healthy nutrition beliefs and behavior that develop into a lifestyle—a healthy nutrition lifestyle. Figure 1–1 depicts the many aspects that the profession of dietetics encompasses (Payne-Palacio & Canter, 1996).

This book is also intended to assist the reader in increasing the activity in the right side of the brain, that part of the brain where creativity takes place. Much of dietetic and nutrition education addresses scientific principles that are primarily a function of the left side of the brain, that part of the brain that specializes in verbal, logical, and analytical thinking. The right side of the brain uses a contrasting method of information processing that relies mainly on visual and spatial functions to perceive the world in holistic or intuitive ways. Although the right brain may be well developed in some people, the right brain has not been as highly utilized as the left in dietetics and nutrition (Edwards, 1986). At the 1995 Annual Meeting of

The Profession of Dietetics

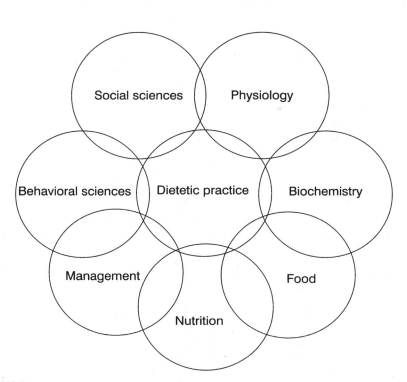

FIGURE 1–1. The profession of dietetics. (From Payne-Palacio J, Canter DD: *The Profession of Dietetics: A Team Approach.* © 1996. Reprinted by permission of Prentice-Hall, Upper Saddle River, NJ.)

the American Dietetic Association, Harry S. Dent, Jr., speaking about "Future Trends in the Marketplace," advised the audience that computers can perform left-brain functions as well or even better than people. What the computer cannot duplicate is creativity, intuition, and holistic thinking—a right-brain function. In essence, he warned that computers are taking over many of the left-brain functions of humans, such as calculations, standardizations, clerical work, and bureaucratic systems. Computers can do that sort of work so much better and more quickly than the human brain that those jobs requiring mostly left-brain tasks are becoming obsolete. What are required and what can never be taken over by computers are all the right-brain functions that humans possess. These include feeling, creativity, sensitivity, and flexibility to changing situations and people.

When it comes to predicting people's success, brain power as measured by intelligence quotient (IQ) and standardized testing (left-brain function) may not be as important as a person's emotional intelligence. Emotional intelligence (EQ), a right-brain function, includes a person's character, understanding of one's own feelings, empathy for the feelings of others, response to stress, and "the regulation of emotion in a way that enhances living" (Goleman, 1995). A cornerstone of emotional intelligence is a sense of self-awareness, of being smart about feelings. Deficient emotional skills may be the reason that more than half of all marriages end in divorce. Human resources executives have been quoted as saying that "IQ gets you hired, but EQ gets you promoted."

When this theory is extrapolated to the field of dietetics and nutrition, the traditional idea of counseling through nutrient calculations, diet instruction, and education can and soon will be the job of computer software (left brain, IQ), which can provide information. Yet it is well known that simply knowing about nutrition often does not bring about changes. It is the motivation to change that brings about change. It is the professional's interpersonal skills, empathy, and the ability to sense clients' attitudes (right brain, EQ) that will endure as motivational tools. The necessary function of the dietitian or nutritionist is not only to know nutrition but also to facilitate behavior changes.

HISTORICAL BACKGROUND

The current profession of dietetics and nutrition evolved from two different roots: university-based nutrition programs and hospital-based medical care. In the United States, the study of human nutrition was largely an outgrowth of efforts to educate American farmers. Land grant colleges were established in every state in the latter part of the 1800s toward this effort. The Iowa Agricultural School was probably the first college to offer cookery courses in 1872. Animal nutrition was an important curriculum entity. During the early 1900s, it was recognized that for the farmers of America to develop fully there was a need for an educational system for the wives of farmers. Human nutrition was essential in this curriculum, which was called *home economics*. Simultaneously, scientists in the medical field were giving more attention to human nutrition and disease in the wake of the discovery of vitamins. In colleges, women scientists were focusing on nutrition; and in hospitals, a specialty in producing scientifically based menus was developing. Although nurses often moved into these fields, nutrition soon was the province of women who had an educational background in home economics at a college or university. These women subsequently completed internships in hospital food service.

In all aspects of nutrition, the focus was on physiological chemistry and biochemistry. A review of the early years of publication of the *Journal of the American Dietetic Association* indicates that 1929 was the first year in which an article appeared that addressed cultural and psychological phenomena in nutrition. World War II provided a breakthrough in the recognition that people choose food not primarily because of scientific knowledge, but because they are used to it or they like it. It was critical that fighting men and women be well nourished, and military personnel (unless starved) wouldn't eat unless they liked the food. In some cases, menus were modified to reflect cultural preferences. The first hedonic scales, measures of pleasure factors, were developed to survey the troops about the pleasures of different foods so that menus might reflect their desires. Billions of cookies, crumbly cakes, and other foods were shipped to fighting men and women to exemplify love, longing, and prayers for a safe return. In a very subtle and unconscious way, a great shift in the scientific understanding of human nutrition was taking place, and the BL aspects of nutrition began to receive closer scientific scrutiny among nutritionists. In 1996, approximately 25 articles addressing the social and psychological aspects of nutrition were published in the *Journal of the American Dietetic Association*. Indeed, several other journals have come into existence that specifically address matters of nutrition education and counseling.

The first hospitals in the United States were founded in Pennsylvania in the 1700s. Mush and molasses was the usual meal in these hospitals, with a pint of beer included for dinner. In the hospitals of the early years of the 20th century, there was little consideration of hedonics in food service, but there was a growing recognition that diet therapy could affect the treatment of disease. Disease-specific special menus began to be used. Some were more scientific than others. Diet therapy as practiced in the early 1900s consisted of various special diets such as the Sippy Diet for ulcers: cream and poached eggs. In many places, doctors prescribed special diets and dietitians were responsible for carrying out orders. Sarah Tyson Rorer (1849–1937) is considered the first American dietitian. She established the first diet kitchen and dietary counseling service, at the request of some prominent physicians. Discharge diets were provided as patients were leaving the hospital. Patients were instructed to eat or not eat certain foods, and compliance was expected. Many times, the process had little effect (Payne-Palacio & Canter, 1996).

In the ensuing years, the health-care community recognized that in a multicultural environment such as exists in the United States, the prescriptive method (the medical model), by which the person in authority tells the patient what to do, with expectation of passive compliance, was not working. Changes in the direction of a guidance model have occurred, and there is a general attitude today that a biopsychosocial model with significant client/patient involvement in treatment is more effective.

More importantly, as we face the 21st century in a multicultural society, it is recognized that there is no one "right way." A health-care professional needs to be proficient in several ways of approaching patients/clients. Flexibility in tailoring messages to coincide with attitudes, beliefs, and values of a wide range of cultures is needed to be effective for people of diverse backgrounds.

Today, in the field of dietetics and nutrition, it is recognized that the reasons most people do not eat what they "should" have little to do with basic science, knowledge, or the information that is available. Nutrition lifestyle is much more influenced by the meanings food has for an individual. Bringing cohesion between these meanings and scientific knowledge is a challenging task. In fact, there is a tendency in our modern world of high technological communication to proliferate so much information or misinformation that it becomes confusing rather than helpful.

WHY PEOPLE DO NOT CHANGE THEIR NUTRITION LIFESTYLE

People often do not change what they eat because it requires changing feelings, attitudes, and cultural habits. One major feeling is love. People show and receive love through food. Most tellingly, infants experience life in all its meanings through nonverbal sensors, especially through food. Giving and taking food remain major social rituals throughout life. There appears to be an array of reasons that people have difficulty changing food habits. These may include, but are not limited to, the following:

▮ Tendencies toward rebelliousness
▮ A way of denying the existence of problems
▮ Psychological illness
▮ General feelings of anxiety and depression
▮ Interpersonal relationships that may be threatened by change
▮ Lack of immediate desirable results
▮ The huge time and energy commitment required to change one's nutrition lifestyle

The last point is significant. Not only is an individual hesitant to make the time and energy commitment (note the many *quick* weight-loss diets), but society is also hesitant. Time and energy translate into money, and our society is currently negative toward extended health-care costs.

The professional needs to have knowledge about how these problems or barriers to changing can be overcome. Individuals with a background in logic, experimentation, and scientific "proof" may, at first, be uncomfortable addressing these problems that are barriers to the development of a healthy nutrition lifestyle. Barriers are often vague, and discovering them requires intervention in the life of the client. The knowledge base underlying social and psychological aspects of nutrition knowledge is more heuristic—more philosophical or opinion-based and less scientific. Theories are much more difficult to prove, which is a real hazard among people used to more provable concepts. Nevertheless, a great deal of study has been conducted on the sociology of food, the anthropology of food, and the psychology of food that has merit, even though heuristic. The reader is urged to look seriously at these for information that can broaden a perspective, especially when there are gaps of data or when a particular approach is not working. Subsequent chapters contain selected information from all of these fields, along with concrete suggestions for combining the information with the scientific principles of nutrition to help people develop a healthy nutrition lifestyle. It is well known that people make changes when it seems in their best interest to do so, and it is up to the medical nutrition therapist to help people recognize what is in their best interests. This is the unique function of the dietetic practitioner. The laboratory scientist can tell us the processes and results of nutrient intake; the psychologist, sociologist, and anthropologist can tell us about people and how to create change. However, it is when all these aspects of human nutrition are addressed that the client is served.

HOW TO USE THIS BOOK

This book can be used in several ways: as a preprofessional systematic way of learning the skills of medical nutrition therapy; by a professional medical nutrition therapist to enhance effectiveness and solve problems when counseling seems to be less effective than desired; or by other people whose responsibilities include nutrition counseling.

The primary target of this book is the upper level undergraduate or internship student in a professional dietetics and nutrition program. It is expected that the student has at least some exposure through general education to principles of sociology, psychology, and perhaps anthropology. A systematic approach to nutrition counseling is presented. There are also activity suggestions for further learning and practicing concepts. Practice is the activity most certain to develop skill.

The secondary target is the professional medical nutrition therapist (MNT) who can use the material as a way to enhance skills in counseling and as a resource in troubleshooting when counseling does not seem to be effective. The MNT can refer to specific parts of the book that address a particular problem that he or she may be facing in practice. It can serve as a review and reference for additional resources if the practitioner needs more in-depth study of some concept or theoretical approach to a client who presents as a puzzling difficulty. It is not intended that an MNT try to become a psychological counselor, but that the client can be approached in ways that are known to be motivating. It is recommended that every MNT work with a psychological counselor as a consultant or on a team in which several health-care professionals pool their expertise to treat the client/patient as a whole person.

It will be noted that the words *compliance, adherence, diet,* and other similar terms are avoided as much as possible in the text. The focus is on clients and on addressing and solving concerns and problems that stand in the way of a desirable nutrition lifestyle. Emphasis is on solutions.

People bring their own personality with them to nutrition counseling and will respond in a variety of ways. An MNT who is flexible in approach will be more apt to reach the motivational levels in different people. These differences are not dependent on the disease entity but on the person, and, as such, there has been an effort to keep the focus on individuals. Effective communication is important whether a professional is working with people who want to stay healthy longer or with people who have a specific disease. Professionals in acute-care facilities do not have the same opportunity for medical nutrition therapy over time, but they will understand patients better and become more effective in guiding patients toward outpatient care that can have long-term success. The adage, "counselor, know thyself" is emphasized throughout the text. In each chapter the reader will be asked to look within; whether it be in terms of ethical issues, cross-cultural counseling, or patterns of assertiveness. If you understand yourself, you will be able to understand and then guide others much more effectively.

The book reviews the general meaning of food, followed by a discussion of the problem-solving approach that is a process for counseling. Following that, theoretical and creative elements that are the essence of counseling are discussed. Disease entities identified as having a psychological basis are addressed in detail. Lastly, specific areas of concern in professional communication and conducting nutrition counseling business are covered.

Chapter 2, The Meanings of Food, is a brief review of the general meanings of food. It is intended to remind the reader of basic human needs. It is very general in tone. The references in this chapter are resources for specific situations in which more depth of understanding is required. This chapter sets the stage for more in-depth discussion throughout the remainder of the book.

Chapter 3, The Problem-Solving Counseling Method, presents a comprehensive process method for problem-solving nutrition counseling that helps to clarify the direction and goals of counseling in a way that guides the counselor toward a desirable outcome with a client. The method also provides a system for monitoring the progress of counseling. The emphasis is on the client and on finding solutions that depend on what the "real" problems and concerns may be for the client.

Chapter 4, Nutrition Counseling Strategies, presents a number of strategies that are particularly useful to the MNT. A few specific techniques are offered that will help the beginner develop skill and confidence in her or his ability to facilitate client change. There are other suggestions for counseling approaches that will add to the flexibility of the MNT and enable him or her to focus more on the individual and draw on a variety of strategies to fit the personality and needs of the client. Empowerment of clients, a goal of nutrition counseling, is discussed at length. The experienced MNT can use this chapter to build her or his own creative approaches to facilitate change. All of the strategies presented have been used successfully in nutrition counseling. It is intended that the reader practice the techniques in simulated experiences or in practice. When she or he feels comfortable with one strategy she or he can begin to learn additional strategies, and even make some up. The long-term goal is to develop creativity and flexibility in interacting with clients.

Chapter 5, Psychological Perspectives, is a brief review of selected theories and models of human psychology that are influential in current psychological counseling practices. Currently, no single psychological theory is successful in satisfactorily explaining individual human psyche. Because of this, the dietetic practitioner needs to draw on different theories. If a client does not fit well in one theory, it can help to look at another theory to see if more insight can be gained about the client. It is intended that each theory add a dimension to the counselor's ability to "read" people, not to say that one or the other theory is more or less correct. Humanist psychology perspectives tells us more about personality structure; behavioral and cognitive perspectives tells us more about cognition and some rather specific counseling techniques that often, but not always, work well. It is well known that in the long run it is not the mechanics of counseling that has the greatest effect, but the interpersonal relationship that develops. The humanists have been more attuned to factors of empathy, trust, and other nontangible aspects of counseling. Behavioral and cognitive psychologists have tended toward tangible, measurable aspects of human psychology.

Chapter 6, Counseling Across the Life Span, offers a review of the context in which nutrition counseling takes place. It reviews human growth and development and provides a summary of the different needs of individuals over the life span. The types of interventions that are most effective for people in different stages of development are discussed. The information is intended to increase flexibility on the part of the MNT.

Chapter 7, Cross-Cultural Counseling, focuses on the differences the MNT will encounter among different cultures. A major variable in understanding cultural differences is an understanding of one's own culture and the bias it presents in the counselor. The overwhelming tendency to stereotype is discussed. To avoid stereotyping, the text contains minimal culture-specific information and a maximum of information on how to go about learning about different cultures. Listening to individual clients and studying the immediate environment is the best way to avoid stereotyping to any degree. In addition, several references are cited that provide very good information about specific cultures. These should be used to study specific situations.

Chapter 8, Emotional Factors, is a discussion of the most common emotional factors that have a bearing on the receptiveness of clients to nutrition counseling. It is not expected that the MNT do anything about people's feelings other than to be supportive and comfortable in the presence of the expression of emotion. It is important that the MNT be able to recognize when emotional issues are so intense that nutrition counseling should be postponed. It is the responsibility of the MNT to access psychological counseling and other health-care or social services as needed.

Chapter 9, Eating Disorders, addresses diseases that have been designated as psychological diseases in which the MNT has a definite role in a team effort to treat patients/clients. It is recommended that the MNT always work with a team in treating these psychological disease states. The MNT needs to work within the theoretical perspective of the medical and psychological members of the team. There are differences of opinion about approach among these professionals. It may be that the approach presented in this text is not the approach that others practice. There are legitimate differences of opinion about the treatment of eating disorders and these must be considered in individual situations. Because treating people with eating disorders is highly specialized, many practical examples and forms are provided for guidance.

Chapter 10, Ethics, is devoted to the ethical issues confronted in dietetics and nutrition practice. Although not directly related to counseling, the ethical considerations of feeding the terminally ill are discussed because questions of feeding often arise in situations in which a dietitian/nutritionist will be called upon to counsel the family of a patient. Ethical codes in general are discussed. Bioethics is then explained in terms of legal, medical, and financial considerations. General business and counseling ethics are also explored. The more exposure to ethical issues a person has, the better his or her ethical judgment becomes (Edelstein, 1992).

Chapter 11, Professional Considerations, addresses issues regarding the counseling setting, payment, and professional communication. These issues are not the essence of counseling but are required if a counselor is to function effectively in the health-care system. Clear and precise communication is necessary for appropriate holistic health care of clients. Additionally, assertive communication is needed to educate other professionals and health-care policy-makers to recognize the function of medical nutrition therapy and nutrition counseling in the cost control of health care. Before medical nutrition therapy and counseling can become an accepted part of health-care treatment, MNTs must not only work effectively with clients but in many cases must also become advocates of the process and advocates for clients in utilizing health-care services. For instance, at a 1996 conference on pediatric nutrition, several speakers mentioned that managed-care organizations (such as HMOs) would expect the medical nutrition therapist to be cognizant of and be able to help solve any problem that might be presented by the client. The therapist does not have to solve the problem personally, but should be able to access the resources needed (Pediatric Conference, 1996).

Although certain individuals under certain circumstances make sudden and significant changes, most people make changes in small segments over time. The problem-solving approach takes this into consideration. The focus is on medical nutrition therapy over several sessions, rather than one session, in an outpatient environment. However, there are still many situations in which dietetic practitioners have only one contact with the patient/client. This should be considered as a nutrition consultation or diet instruction, not as counseling. Nutrition consultations are best utilized for providing information and helping patients/clients access additional medical nutrition therapy. However, effective communication is as important in nutrition consultation as in nutrition counseling. The only aspects of counseling that usually are not effective in nutrition consultations are confrontational strategies. An effort is made at certain points in the text to provide examples of ways in which effective communication concepts can be applied to the various settings and circumstances in which dietetic practitioners work.

Summary

The art and science of nutrition counseling is very young, and it is only recently that interdisciplinary considerations in human nutrition have become appreciated. The medical nutrition therapist is the major professional to bring interdisciplinary knowledge to bear on efforts to influence nutrition lifestyle, by the translation of nutrition knowledge into specific action behaviors. Interpersonal communication skill is essential in this role. The development of skill is equal to the acquisition of knowledge in professional competence. Each reader is urged to take ideas from this book and let the right brain work on them creatively to enhance professional competence. Enjoy the rest of the book!

Suggestions for Further Learning

1. Define the role of the medical nutrition therapist (MNT).

2. Interview professionals in the field of dietetics and nutrition to discover their approaches to counseling patients.

3. For professionals already practicing, define your own role as a counselor as you saw it 5 years ago, today, and 5 or 10 years in the future.

4. Read the rest of this text with an open (right) mind and be willing to experiment with some of the ideas that are new to you.

CITED REFERENCES

Barer-Stein T: *You Are What You Eat: A Study of Ethnic Food Traditions.* Toronto: McClelleand and Stewart Ltd, 1979.

Conference on Pediatric Nutrition for Children with Special Needs. Denver, Colorado, Sept. 23, 1996.

Dent HS: Future Trends in the Market Place. American Dietetic Association Annual Meeting, Orlando, FL, Oct. 24, 1995.

Derelian D, Gilbride J: President's page: Positions—an important means of fulfilling our mission and vision. *J Am Diet Assoc.* 1995;95(1):92.

Edelstein S: Development of moral judgment and its relationship to the education and training of dietitians. *J Am Diet Assoc.* 1992;92(8):938–941.

Edwards B: *Drawing on the Artist Within.* New York: Simon & Schuster, 1986.

Goleman D: *Emotional Intelligence.* New York: Bantam Books, 1995.

Payne-Palacio J, Canter DD. *The Profession of Dietetics: A Team Approach.* Englewood Cliffs, NJ: Prentice-Hall, 1996.

CHAPTER 2

The Meanings of Food

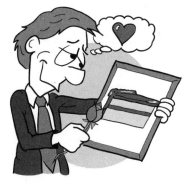

GOALS

The goals of this chapter are (1) to review generally the wide range of viewpoints regarding the meaning that food has for humans and (2) to interest the reader in probing clients to discover individual meanings of food in the process of counseling.

Learning Objectives

At the end of this chapter the reader will be able to:

1. Articulate the personal meaning food has for him or her.

2. Identify various ways in which the meaning of food influences food choices.

3. List ways in which various researchers study food meanings.

4. Effectively question others about the meaning of food.

Air, water, food, shelter, reproduction: these are the physical necessities of life. But of these, none seems to symbolize the essence of life more than food. Life is organized around obtaining food and eating. In areas of the world where food is less abundant, physical survival is paramount. In this part of the world, where food is abundant and threats of starvation are diminished, true to Maslow's hierarchy of needs, food is used to help fulfill our higher psychological needs, such as the need for love, belonging, status, and self-fulfillment (Kittler & Sucher, 1989). Food means life, love, and the pursuit of happiness. Food means danger, passion, and identity. "Soul food" feeds our spirituality as well as our bodies. Food is power, and giving of food is a most prestigious exertion of power. Food is hospitality, romance, pleasure, and security. Food is health, and food is death. All of these descriptions of food can be found in scientific literature, novels, poems, advertisements, music, art, language, and human memory.

One of the unique attributes of humans is the fact that, unlike for other animals, for us there is a difference between feeding and eating. Feeding is instinct-driven consumption. Human eating behavior is social and depends as much on learning, motivation, attitudes, values, social factors, and emotions as on physical needs. Interactions among these factors are involved in why people eat what they eat and why food habits are extremely resistant to change (Fieldhouse, 1995). Both the point of view, "we are what we eat" (physical transformation) and "we eat what we are" (cultural determination of food choice) have been expressed by students of human eating phenomena.

Eating and feeling seem to be primal links between physical survival and psychosocial growth. First one must survive, then psychosocial growth embellishes the meaning of food and intertwines it with meanings of love, one's place in the world, and consciousness of the pleasure of eating. The exact nature of the interaction between food and feeling is elusive and has been studied only rudimentarily. However, in the very recent past there has been increased interest in why people eat what they do and why their food habits are so resistant to change (Axelson & Brinberg, 1989).

The purpose of this chapter is to review, briefly, current knowledge and speculation about the meaning that food has for humans and the implications this has for dietetic and nutrition professionals, especially those engaging in nutrition education and counseling in wellness and medical nutrition therapy. The possibilities for meanings of food are almost endless. The only way to know the mix of meanings that any one client has accumulated is to listen to each client. This chapter looks at more personal meanings. The influences of culture on the meaning of food for clients is addressed in Chapter 7, Cross-Cultural Counseling.

FACTORS AFFECTING FOOD CHOICES

It is ironic that there are few topics which elicit more emotional responses and on which people have stronger opinions than food, yet this topic is so little studied (McIntosh, 1995). Perhaps this is because human beings have always found it much more difficult to study themselves than any other subject. Scientific inquiry into nutrition is little more than 100 years old, and scientific inquiry into the links between human psychology and eating is in its infancy. Most of what we know or believe about the psychosocial aspects of eating has not been rigorously tested. Yet in the practical world of nutrition counseling, we know that habits and lifestyle, including nutrition lifestyle, are the means to the goal of optimal nutritional status. Nutrition concepts are only a small part of the influences on nutrition lifestyle, as shown in Table 2–1.

Other factors affecting the selection of food include biological needs, individual experience, and culture. These factors interact as determinants of food choices at any given time (Barker, 1982).

Biological Needs

Mammals, including humans, have receptors that respond to chemicals, and the result is similar in most animals. Sugars are accepted, bitters rejected. Some proteins stimulate some receptors. Some receptors are stimulated by various salts and acids. Genetics also affects what foods an individual can tolerate.

TABLE 2 – 1

Factors Affecting Food Choices

Biological Factors	Cultural Factors
Nutritional needs	Education
Heredity	Understanding of nutrition/health concepts
Special physiological conditions (eg, pregnancy)	Income
	Social class, status
Special diseases or abnormal conditions	Traditions, beliefs, values
Taste preferences (genetically determined)	Ideology (worldview, religion)
Individual cravings or idiosyncrasies	Communication
	Influence of business, government, professionals
Environmental Factors	Politics
Geography, climate	
Season	
Economics	
Transportation	
Technology	
Fuel availability	

From McIntosh EN: *American Food Habits in Historical Perspective.* Copyright © 1995 by Praeger. Reproduced with permission of Greenwood Publishing Group, Inc, Westport, CT.

Personal Experience

In humans, personal experience can be perceived even in infants. Sweets are especially liked. Sugar remains important throughout life, and many psychological meanings are accumulated. The physiopsychology of food is expected to produce much information about how the human organism controls food intake. Individual experience includes the availability of food. Many factors impinge on the availability of food, such as economics, wars, geography, early feeding experiences, health and illness, and various habits such as the amount of salt used in food. The feelings of satiety or stomach distress are also influential personal experiences.

Cultural Factors

Cultural factors are a major influence and include the rules of the culture in which a person grew up. People who move into different cultures necessarily change if previously accepted foods are no longer available. People may choose to make changes in their nutrition lifestyle as they become acculturated into another society (Kittler & Sucher, 1989). However, flavor remains an overriding variable (Barker, 1982).

Effective counseling relationships that open the door to nutrition education and the MNT's influence on clients depend upon understanding and accepting not only the importance of food as a biological need, but also food's centrality to life and its role in meeting psychosocial needs. A major aspect of nutrition education, counseling, or medical nutrition counseling is discovering both obvious and less obvious meanings attributed to food by the individual client and utilizing these meanings to influence change.

EATING AND FEELING

It has been said that only two things are inevitable in life, death and taxes. The person who said that missed two other major inevitabilities—eating and feeling. They, too, are inevitable throughout life, the two inexorably linked from earliest childhood. Interactions between the two play a role in our growth and development in stature and in mind. Beginning with the first feeding, the connections and linkages between food and the fulfillment of human needs are being established. Not only are biological needs being met, but also identity and perceptions of the relationships between the child and the world. Throughout life, meaning is added, often unconsciously, rituals are formed, and invisible threads stitch together food and self. Upon superficial examination they may seem unconnected, but they do produce "tenacious biases regarding food habits, which reflect our cultural conditioning and experience" (McIntosh, 1995).

Early Childhood

In early childhood, two developmental events have a strong influence on the union of eating and feeling in our lives. First is the dependence on our caretakers for nourishment, and second is our need for independence. The newborn baby eats, feels, and sleeps, and thus an inescapable fusion of eating and feeling begins. The baby learns about its world, its caretakers, its place in the world. Lifelong attitudes are formed by the quality of this interaction (Satter, 1987). Within a few months, however, dependence is recognized as a burden and the slow, lifelong drive for independence begins.

Dependence

The infant is totally dependent on caretakers to meet his or her needs. The quality of the caretaking will set the tone of life. Feeding is probably the most important, with warmth being second. A large proportion of the human contact the baby has is during feeding time.

The way in which a baby is held during feeding, stroked by voice or hand, provides the child with information as to her or his place in the world. The process of feeding relays different messages, depending on the treatment of the child. For instance, a baby who is fed on demand, with accompanying petting and cooing, is likely to make different connections with food than one who is fed on a strict schedule, cries from hunger for a period of time, and is too tired to eat when food is presented. The feeding relationship can be loving and comforting, relieving stress, or it can be a struggle. The normal child who eats well generally will feel well, and a child who does not eat well may not feel well and in response eat poorly (Satter, 1987).

Feelings of Well-Being

Anyone who has ever heard a newborn baby cry is acutely aware of the intensity and urgency of feeling embodied in the communication—a demand for immediate attention. We recognize a pressing need and translate the message to "feed me," "warm me," "love me," "make me comfortable." When we hear the stress in the infant's cry, we might characterize the crying as indicating anger, fear, or physical pain. We see stress in the little body—tight fists, tense body, a flushed face.

Unless we have evidence to the contrary, our first thought upon hearing the cry of demand is that the baby is hungry, and so we offer food. If this works, everything is OK and the baby learns that food relieves stress (so does the caretaker). We can recognize by the relaxation of the body and perhaps by some cooing sounds as that the baby is happy, content, and calm. The message to the baby is clear and linear: feel stress, get food, feel good (within and about myself).

Feelings of Discomfort

Positive relationships between food and self are generally assumed, yet there may be negative relationships of deep significance being developed among children who have unpleasant feeding experiences in infancy. For instance, forced feeding, pinching the cheeks, and thrusting a hard spoon into a baby's mouth are probably as unpleasant to a baby as to an adult. Trying to make people understand what you want with such a rudimentary communication system (only being able to push the food away when you do not want it, or fussing and crying) is undoubtedly frustrating to a baby. When feeding experiences are negative, neurotic problems can result. Eating disorders can have roots in early feeding experiences (Satter, 1987).

When feeding does not relieve stress, the resulting message is negative (discomfort—eat—no relief). There are many possible reasons for unpleasant consequences of eating. Indigestion or colic may produce an undesirable link between eating and feeling bad. A suboptimal caring environment may create negative or confused eating-and-feeling messages. A caretaker might not recognize a baby's satiety level, for instance, and overfeed or underfeed a baby, perhaps reducing the natural biological hunger/satiety mechanisms. A nervous mother may transfer her feelings to a baby, or an irritated father may transfer his feelings.

Independence

A second emotional entanglement with food results from our efforts at self-control and independence. Even the very small infant soon learns to accept or reject the nipple at will. Erikson identified biting the nipple that fed him or her as the child's first social task of independence (Erikson, 1963). Soon the baby wants to hold the bottle and just as soon (or even before) motor skills are developed for self-feeding, the little people are in a control battle to feed themselves. The following case example illustrates such a battle.

CASE EXAMPLE ·

A young mother became quite worried about the nutrition status of her 9-month-old who ate little more than green beans for about 3 weeks. He absolutely refused to let anyone feed him. He couldn't manage a spoon and he couldn't pick up any food with his fingers except green beans or some properly cut up potatoes, carrots, and so on, but he liked the green beans best. The MNT reassured the mother that her child's nutritional status would survive this psychological growth and he would develop into a more independent person.

· ·

The need for independence does not diminish throughout life and often consti-
tutes the one aspect of life most easily and lastingly controlled by the individual.
The area of growth for a child striving for adulthood is an eternal shift from dependence to independence with each accomplishment. And, although we do not
live in this world alone and isolated from other living things, independence and the
acquisition of the ability to be self-sustaining and self-nurturing is a critical aspect
of an individual's ability to survive and thrive.

Later Childhood

As children become toddlers, begin school, and become teenagers, feelings about
food continue to develop, likes and dislikes form, and more independence of
choice occurs (or does not occur). For most young children, a certain fear is connected with trying new things, including fear of the unknown. When this is handled properly, the child learns to enjoy new foods. Both structure and freedom of
food choice develop positive feelings about food. Restrictive or laissez-faire environments are likely to result in confusion about food, just as they contribute to
confusion about other aspects of life. Satter said: "Parents (and children) get into
trouble when they cross the lines in the division of responsibility" for eating. Parents are responsible for presenting nutritious and enjoyable food; children are responsible for what they eat (Satter, 1987). Life can become a hodge-podge of do's
and don'ts, confusing and angering to a child (McIntosh, 1995). Satter discussed
the love of eating, citing a child whose happy feelings were so intense that they resulted in audible moaning as she ate. The concern in this case was that when such
obvious feelings are not accepted in a child (or adult, for that matter) they can be
pushed "underground" and be part of the cause of disordered eating.

As children become teenagers, independence becomes a major developmental
issue, and food is again a tool of identity. One study reported that adolescent
women divided foods into two groups, health foods and junk foods. The subjects
attributed meaning such as weight gain, pleasure, friends, independence, and guilt
with junk food, and weight loss, parents, and being at home with healthy food
(Chapman & Maclean, 1993). Controlling what one eats becomes a major issue,
and many times control of others is manifested through one's food selection (Lyman, 1989).

Adulthood

The love symbolized by food becomes more apparent in adulthood. Food is not
only received by adults, but is also given. Special foods are given to signify love.
Eating activities are used, such as a trip to a fast food restaurant, to express caring
to a child. Going out to a nice restaurant with another adult can also symbolize
love. There is speculation among some researchers as to the possibility that food
not only symbolizes feelings, but actually becomes a substitute for feeling. Instead
of saying "I love you," food is substituted (Mintz, 1982).

In adults, stress and calmness, unlike the simplicity of feelings in a infant, have
a whole range of descriptor words—fear, anxiety, depression, grief, joy, elation,
anger, frustration, annoyance, love, hate—and food often remains a primary
source of relief from and perhaps a cause of these emotions. Logue identified 31

different emotions that people related to eating. The preponderance of evidence points to little physiological "cause" for these emotional ties, but rather to the memories of feelings from previous experiences with a food (Logue, 1986). For instance, if we feel good when we eat ice cream, then the ingestion of ice cream can make us feel good. Based on this premise, the use of food has been tried in psychotherapy (Lyman, 1989). We often make connections between food and the events that follow eating the food even though the two are, in fact, unrelated. This creates confused connections with food. For most people the connections between eating and feeling have become very convoluted by the time they reach adulthood.

The young adult is also transferring meaning to the next generation. Children are being taught the rules of eating. Food for "us" is defined, and customs in preserving identity are emphasized.

Later Adulthood

As later adulthood and old age approach, memories about food have a strong impact on food intake (Barker, 1982). Almost everyone remembers special foods with fond memories. Tastes of childhood become nostalgic; for instance, Mom's apple pie and chicken soup become sacrosanct memories. Food smells will stimulate memories of the past.

Simultaneously, bodies are changing. Keeping old food habits begins to have new and negative consequences, such as increased weight, or the discomforts of intestinal gas. Results may affect a sense of well-being. Resistance against changing food habits may be a resistance against aging. Among the very old, a downward spiral in health may result from social isolation and poor eating habits. The old may accept stereotyped beliefs about what the old eat and severely restrict their food variety.

SOCIAL MEANINGS OF FOOD

Attitudes toward food become deeply and subtly formed in the acculturation a child experiences in early years. Almost everyone can remember comments about the "proper" foods, or "reward foods" ("If you are a good boy, I'll give you a lollipop!"). Anthropologists report countless culture-food relationships. Many classifications of food exist: edible/inedible, male foods/female foods, foods for children/adults/old people, scientific classifications, food for the rich/poor, food for us/them, and so on.

Rules of Eating

Secular

Eating is essentially a social activity. Proper times, places, companions, ways of preparing food, and appropriate types of food are part of the acculturation process for children. They are important in the total identity of an individual and of groups. In the adult, these factors impinge on food choices for everyday food intake, holiday foods, and foods deemed appropriate for stressful and emotionally charged situations. All major, and most minor, social occasions include food. Rituals are replete with rules and regulations about food. Certain foods are accepted (even when the lack of a scientific basis is recognized) as assuaging or enhancing strong feelings or causing feelings. Psychology, sociology, anthropology, literature, religion, and history all document the central position of food in a holistic understanding of humanity.

Religion

Almost all ritualistic events include rules about acceptable or unacceptable food. Religious food proscriptions may influence food intake on special occasions or can become an entire nutrition lifestyle. Jewish food laws, Muslim food laws, and vegetarian tenets of Seventh Day Adventists are important social factors for individuals belonging to these religions (Lowenberg et al, 1979). Religious food customs have meanings as mediating communication with God (Fieldhouse, 1995), as in the example of eating a communion wafer in a Christian church.

Food and Personal Values

Food is often symbolic of personal values. It can be related to a person's beliefs about what is good for himself or herself, versus what is non-food or is food for others. There is hardly any food that is not a favorite for one person and repugnant to another. If a client repeatedly consumes a food that is less desirable, it should be assumed that a significant value is placed on that food. There are many examples of the symbolism of food for other values: chocolate candy and love, chicken soup and caring, cake for enhancing joy, beef and manliness. The more primary the value, the more difficult it will be to change the food habit. Foods related to religion, ethics, and survival are probably the most ingrained. The association a person makes with food may be irrational to the nutrition counselor. To work effectively with clients, it is often necessary to trace their mental associations, to determine underlying meanings, and to accept them.

Nutrition Lifestyle and Health Beliefs

Living long and well is becoming a cherished value in America. It is also becoming accepted that one's way of life, lifestyle, has an important impact on living well and long. People's attitudes toward the quality of life in general are usually predictive of the attitudes they will have toward nutrition and their eating habits, which we are titling *nutrition lifestyle.*

Psychosocial factors differentiating those who made desirable dietary changes from those who did not have been studied. Subjects responded to items about outcome and efficacy expectations. Results indicated that changers and non-changers were different in the following areas:

1. Their perception of personal susceptibility to diet-related diseases
2. Their perception of benefits from taking preventive health actions
3. Their overall health concern
4. The beliefs of those people who are important to them
5. Cues to action
6. Locus of control (Contento & Murphy, 1990)

Social food and nutrition messages to the ill are somewhat mixed. Especially in the current environment, there is a tendency to blame the victim for degenerative diseases, implying that the person did not eat right in the past. Such a societal attitude does little to aid the patient.

Often, "bad" food choices were "good" choices according to nutrition experts at some time in the past. Food choices play an important role physically in many disease states and emotionally in almost all illness. Meanings do not suddenly go away because of illness, and the way food is handled is significant in overall care. The first emotions expressed by patients/clients who have been told of the need for changes in food intake may range from anger to sadness, anxiety, depression, and so on. Later, reason will again return.

Miscellaneous Meanings

As the 21st century approaches, we find ourselves in a milieu in which a wider and wider segment of the population is beginning to recognize the importance of nutrition. Lip service is given to a healthy lifestyle, whether or not it is put into practice. The environment has never been more positive for influencing both the public and private individuals to eat in a healthful manner. Professionals who understand and use the various meanings of food as a tool in rendering healthy food choices and meaningful food choices equivalent are also those who will become the nutrition leaders of tomorrow.

There are *core foods* that are such staples for individuals or cultures that people expect to eat them at least once a day. Among the Irish, for example, potatoes may be a part of every meal. For many people, rice is part of every day or every meal. Salt, fat, and sugar are foods that seem to have particular *gustatory significance* for people. Although there has been taste research involving fat and sugar together, it is noteworthy that research has not included salt, fat, and sugar studied together. Different meals and foods have *relative emotional weights*, which are significant in attempting to change food habits. The meal with the least emotional weight is "the first meal of the day. This is also the one least likely to be eaten with other members of the family" (McIntosh, 1995). It is very likely that this meal is more susceptible to change than are meals that have more emotional weight.

As infants grow, food memories accumulate and become part of the psychological response to food. No one knows exactly how memories are made in the brain, but smell and taste are active brain stimulants. More information on these relationships will be of immense value in better understanding of individual nutrition choices (Lyman, 1989). Socialization and learning influence food choice in many ways.

Methods for Studying the Meanings of Food

Many disciplines study foods, and each has its own viewpoint. Listed here are some of the ways in which research is currently conducted.

Measures of food intake
24-hour recall
Conservation of beliefs
Attitudes

Knowledge
Sociodemographic determinants of food choice, ie, ethnicity, race, religion, education
Physical stimulation of senses
Anthropological measure
Sociological measures

More interdisciplinary studies are needed, especially those that include dietetics and nutrition research.

Summary

Food has meaning for humans, for both physical and emotional survival. Food is central to culture. Food has general meanings, both in a personal sense and sociologically. However, the type and strength of meaning is individualistic, and the MNT needs to probe the specific meanings of food for each client in order to effectively address these meanings in nutrition counseling.

Several disciplines conduct research into the meaning of foods. The dietetic practitioner can use findings from other disciplines to supplement concepts learned within the field of dietetics and nutrition. The addition of specialists in the field of nutrition and dietetics would also serve to enhance research into the meaning food has for people.

Suggestions for Further Learning

1. Discuss in class the different meanings food has for class members.
2. Write a paragraph about one or both of the following:
   a. what food means to me
   b. my favorite food
3. Read one or more of the suggested readings.
4. Interview people of different ages to investigate what food means to them.

CITED REFERENCES

Axelson ML, Brinberg D: *A Social-Psychological Perspective on Food-Related Behavior.* New York: Springer Verlag, 1989.

Barker LM (ed): *The Psychobiology of Human Food Selection.* Westport, CT: AVI Publishing Company, 1982.

Chapman G, Maclean H: "Junk food" and "healthy hood": Meanings of food in adolescent women's culture. *J Nutr Educ.* 1993;25:108–113.

Contento IR, Murphy BM: Psycho-social factors differentiating people who reported making desirable changes in their diets from those who did not. *J Nutr Educ.* 1990;22:6–14.

Erikson EH: *Childhood & Society.* 2nd ed. New York: WW Norton & Co, 1963.

Fieldhouse P: *Food and Nutrition: Customs and Culture.* London: Chapman and Hall, 1995.

Kittler PG, Sucher K: *Food and Culture in America: A Nutrition Handbook.* New York: Van Nostrand Reinhold, 1989.

Logue AW: *The Psychology of Eating and Drinking.* New York: WH Freeman and Co, 1986.

Lowenberg ME, Todhunter EN, Wilson ED, et al: *Food and People.* 3rd ed. New York: John Wiley, 1979.

Lyman B: *A Psychology of Food: More Than a Matter of Taste.* New York: Van Nostrand Reinhold Company, 1989.

McIntosh EN: *American Food Habits in Historical Perspective.* Westport, CT: Praeger, 1995.

Mintz SW: *Choice and Occasion: Sweet Moments.* In Barker LM (ed): *The Psychobiology of Human Food Selection.* Westport, CT: AVI Publishing Co, 1982.

Satter E: *How to Get Your Kid to Eat: But Not Too Much.* Palo Alto, CA: Bull Publishing Co, 1987.

ADDITIONAL REFERENCES

Camp C: *American Foodways: What, When, Why and How We Eat in America.* Little Rock, AR: August House, 1989.

Capaldo ED, Powley TL: *Taste, Experience and Feeding.* Washington, DC: American Psychological Association, 1990.

Gallagher CR, Allred JB: *Taking the Feat Out of Eating: A Nutritionists' Guide to Sensible Food Choices.* New York: Cambridge University Press, 1992.

Hirschmann JR, Munter CH: *Overcoming Overeating.* New York: Fawcett Columbine, 1988.

Iggers J: *The Garden of Eating: Food, Sex and the Hunger for Meaning.* New York: Basic Books, 1996.

Kadi J: *Food for Our Grandmothers.* Boston: South End Press, 1994.

Kuper J (ed): *The Anthropologists' Cookbook.* London: Routledge and Kegan Paul, 1977.

Levenstein H: *Paradox of Plenty: A Social History of Eating in Modern America.* New York: Oxford University Press, 1993.

Lupton D: *Food, the Body and the Self.* London: Sage, 1996.

Mennel S, Murcott A, Van Otterloo AH: *The Sociology of Food: Eating, Diet and Culture.* London: Sage, 1992.

Roth G: *When Food Is Love: Exploring the Relationship Between Eating and Intimacy.* New York: Plume, 1992.

Yagley R: *Poems from the Table: The Fruits of the Earth in Verse.* New York: Barnes & Noble Books, 1995.

CHAPTER 3

The Problem-Solving Counseling Method

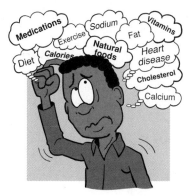

GOALS

The major goals of this chapter are (1) to explain the concept of nutrition counseling as a facilitative process, (2) to introduce a problem-solving approach to nutrition counseling, and (3) to provide a step-wise model for medical nutrition therapists to follow in practice.

Learning Objectives

At the end of this chapter, the reader will be able to:

1. Describe the MNT's role and the client's role in counseling.

2. Define the counseling process as an internal process, as a sequence of events, and as an interpersonal relationship.

3. Outline the stages in the problem-solving method and give examples of dialogue in each stage.

4. Begin to practice this method of medical nutrition therapy/nutrition counseling.

Key Terms

▶ **Problem-Solving Approach:** an approach to counseling that addresses individual client problems; focus is on identification of problems and their solutions in a client-centered manner.

▶ **Problem:** synonymous with *issue* and *concern*. The term *problem* is used for uniformity in this text. The terms *issue* and *concern* are alternate words that may be used with clients as appropriate.

Webster's dictionary defines "to counsel" as "to give advice or guidance." Historically, giving advice has been the operative definition used among authoritative medical professionals. However, modern theories of psychology suggest that guidance rather than advising is more effective in bringing about changes in people, including changes in health habits. Giving advice is often regarded as appealing to the unmet needs, perhaps unconscious, of the advice giver rather than the person receiving the advice. Current counseling modalities emphasize the guiding role of counselors, and health-care professionals are beginning to see themselves in this light as the function of health care changes from curative to emphasizing wellness and the prevention of disease. Wellness places responsibility for a healthy lifestyle squarely on the shoulders of the individual. The professional's role has become one of helping people to select healthy lifestyle goals, including nutrition lifestyle, and to solve their health problems.

Most people in the "helping professions" today consider counseling to be an interpersonal relationship between a helper/facilitator and individuals seeking support and guidance in making changes in their behavior and their attitudes toward life, with the goal of achieving a more satisfactory life. More lasting results are seen when all helping professionals, not just psychologists and psychiatrists or other extensively trained professionals, increase their awareness of, and their ability to use, counseling strategies that facilitate change and personal growth in patients and clients (Brammer, 1985). The dietetic professional also needs to consider that the purpose of medical nutrition therapy/nutrition counseling is to guide clients toward healthy nutrition lifestyles and solve nutrition-related problems.

This chapter covers concepts involving the participants of counseling, the MNT and the client/patient, as well as defining the actual process of counseling. The authors' problem-solving approach is described in a method that can be practically adapted. Many case examples and dialogues are provided to assist in practical application.

CONCEPTS OF NUTRITION COUNSELING

In their book *The Dynamics of Clinical Dietetics*, Mason and coauthors recognize nutrition counseling as assisting individuals with nutrition problems by helping them gain knowledge or motivation, or both. An especially important part of this observation is the inclusion of the idea of helping people gain motivation as well as knowledge. The notion of counseling as practical application of knowledge has also been supported by Snetselaar (1989). She described nutrition counseling as translating theory into practice, suggesting the motivational and helping function of the counselor. Both of these views recognize the importance of psychological factors in good nutrition.

To be fully effective, an MNT must not only instruct clients on the principles of basic nutrition and nutrition therapy, but also build a relationship that will facilitate changes in behavior and enhance problem-solving skills. It is very important that MNTs not only know nutrition but also have a basic understanding of human psychology and communication skills. A professional educated only in nutrition science or only in psychology has some gaps in the knowledge needed to facilitate change toward desired nutritional behaviors on the part of clients. Facilitative skills require a reasonable knowledge of human personality and interactions and of motivation and behavior principles beyond that gained by everyday experience.

Nutrition counseling in the context of facilitating change focuses on clients and their lifestyles, not on a diet or a disease entity. In this context, the way in which people nourish themselves is their nutrition lifestyle. A diet, as specific food intake, is simply part of a nutrition lifestyle. When a person becomes aware, or is told, that there is a health reason for changing his or her nutrition lifestyle, problems usually arise. Assistance is often sought in the form of medical nutrition therapy/nutrition counseling to solve these problems.

Even though certain problems may be common in conjunction with a particular health condition, each individual presents a unique mix of problems, motivational forces, and acceptable solutions. No particular personality trait or behavior is connected uniquely to one disease or other or to the complexity of a particular diet. People with diabetes, for instance, do not have unique psychological characteristics because they have diabetes. Their responses to the restrictions in their nutrition lifestyle vary according to their personalities. One person may learn easily and be easily motivated whereas another may learn easily yet have many personality barriers to change. A disease might have a rather simple medical nutrition protocol, and yet a complex and resistant personality might have difficulty with its restrictions. *It is a mistake to categorize clients according to their disease, or to assume that a method of teaching or counseling suits one disease state and not another unless the nutritional problems are directly related to mental illness.*

The Challenge of Medical Nutrition Therapy/Nutrition Counseling

Nutrition counseling is not psychotherapy, although emotional issues sometimes must be resolved before nutritional behavior can be changed. In many situations, the counseling skills outlined in this book or those derived from short-term training programs are sufficient to facilitate problem-solving. If a client has serious emotional problems, however, consultation with a psychological specialist or a similar referral is appropriate.

An outpatient setting, where the assumption is that a number of counseling sessions will occur, is the most appropriate place for medical nutrition therapy/nutrition counseling. In most instances, behavioral changes are recognized as normally occurring slowly over time. Changes in nutrition lifestyle are no exception. Therefore, treatment is much more likely to be effective if the MNT can follow a client over several sessions. The environment needs to be businesslike and comfortable and must be able to accommodate the handicapped (ie, ramps for wheelchairs). It may be necessary to explain the client-centered problem-solving style of counseling because many clients will have stereotyped impressions of a dietetic practitioner as one who hands out lists of foods that one "should" or "should not" eat.

In short, the concept of nutrition counseling encompasses facilitative techniques, interpersonal skills, expertise in nutrition in health and disease, and the ability to guide clients in solving nutrition-related problems. Understanding of the psychology of food habits and other nutrition behavior is needed before significant improvement can be made in the success record of counseling efforts. Neither the public nor most professionals have appreciated the difficulty of changing food habits and lifestyles and the length of time needed to bring about long-lasting changes. It is hoped that understanding will deepen and that new research will suggest better strategies for influencing people so that the process of counseling can be shortened.

All people have some psychological needs that are fulfilled through food, often outside their awareness. These were summarized in Chapter 2, The Meanings of Food. In general, it can be expected that psychological needs will exert more influence on food habits than will logic and knowledge of nutritional needs. The major distinction between merely providing advice and being a counselor or therapist is that counseling includes bringing to the client's awareness the social and psychological connections he or she has with food and reconciling those needs with physiological needs. This takes time—weeks, months, or years. Individuals differ in the negative or unhealthy psychological connections they have made with food. Some need the help of specialists in psychotherapy, while others simply need someone who can facilitate problem-solving. The challenge facing the MNT is to be a true counselor and to address those psychosocial issues that have an impact on nutrition and physiological needs. Once these are addressed, changes in nutritional behaviors can enhance clients' lives as well as improve nutritional status.

The Role of the Medical Nutrition Therapist

The dietetics and nutrition professional has emerged from a role as technician to assume the role of nutrition expert. She or he is expected to bring about change in public and individual food habits as a counselor and as an agent for change. In the realm of nutrition counseling, the responsibilities have expanded to include not only provision of nutrition knowledge and advice, but also facilitation of client change. This role exemplifies a goal of the dietetics and nutrition profession *to translate nutrition knowledge into desirable nutrition behavior.* This is a unique function of the profession of dietetics and nutrition.

A comparison of psychologists and MNTs clarifies the background necessary for effective nutrition counseling. Psychological counselors have successfully provided counseling to those who have wished to change nutrition behaviors for years. Their strategies focus on problem-solving and client growth. They have not always recognized the importance of nutrition knowledge in selecting healthy food habits. The MNT, on the other hand, knows nutrition and its importance in health and in a high quality of life, but may not understand people, how people grow psychologically, or how to improve problem-solving skills. Psychologists and MNTs will perform better if they seek information and counsel from one another and enhance their knowledge in each other's field. Success as an MNT lies in knowing not only nutrition, but also enough about human psychology to approach clients in a way that facilitates change and encourages them to learn nutrition and to become motivated to solve their problems based on sound nutrition knowledge. If an MNT makes a commitment to invest time, energy, and attention to help someone solve a personal problem, then a positive therapeutic relationship can exist because the client experiences that his or her problems are important to another person (Stuart & Simko, 1991).

Viewing the dietetic practitioner in the role of expert and counselor (MNT) is relatively new to both professionals and the lay public. Because the role previously was seen as that of an advisor, clients are sometimes surprised by the use of facilitating techniques. The MNT often needs to explain that a problem-solving modality is one in which the client takes an active role in solving his or her problems. Client and counselor are a team with the aim of establishing a nutrition lifestyle, not trying to get the client to "stay on a diet." The role of facilitator will grow as

MNTs are able to help people solve nutritional problems and as clients see positive changes in their quality of life.

The role of a facilitator is not an entirely comfortable one for many dietetic practitioners. There are several reasons why. They may respond to stereotyped older views of dietetic practitioners as technicians or as laboratory scientists and be unsure that they are correct in taking professional responsibility for counseling. Another difficulty arises in giving up the medical model of intervention in which the professional tells patients what to do and expects acquiescence. When underlying issues in changing one's nutritional lifestyle are addressed, emotions inevitably must be addressed that may create discomfort for an MNT. In addition, some dietetic professionals may not know enough about people, and themselves, to effectively interact in a facilitating manner. However, all of these things can be learned.

Role of the Counselee/Client/Patient

Some people seek nutritional counseling when their eating behaviors are symptoms of emotional distress, such as a person who is gaining or losing weight in response to some stress in his or her life. Other people need medical nutrition therapy because of a change in health status or the wish to prevent early onset of nutrition-related diseases. Some come willingly, others reluctantly. Whatever the reason that causes people to seek nutrition counseling, they are assuming the role of counselee/client/patient.

In most cases, individuals who decide, or are advised, that they have a physical condition that must be treated by medical nutrition therapy feel disappointed about the situation. They undoubtedly feel ambivalent toward talking to someone about their problems. They may even be hiding some emotional problem by focusing on changing their food habits. They bring with them all their fears, angers, biases, and guilt, as well as their strengths, hopes, and desires for a good life. Each person brings his or her typical ways of coping with life and solving (or not solving) problems. If an individual generally approaches life in a problem-solving manner, the role assumed in counseling likely will be that of a problem-solver. Many individuals are very motivated and think that by changing their nutrition lifestyle they can forgo surgery, medication, or other undesirable and costly procedures. If an individual is not motivated, she is likely to approach nutrition counseling with a defeatist attitude and be a difficult counselee. Another person will assume the role of a good child and do as he is told and be compliant, telling you what he thinks you want to hear, then doing what he wishes out in the "real world." Whatever role the client assumes will be unique, yet there are a few general assumptions that can be made about clients that can be useful until you get acquainted with each one personally.

Clients are a product of their culture. Their behavior as counselees will be heavily influenced by their cultures' attitudes toward nutrition and toward counseling. Many clients will be somewhat depressed by the idea of needing to change their food habits. Depression, when looked at closely, includes some anger and resentment. There may also be some anxiety. These emotions can make a person resistant to change. These feelings may be mixed with relief for having taken a step toward solving a problem. Their feelings are probably ambivalent, resisting and wanting change at the same time. On the other hand, some clients are highly motivated, and this energy can be used to make productive changes.

Clients are fully capable of making their own decisions, but they often need more information or motivation, or both. They have goals, ambitions, and expectations of life that make it important to them to change their nutrition behavior. Many clients want to learn and change, even if they do not show it. A variety of factors influence a client's ability to achieve behavioral change goals, including knowledge base, current practices, sense of personal empowerment, and environmental support systems (Schwartz, 1996).

DEFINITIONS OF THE COUNSELING PROCESS

Counseling has been variously described as (1) an internal process for the client, (2) a sequence of events, and (3) the elements of the interpersonal relationship between the counselor and client. All of these definitions are relevant in a comprehensive understanding of nutrition counseling.

Counseling as Internal Processes

Carl Rogers, the founder of client-centered therapy, saw counseling as a systematic internal change during which a client begins to see himself or herself and the world differently. As sessions continue, self-esteem rises, and statements made by the client reveal more self-awareness, indicating internal change. Rogers described counseling as "a unique and dynamic experience, different for each individual, yet exhibiting a lawfulness and order which is astonishing in its generality" (Rogers, 1961, p. 740). In addition, he noticed that as clients change, there is also more evidence of positive attitudes and more maturity in reported behavior. Clients become more accepting of themselves and become more controlled. Physiological changes for the better occur.

Although nutrition counseling is not aimed directly at changing personality, an effect on the personality of individuals who significantly change their nutrition lifestyle is inevitable. The MNT will note changes in a number of areas mentioned by Rogers. For instance, there is a shift from outer-directed to inner-directed behavior (locus of control) when an individual learns to maintain desirable nutrition behaviors even in the face of pressure to "break down" and participate in unwanted behavior. The following case example provides an illustration of changed locus of control.

CASE EXAMPLE ·

First Counseling Session

Rapport has been well established, and problems are being explored.

M N T: "What situations seem to create the most difficulty for you in following a low-fat food intake?"

C L I E N T: "Well, one of the hardest times I have is refusing desserts from my Aunt Millie, especially when Mother is around. Mother always taught me that I shouldn't refuse because Aunt Millie had put all her love into making desserts and would be hurt if we didn't eat the food she prepared. Isn't there a way to adjust the diet so I can keep Aunt Millie happy?"

M N T: "That's a possibility. How often do you see Aunt Millie"

C L I E N T: "At least once a week."

M N T: "Do you think you can reach your goals and work Aunt Millie's desserts into your menu every week?"

C L I E N T: "Seems like it would be hard to do."

The client made a commitment to say "no, thank you" to dessert the next time Aunt Millie offers it.

Second Counseling Session

M N T: "Good morning, Sue, how have your efforts to follow a low-fat food intake worked out since our last session?"

C L I E N T: "Great! Do you know what I did? Twice I told Aunt Millie 'no thank you' when she passed out dessert. She sort of pouted the first time, and I was tempted to give in, then I said to myself, 'I'll feel a lot better if I don't eat dessert and it is more important for me to feel good than to placate Aunt Millie.' I do feel proud of myself. It's not easy to say 'no' to Aunt Millie."

M N T: "I feel proud of you, too. Not only are you following your plan, but also I see that you are becoming more confident and assertive!"

· ·

Gestalt therapists consider the counseling process to be one of developing internal changes in the view of the world held by the client. Perls, the founder of Gestalt therapy believed that changes do not occur on purpose but are the result of changing awareness. Strategies of therapy focus on awareness and nothing else. During a counseling session, the counselor and the client "work" on awareness of what the client is experiencing in the here and now. The internal process is described as the development of maturity by becoming more aware of oneself and the relationship between the self and the world. An example of this would be the discovery, by the client, of the way she or he makes decisions about what food she or he eats. The following case example shows this kind of discovery by a client who bordered on anorexia nervosa as she gained a new awareness, or *gestalt*.

CASE EXAMPLE ·

C L I E N T: "My mother leaves food cooked for me each night when I get home late, but I don't eat it."

M N T: "Are you hungry when you get home?"

C L I E N T: "Starving!"

M N T: "How is it you choose not to eat when you are starving?"

C L I E N T: "I don't know. Well, I guess I don't like the pressure Mother is putting on me to get me to eat."

M N T: "You refuse to eat to rebel against your mother?"

C L I E N T: "Uh, well, yes, I guess I do. Yes, I feel angry when I see that food, as if she's scolding me for not eating enough. I never thought of that before."

• •

Psychological theories are discussed in more detail in Chapter 5.

Counseling as a Sequence of Events

Psychologists who deal in behavior modification think of behavior changes as a process by which one behavior is eliminated and another is instituted. This change takes place in response to manipulation of the environment and through a system of reward and punishment. Clients discuss what they want to do and often outline the process by which they will incorporate new behaviors into their lives.

Descriptions of nutrition counseling have tended to focus on the sequence of events. Snetselaar (1989) describes the process of nutritional counseling as encompassing the functions of assessment, treatment, and evaluation. Mason and coauthors (1977) present a system of client-centered processes that includes the assessment component, the planning component, the implementation component, and the evaluation component. These two descriptions are oriented toward the problem-solving nature of nutritional counseling and the sequence of events in the process.

Theorists generally define problem solving as including the following steps:

■ Defining the problem
■ Searching for alternative solutions
■ Selecting one to implement
■ Evaluating results

The *problem-solving nutrition counseling method* described in this book is a process method based on these concepts. It is modified somewhat to include a stage of building a foundation of interpersonal trust and gathering basic data that is necessary in nutrition counseling before embarking on the task of solving problems. The stages for this method are defined as follows and will be described in detail later in this chapter:

■ Build the counseling foundation
■ Define problems multidimensionally
■ Select alternative solutions
■ Plan for change
■ Reach commitment
■ Evaluate progress

This type of methodology tends to emphasize the intellectual aspect of counseling. However, an effective counselor must always keep in mind that the interpersonal relationship that occurs between counselor and client is the crux of successful counseling (Brammer, 1985). If only the intellect is engaged, the steps could be followed but the purpose never fulfilled.

Counseling as the Interpersonal Relationship Between Client and Counselor

The concept of counseling as the interpersonal relationship between client and counselor focuses on the dynamics of communication. The need for long-term psychological training on the part of the counselor is not as important as the development of trust between the counselor and the client. Research indicates that a caring, sincere, lay person can be as successful as a highly trained professional in guiding people to make changes in their lives. The essential ingredient is the establishment of trust between two individuals (Brammer, 1985).

Everyday experience tells us that when we think another person is trustworthy we become more open to suggestions from them. Generally, trust means that we believe the other person basically likes us, believes that we are competent, will not belittle us for our weaknesses, will not talk about us behind our backs, and will not use the information we give them to take advantage of us. When we feel safe with another person, we also tend to develop a wish for them to continue to approve of or like us, and in so doing we give them power to influence our behavior. In the case of nutrition counseling, the client wants the MNT to approve of his or her nutrition lifestyle and is motivated to exhibit desired behavior in order to gain this approval.

Counseling begins with the establishment of a counseling relationship. Even before the first meeting, a counseling relationship begins between the counselor and client in anticipation of what is going to take place. The following case example illustrates the thoughts and feelings a person might have as she anticipates adopting the role of a counselee and of a counselor. (Contributed by S. Himburg.)

CASE EXAMPLE ·

The Client's Thoughts Awaiting Her First Counseling Session

I want help. I wonder what will happen here. I am afraid of her. I want to change the way I eat and the way I look, but I don't want to change *me*. I don't know if this will work. Oh, I hope it will work. But, I don't know whether to trust her. She will see things that I try to hide—frightening and bad elements. I can see many things about myself that could be different, yet there is a force that seems almost to prevent me from changing. I am afraid of exposing a part of me that even I have never seen before. Do you suppose that is how I really am?

The MNT'S Thoughts About Each New Patient

I am glad that this new client is coming. I feel some apprehension with a new relationship. There is a lot of responsibility in caring for another human being. She may need to trust me with secrets about herself that she may never have told anyone else. I think we can develop a close relationship in which she will be comfortable and be able to make nutritional behavior changes, and grow as a person, too.

· ·

Other clients and counselors may have similar thoughts or they may have other thoughts. Each client brings to the first counseling session a unique combination of feelings and attitudes and anticipation of what this relationship will mean.

The initial contact is the moment when counselor and client "size each other up." Each observes the other and makes a tentative judgment about how the relationship feels. A connection is established, which is called *rapport* (Berne, 1966). It is possible to have poor rapport, but the word generally refers to a positive relationship and a sense of trust between people. The counselor's self-confidence and acceptance of clients is the most important factor in the establishment of a successful counseling relationship. Other communication skills and strategies are explained in depth in Chapter 4, Nutrition Counseling Strategies.

Each of these descriptions of counseling has merit, and, in the practical world, aspects of each of these three views of counseling can be incorporated into a successful counseling style. Nutrition counseling, although focused on one aspect of a person's life, impinges on all aspects. General counseling models have relevance for developing nutrition counseling skills.

A PROBLEM-SOLVING NUTRITION COUNSELING METHOD

In *Theories and Strategies in Counseling and Psychotherapy*, Gilliland and coauthors (1989) present an eclectic counseling model that combines the best elements of several concepts and theories of counseling. The authors recognize that no one concept of counseling holds all the answers and that the counselor's personal and professional judgment is crucial to success. The book is practical, is developed on a strong scientific basis, and recognizes the essential goals desired in a counseling environment. A problem-solving model is described with clarity and lends itself to adaptation to nutrition counseling. The model has underlying assumptions that exemplify true regard for clients, their goals and lifestyles, and their ability to make decisions for themselves. These assumptions are so valuable for an MNT that several bear repeating in Box 3–1.

The nutrition counseling method presented in this chapter is based on these assumptions and on the additional assumption that food habits and nutrition behaviors are an integral and central part of personality. Clients can grow and develop as whole individuals as they become aware of and make changes in their nutrition lifestyle through effective counseling.

Human nutrition is unique because not only physiological but also emotional and social needs are met by our nutritional behaviors. In the wild, animals do not appear to make food choices based on social or psychological factors to the extent that humans make them. Animals raised for food or as pets are usually fed according to scientific principles of nutrition and have little part in deciding what they will eat. In contrast, within a year or so of birth, human food intake usually becomes largely the province of individual choice and becomes very much associated with social beliefs and psychological needs. The need and ability to choose creates problems when free choice results in unhealthy lifestyles or when a medical problem necessitates change. A systematic approach to these problems makes them easier to solve.

Box 3–1

Assumptions of a Problem-Solving Model

1. No two clients or client situations are alike.
2. Each client and counselor is in a constant state of change and flux—no person or situation in counseling is or can ever be static.
3. The counselor uses all the available personal and professional resources in the helping situation but is fully human in the relationship and cannot ultimately be responsible for the client.
4. Competent counselors are aware of their own personal and professional qualifications and deficits and take responsibility for ensuring that the counseling process is handled ethically and in the best interest of the client and of the public.
5. Client safety takes precedence over need fulfillment of the counselor.
6. Many problems in the human dilemma appear to be insolvable (and, indeed for some problem situations we sometimes believe we can find no satisfactory options), but there is always a variety of alternatives, and some alternatives are better for the client than others.
7. The client is the world's greatest expert on his or her problems.
8. The effective counselor exhibits a flexible repertoire of activity on a continuum from nondirective to directive.
9. Counselors and the counseling process are fallible and cannot expect to observe overt or immediate success in every counseling or client situation.
10. Many different approaches and strategies are available for conceptualizing and dealing with each problem—there is probably no one best approach or strategy.
11. Generally, effective counseling is a process that is done *with* the client rather than to or for the client.

From Gilliland BE, James RK, Bowman JT: *Theories and Strategies in Counseling and Psychotherapy.* Englewood Cliffs, NJ: Prentice-Hall, 1989, p. 299.)

Problem-Solving Nutrition Counseling

A problem-solving approach, using sound facilitating strategies selected from various counseling therapies, is appropriate for nutrition counseling. The problem-solving nutrition counseling method is a scientific, practical, systematic approach to counseling. It can be used to guide people toward healthy food habits and lifestyles for wellness or for disease treatment. It provides a framework within which to focus on solutions to nutrition-related problems, issues, and concerns. The goals of the problem-solving nutrition counseling method are as follows:

1. To help clients become aware of solutions to problems they face.
2. To help clients consciously and intentionally choose to control nutritional behavior based on valid nutrition principles and their own lifestyles.
3. To help clients reach a higher level of personal integration through assertive nutrition decisions.

As mentioned earlier, there are six stages in the problem-solving approach to nutrition counseling:

I. Build the foundation
II. Define problems multidimensionally
III. Select alternative solutions

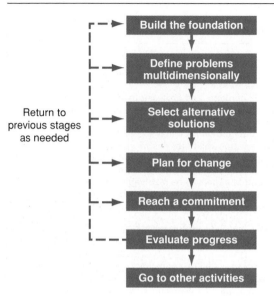

Return to previous stages as needed

FIGURE 3–1. Problem-solving nutrition counseling method.

IV. Plan for change
 V. Reach a commitment
VI. Evaluate progress

These stages provide the framework for the interpersonal relationship that will facilitate (or have the potential to hinder) changes in nutrition behaviors. The MNT guides the client through the process, moving between stages in a forward manner but not usually in a straight line. As movement occurs from one stage to another, the challenges of the new stage may bring awareness that the previous stage was not completed. For instance, when beginning Stage III, "Select Alternative Solutions," dialogue may reveal that the "real" issue had not been identified in Stage II and a return to Stage II is warranted. Figure 3–1 shows the dynamic nature of the method, indicating movement between stages as situations demand, recycling through the process when evaluation directs it, and moving out of the cycle when the identified problems are resolved or other priorities evolve in the life of the client. In the application of the method, attention is given both to the internal processes being experienced by clients and to the interpersonal relationship that develops between counselor and client.

This approach lends itself to the incorporation of new behaviors in small increments over a period of time. Complex changes are accomplished in small steps and require a fluid yet systematic process, not a sudden traumatic attempt to institute an entire dietary regimen. Movement forward through the steps of problem-solving is accomplished as quickly as clients are willing for it to occur.

Stage I: Build the Foundation

The initial identification of nutrition problems generally occurs as a prelude to determining that a person will seek nutrition counseling. Most often, a medical professional advises a patient of the need for medical nutrition therapy. Sometimes an individual decides to seek nutrition counseling without medical consultation. In either case, the counselee appears before the counselor with a "nutritional concern."

Establishing Rapport. When the client appears at the counselor's door, the early interaction generally determines the kind of interpersonal relationship the client and counselor establish. The first few minutes are of great importance in establishing a working rapport. It is important to remain *nonjudgmental* and *nonconfrontational* in this initial stage of the counseling relationship. If rapport is not being built at this point, it is unlikely that the problem-solving process will proceed to its fullest potential.

Gathering Data. Most people begin nutritional counseling after referral from a health-care professional as part of disease treatment or prevention. In these cases, professional nutrition screening is a prelude to medical nutrition therapy. Nutrition screening may occur in a medical office, an inpatient setting, an outpatient setting, a public health facility, or an MNT's office. The Nutrition Screening Initiative encourages individuals to do their own nutrition assessment. This initiative was developed in 1990 and includes three screening tools. The first one, "Determine Your Nutritional Health Checklist" is available in English and Spanish. It is a public awareness tool that can be self-administered. The two other tools are used as a follow-up and when the screens indicate a potential problem (Helm & Klawitter, 1995). These forms are available from the Nutrition Screening Initiative in Washington, DC (202-625-1662). This program also has an impact on the methods used to identify the need for nutrition counseling. See Additional References for more information on the Nutrition Screening Initiative. If a person has not had previous nutrition screening or has not brought a referral from a physician, the MNT generally needs to obtain a referral before counseling the client if reimbursement is desired or if a potential medical problem is evident.

As Stage I progresses, the MNT, ever mindful of the rapport between himself or herself and the client, gathers the data needed to determine problems. She or he begins to explore the issues internally, not verbalizing them, as information is being relayed by the client. Questions and comments are aimed at encouraging the revelation of food intake, nutritional status, presence of a support system, and thoughts, feelings, beliefs, and attitudes about food. Any sense of judgment picked up by the client will reduce client candidness. Data gathering may include all or some of the following sources of information:

Medical data—current and past medical history, laboratory data, food allergies, medications, weight, height, weight change, and other information from medical records.

Food history data—food preferences, eating habits (where, when, with whom), who cooks, who purchases, 24-hour recall, previous special diets, client knowledge about nutrition.

Lifestyle data—exercise, stress level, living situation, marital status, smoking/drinking/drugs, significant life events (losses, gains).

In summary, Box 3–2 lists nutrition counseling criteria and examples of interventions for Stage I.

Box 3-2

Nutrition Counseling Criteria and Examples: Stage I

STAGE I: BUILD THE COUNSELING FOUNDATION

Introduces Self to Client

"Good afternoon Ms. X; I'm Mary Doe, student dietitian from University Y."
  Include full name, title, school affiliation.
  Address client by courtesy title and last name.

Establishes Rapport—May Include "Small Talk"

"Did you have any problems finding the office?"
"It's so nice to finally have a sunny day."
"It sounded hectic in your house when we spoke on the phone. How many children do
  you have?"

Addresses Client Appropriately

Use courtesy title (Mr., Mrs., or Ms.) unless otherwise directed by the client.
Smile—hand shake, if appropriate.
Avoid closed positions (arms folded, legs crossed, hunched over).
Shoulders comfortable, back; good posture.

Explains Purpose or Allows Client to State Reason for Visit

"What can I do for you today Mr. X?"
"As I explained to you on the phone briefly, my approach with working with people is
  just that. I will work *with* you to solve these issues, not just give a diet to follow,
  which means I'll need your active participation in this process. Is this okay with
  you?"
"I'm going to talk with you about foods you normally eat; this is called a diet history.
  I'm going to write this down, so we can refer to it later."

Determines Readiness of Client to Begin Session

"This will take about 30 minutes. Is that okay with you?"
"Is this a good time for you?"
"Are you ready to tell me about your food intake?"

Obtains Accurate Information from Client

"One slice of white toast with 1 teaspoon grape jam" versus "toast and jam."

Obtains Complete Information from Client as Needed

Asks all questions needed to help clarify the problem.

Asks Only Pertinent Questions Related to the Problem

Detailed questions about fruit intake may not be important for a person on a sodium-
  restricted diet.

What clients have to say is, in the long run, the most important source of data for the MNT. For example, a physician refers a client for weight loss, but the client does not really agree and has come for counseling only to placate the physician. The counseling session could proceed as follows:

CASE EXAMPLE ·

A male client, obviously overweight, is being interviewed.

CLIENT: "My doctor sent me here to see you."

MNT: "What reason did he give you?"

CLIENT: "Something about my weight and blood pressure."

MNT: "What do you think he meant, specifically?"

CLIENT: "Well, I know I have high blood pressure and he thinks I'm overweight and that's making it worse."

MNT: "Do you think you are overweight?"

CLIENT: "Well, my wife thinks I am."

· ·

In this example, please note that the counselor is simply asking questions, clarifying information, and collecting data from the client. There is no attempt at this point to do anything about what the client reveals, although the counselor has gained quite a bit of information. He knows that the client has a diagnosis of high blood pressure and is overweight. The client does not seem to accept the information himself and refers to what the doctor or his wife thinks as an avoidance of addressing the issue. The MNT needs to verify some of this information with medical records.

At times it is better not to collect a lot of data at once. A client may become bored with answering questions and lose interest. An uncomfortable counselor may avoid confronting the client by asking many questions. (Confrontation is an intervention strategy explained in detail in Chapter 4, Counseling Strategies.) It can be seen in the continuation of the dialogue that even though there may be more information to gather about food intake, progress can be made by moving to Stage II: "Define problems multidimensionally."

MNT: "What do *you* think?" (a confrontation)

CLIENT: "I suppose I am, but I can never seem to take it off. It's too hard."

MNT: "That's probably why your doctor sent you to me. I'm sure I can help make weight loss easier. Tell me the problems that make it hard to lose weight."

The client has expressed a problem: "It's too hard to lose weight." There will be time later to return to gathering data, but this point offers an opportunity to discuss problems. There are several dimensions to the problem expressed by this client that need to be addressed.

It is sometimes tempting for both client and MNT to remain in the data-gathering phase of Stage I. It is much more comfortable to gather data than to get to work solving the problems faced by the client.

Alternatives to the verbal method of gathering data could include written questionnaires and computer-assisted data gathering. These methods allow precious counseling time to be used for the more difficult aspects of problem-solving.

Stage II: Define Problems Multidimensionally

In Stage I, data are gathered and the counselor and counselee begin to recognize nutrition problems from several angles, or *dimensions*. There are at least four dimensions: the MNT's dimension, the client's dimension, the physiological dimension, and the psychosocial dimension. All of these dimensions impinge on the outcome of counseling, and issues and concerns may arise in any or all dimensions at the same time. In Stage II, dialogue begins to probe the many variables impinging on food intake and barriers that may inhibit change, including lifestyle, attitudes, beliefs, feelings, and nutritional needs. Awareness will begin to arise regarding many subtle aspects of a client's life that influence his or her eating and how these aspects may be problematic. Discourse begins on broad issues and then focuses on specific problems. For instance, a client whose "problem" is overweight may discover that eating too many desserts is a major problem with his overweight condition. Probing may reveal that part of his problem not only entails liking the taste of desserts but also entails his inability to say "no" to his wife's desserts. The "real" issues may have to do with his feelings and his assertiveness patterns. Facilitation of problem-solving by this man's MNT must include addressing problems that are not direct nutrition issues. It is usually necessary for the MNT to take the initiative to confront the client's lack of awareness of concerns within the area of feelings, attitudes, and belief systems.

Some questions for eliciting feelings about the stated problem include, "What is going on in your life right now?", then, "How do you feel about it?", "What troubles you about that?" and "How are you handling that?". Empathy is also needed, for example, "That must be very hard for you" (Stuart & Simko, 1991).

The less defining of problems by the MNT and the more by clients, the more successful the outcome. Problems that may seem trivial to an onlooker may be big stumbling blocks to clients. It is necessary to have dialogue about issues and concerns until agreement is reached between counselor and client on problems relevant to establishing the desired food habits. Sometimes clients do not see problems that the counselor sees. The counselor who is wise does not force a client to accept his or her views. Arguing with clients is usually damaging to the rapport and the counseling relationship. For instance, the counselor may think a client's weight loss goal should be 100 pounds, while the client's goal may be 50 pounds. Certainly, the client will be better off losing 50 pounds than none. If tension is created from conflict between client and MNT, there is likely to be no problem-solving. In the final analysis, the problems that the client believes stand in the way of meeting his or her life needs and goals are the ones the client will be motivated to solve. He or she is not likely to be motivated to do what another person thinks should be done. Lack of agreement over the definition of problems or failure to uncover real problems prevents forward movement, and attempts to identify alternative solutions will be a frustration.

The more precise and concrete the problem definition is in Stage II, the easier it will be to move on to Stage III, "Select Alternative Solutions." If the MNT and the client are unable to agree on a definition of the problem, the process should be returned to Stage I. The MNT may not have enough data to clearly define the problem.

Almost always, Stage II results in redefining nutrition-related problems from the original statement of the problem. Problems range from simply a lack of nutrition knowledge to deep-seated problems in the social and emotional realm. Knowing what eating patterns will bring about desired physiological changes within the body is relatively simple compared with knowing how they will become a lifestyle for the client.

Goals. As problems are defined, they seem to naturally evolve into goals. The client needs to be guided toward establishing both long-term and short-term goals. Goals are an important measure of expected client outcomes. Long-term goals need to state clearly what the client will be able to do or achieve as a result of the counseling process (Helm & Klawitter, 1995). A part of the problem might be "I don't exercise enough." This can become a short-term goal of exercising three times per week for 20 minutes. The problem might be the risk of another heart attack. This might then be termed as a long-term goal such as "maintain a nutrition lifestyle to reduce the risk of another heart attack." Long-term goals can be generally ascertained. Then it is important to set short-term goals that can be worked toward in the time frame between counseling sessions. Psychologically, long-term goals may be too overwhelming and discouraging. Short-term goals need to be attainable, realistic, timely, measurable, and within the person's control.

In summary, Box 3–3 lists nutrition counseling criteria and examples for Stage II.

One major obstacle that prevents definition of the real issues and problems is avoidance of feelings by the MNT, the client, or both. Discussing too many nutrition facts may be used as a defense against dealing with feelings, so the counseling reverts to Stage I or flounders. Clients may keep asking questions about nutrition facts to avoid confronting psychosocial issues. MNTs uncomfortable with the emotional aspects of counseling, or those untrained in nutrition counseling methods, may continue to instruct rather than counsel. In many cases, there is no need for the MNT to do anything more with feelings than simply allow their expression while sitting quietly and listening. Release of emotion is often an important step in releasing tension and thus increasing the ability to think productively. Thinking is essential to define problems accurately and begin the task of planning solutions.

CASE EXAMPLE ·

A woman who has been sent for weight loss is in Stage II.

M N T: "What do you see as the major problem?"

C L I E N T: "I guess I just need to lose weight." (suggests avoidance or pressure of some other problem)

MNT: "You guess? Do you have any other guesses?"

CLIENT: "You bet. My husband is the problem. He nags at me about going on a diet, then when I do he brings home candy all wrapped up pretty, and he *knows* that's temptation." (by the end of the sentence the client is virtually screaming)

MNT: "Do you feel like screaming when he does that?"

CLIENT: "Yes."

MNT: "How else do you feel?"

CLIENT: "Angry." (more calmly)

MNT: "Do you want to tell me more about that?"

CLIENT: "Well, no, I'm calmer now. It is a problem, though."

MNT: "Is there a solution to this problem?" (moving into Stage III)

· ·

Box 3–3

Nutrition Counseling Criteria and Examples: Stage II

STAGE II: DEFINE PROBLEMS MULTIDIMENSIONALLY

Allows Client to State Problem in His or Her Own Words

"What I am hearing from you is that you think you are 50 pounds overweight. Is that right?" (to be sure client sees this as the problem)
"What do *you* see as the problem?" or "How do you see this as a problem in your life?"

Elicits the Real Issues/Problems from the Client

Determine patient's knowledge. For example: "What medical nutrition therapy has your doctor prescribed for you?"
Non-verbal clues to accuracy of patient information can be body language, eye contact. For example, if patient appears uncomfortable or avoids eye contact, s/he may not be providing accurate data.
Include questions on exercise, finances, social situation, life changes, etc, not just food-related questions.

Allows Client to State Feelings as Well as Factual Aspects of the Problem

CL: "I feel out of control with my food intake."
MNT: "Tell me more about that."

Offers Own Idea of Problem and/or States Agreement with Client

"I suspect there is a problem with your body image as well."
"I agree that it would be healthy for you to lose 20 to 25 pounds to help you control your diabetes."

Allows Client to State Own Short- and Long-Term Goals

MNT: "What would you like the outcome of counseling to be?"
CL: "I want to lose 6 pounds this week, 20 pounds this month and 45 pounds in 3 months."

Nutrition Counseling Criteria and Examples: Stage II *(Continued)*

Offers Own Idea of Goals and/or States Agreement with Client

"In my experience, a weight loss of 1 to 2 pounds per week is more realistic and healthy
for most people. It also provides insurance that the weight will stay off. To lose 45
pounds in 3 months, you would need to make drastic changes that I probably
couldn't support. Let's take a closer look at your weight goals."

Allows Client to Move Into Other Areas if Needed

CL: "My mother always made me clean my plate at mealtimes."
MNT: "How does that affect your eating habits now?"

Keeps Client From Avoiding Issues by Changing the Subject

MNT: "Do you like the way you look now?"
CL: "Are we almost finished?"
MNT: "We have 15 more minutes; do you like the way you look now?"

Determines Nutrition Education Level of the Client

"Tell me what you know about cholesterol."
"Which of the foods in your nutrition history are high in sodium?"
"What has your doctor already explained to you?"

Provides Instructions as Necessary

Review medical nutrition therapy principles, for example, nutrition management of
    diabetes.
Obtain information applicable to adjusting nutrition planning to patient; for example,
    meal pattern, food preference, cultural needs, socioeconomic status, activity level.

Uses Audio-Visual Aids Appropriately

Audio-visual aids are able to be used by client. For example, do not give small print diet
    instruction sheet to a person with visual problems.
Audio-visual aids relate to person's eating habits, cultural habits, socioeconomic level.
    For example, avoid using steak/meat charts when counseling a vegetarian.
Audio-visual aids contain information that agrees with data being given. For example,
    do not give a sodium-restricted diabetic patient a handout that lists bacon after
    telling him or her that bacon is forbidden.
Ensure that audio-visual aids are at appropriate level. For example, pictures of digestive
    system are not appropriate for a young child.
Make sure audio-visual aids are practical in the situation. For example, size, weight,
    availability of auxiliary equipment are appropriate.
Be sure audio-visual aids are legible, attractive, appealing, interesting. For example, use
    colorful plastic models rather than faded charts.

Nutrition instruction is often accomplished during this stage when knowledge is
needed before appropriate alternatives can be elicited.

Stage III: Select Alternative Solutions

Stage III, selecting alternative solutions, is intended to explore as many alternatives
as possible for addressing problems. A nonjudgmental and creative MNT can guide
a client through a wide range of alternatives. Many potential goals, solutions, and activities are subject to exploration. They include changes in food choices as well as

changes of feelings, attitudes, beliefs, and perhaps interpersonal relationships. Stage III is a brainstorming session. Even the alternative of doing nothing about the problem can be explored. Creativity is the key to success in selecting alternatives. The expression of many thoughts and feelings should be encouraged and explored. If there is difficulty in eliciting alternatives, the MNT can make a tentative suggestion such as, "Have you considered exercise?" and then let the client verbalize a specific exercise alternative. Avoid the tendency to come up with all the alternatives and thereby do the work for the client to solve the problem. The client needs to be the more active participant in this process. The fewer alternatives you offer, the better for the client. Experience has shown that in most cases, the client will choose to put into action alternatives that were determined by himself or herself. No ideas should be disregarded. Sometimes an alternative at first unappealing will become attractive later. Both client and MNT will have ideas, the more the better. Ridiculous ideas can make the process fun, and the more fun it becomes, the more good ideas will surface. Finally, workable alternatives that are reasonable, attainable, appropriate, and "ownable" by the client must be considered. "Owning" an alternative means accepting responsibility for the consequences of an alternative put into practice. If the client does not accept responsibility for an alternative, one of two undesirable events will result; the client will feign compliance or the client will openly rebel. Rapport then deteriorates and failure is imminent.

In summary, Box 3–4 lists nutrition counseling criteria and examples for Stage III.

Box 3–4

Nutrition Counseling Criteria and Examples: Stage III

STAGE III: SELECT ALTERNATIVE SOLUTIONS

Allows Client to Think of His or Her Own Alternatives to the Problem

"Maybe I could count calories and ignore my weight on the scale."
"I could do my own grocery shopping, instead of having my sister do it."

Offers Tentative Suggestions to the Client

"How about increasing your exercise in some way?"
"What about portion sizes?"

Creates an Atmosphere of "Brainstorming"

Assure the client that she or he is not committed to any suggestions made at this stage and should just say anything that comes to mind.

Alternatives Chosen Are Reasonable, Appropriate

Once a list has been generated, it can be fine-tuned. Pick one alternative. Begin thinking of all the different ways to implement the alternative.
"When you are out shopping, what things do you think you can do to attain low cost meals?"

Alternatives Chosen Are "Ownable" by the Client

Make sure that alternatives are reasonable for the client's lifestyle. Sometimes "ownability" is not recognized until the planning and/or action commitment stages occur.

Stage IV: Plan for Change

Incorporating a few or even one change in food intake does not overwhelm a client as readily as does an attempt to incorporate an entire change in nutrition lifestyle. MNT and client together look at alternatives and select one or two as appropriate for implementation. Alternatives for solving nutrition problems fall into two categories—nutritional needs and psychosocial needs. If lack of nutrition knowledge has been determined to be a problem in food choices, nutrition instruction is the solution. For clients who already understand their nutritional needs, do not spend too much time reiterating information. Begin to plan coping mechanisms for difficult situations and ways to solve the problems that prevent the client from putting his or her knowledge into practice. If a client is showing a high level of emotional involvement, it is necessary to address emotional issues before the client will be willing to listen to nutrition information. The MNT who listens carefully to clients finds that a client who has been heard becomes a willing listener.

Even though most people can understand nutrition, they usually cannot incorporate an entire nutrition plan into their eating habits at one time. A plan that is too comprehensive and overwhelming becomes part of the problem rather than a solution. Early in the counseling process, making plans that have a high probability of success are important in the overall success of problem-solving. Attaining one small goal is powerful motivation in guiding clients toward reaching the next goal and the next after that. Positive feedback to the client, affirming his or her ability to make the changes, is necessary and vital for the initial step and for the entire counseling process. Client affirmation is discussed in detail in Chapter 4, Counseling Strategies.

In the United States, where food and information about food are abundant, it is important to remember that for the majority of clients' *lack of information is not the problem.* Problems are more likely to lie in attitudes, interpersonal relationships, self-concept, or emotional factors.

In summary, Box 3–5 lists nutrition counseling criteria and examples for Stage IV.

Box 3–5

Nutrition Criteria and Examples: Stage IV

STAGE IV: PLAN FOR CHANGE

Selection Is Made of One or Two Alternatives Upon Which to Focus Implementation

Assuming a goal has been determined, "Which alternatives would you like to work on from now until the next time we meet?"

Affirms Client's Ability to Make Desirable Changes

After observing menu selection for several days for weight reduction plan:
MNT: "I can see by your weight loss and observing your menu selections for the past several days that you're well on your way toward reaching your goal."

Include Coping Mechanisms for Difficult Situations Related to the Stated Problem

It has been determined that a client with diabetes finds it difficult to refuse candy bars when a crowd goes to the movies.
MNT: "How will you handle that?"

Stage V: Reach a Commitment

The purpose of Stage V, reaching commitment, is to bring about genuine commitment to the action steps on the part of the client. Commitment to specific behaviors during a specific time period helps make the nutrition plan feasible, reasonable, and attainable. Some clients respond well to rigid plans; others resist regimentation. It is in Stage V that the MNT needs great flexibility to support clients in doing things their own ways. Sincere involvement and support from the MNT are important, but the commitment to action must be the client's commitment.

The dialogue in Stage V determines with exactness how the plans in Stage IV are to be put into practice. Often a contract form can be used to help document plans and can serve as a reference for the client after the session is over. Exact behaviors to be exhibited, or specific thoughts and feelings to be practiced, and the structure the client needs to support the desired changes will be determined. When the client is very sincere about a commitment, that commitment will be easy to keep. If resistance is discovered, a return to an earlier stage is required to probe the resistance, overcome it, or take another direction for the moment. Frequently at this late stage, the client becomes acutely aware that alternatives to which she or he has given lip service are not the ones she or he is willing to implement. It is then necessary to retreat to earlier stages and search for an alternative to which the client will commit himself or herself. The step the client does take, *committing* herself or himself to action, no matter how small, is the beginning of success.

Contracting Procedures. The process of developing a contract for change can guide clients through the stages of counseling, confront problems, and culminate in the formal commitment to action that comes in Stage VI of the problem-solving counseling method. A contract at this stage results from the answers to the questions that are discussed between the counselor and the client in Stages II, III, and IV. It is important to remember that each question can be stated in several ways, and each MNT develops his or her own style. Nevertheless, in one style or another these questions need to be answered if a sincere commitment is to be achieved.

1. What are you going to do? Goals.
2. How are you going to go about doing it? Plans.
3. What will be the consequences of the change? Consequences that are realistic expectations as well as devised to reinforce change must be included in the answers. The importance of reinforcement is discussed in Chapter 5, Psychological Theories.
4. What are the barriers to change? This question almost always results in confrontations that are productive. Many times the answer to this question creates awareness of client thoughts about ways to avoid making changes, or reasons for failures in past attempts to change.

The process is rarely as simple as this list suggests. Most often the questions lead to confrontation of the problems in making changes in nutrition lifestyle. The dialogue flow is analogous to a road map where crossroads appear and decisions are required as to the direction to take. The counselor must decide on interventions at each juncture, and each client decides the path she or he is really willing to take. Careful listening is required to select facilitating interventions. The listener listens to learn and understand, and from this listening develops the basis for reassuring, guiding, consoling, interpreting, and supporting the client. Box 3–6 pro-

Box 3–6

Responses That Support Development of Specific and Firm Contract for Change

QUESTIONS	FIRM RESPONSES	UNSURE RESPONSES	CONFRONTATIONS
What are you going to do this week?	I am going to limit ice cream to ½ cup two times a week.	I'm not going to eat any ice cream.	Is that realistic for you?
		I'll try not to eat ice cream.	"Try" sounds unsure to me. **or** That is what you are not going to do. Would you change the statement to a positive statement?
		Maybe I should leave ice cream alone.	*Counselor has the choice to confront the "maybe" or the "should."* You have said "maybe I should leave ice cream alone." Let's examine that. What do you want to do? *Client can discuss shoulds, wants and the decision of what to do.*
How are you going to plan for eating ice cream 2 times per week?	I'll have it for lunch on Tuesday and dinner Saturday night.	I don't know.	Make a guess. *The client does know how to plan.*
		Maybe.	Will you change the "maybe" to a firm statement?
How will you and I know you have succeeded?	I'll tell you. I could mark it down on the calendar.	I guess I could tell you.	You guess?
How will you reward yourself for success?	First of all, I will feel good. I will watch my favorite TV show Sunday night.	I'll have some ice cream.	Is that a reward that will bring about lasting change?
How will you prevent yourself from keeping this contract?	I could forget I ate the ice cream Tuesday night and eat more Wednesday. I won't do that.	I could just ignore this contract.	Are you going to do that? Perhaps this isn't the right contract for you this week.

Nutrition Counseling Criteria and Examples: Stage V

STAGE V: REACH A COMMITMENT

Introduces Concept of Contract Effectively

A contract is an agreement made by the client with himself or herself to change a specific behavior or feeling. It is meant to help motivate the client and serve as a reinforcer after the session is over.

Determines Willingness of Client to Execute Contract

"Are you willing to create this contract for change for yourself?"

Allows Client to Complete Own Contract

Let client read and fill in all the spaces, as appropriate.

Works with Client to Complete Contract When Questions Arise

CL: "What do you mean by reward?"
MNT: "It's a reinforcement for yourself. It could be something you buy for yourself, or do for yourself, like buying a shirt, getting a manicure, or going to the beach."

Makes Steps in Contract Workable and Feasible

First go over verbally what the client wants to put in the blanks. Then, after your agreement, have him or her write it in. If a client resists writing a contract, do not argue.

Makes Steps in a Contract Specific

Reward: "I'll be nice to myself."
Clarify what this means to the client and have him or her write that in.

Obtains Feedback from Client that He or She Is Satisfied with Contract and His or Her Own Projection for Success

"How do you feel about this contract? How do you think you'll do?"

Offers Verbal Affirmation, Enthusiasm, and Support for Client's Commitments

"This contract is great! I know you'll do really well to accomplish these changes this week!"

Client Summarizes Plan and Commitment for the Time Between Session

Ask client to summarize his or her contract verbally to ensure comprehension.

vides some examples of responses that support the development of a specific and firm contract for change. Figure 3–2 shows an example of a contract form. Figure 3–3 shows a completed contract form.

In summary, Box 3–7 lists the nutrition counseling criteria and examples for Stage V.

Stage VI: Evaluate Progress

Session Evaluation. To a certain extent, each response to the client is evaluation, and the end of a counseling session is simply a final summation of what has transpired during that session. The last few minutes of the session are spent evaluating

Short–Term Goal_____

My commitment is to _____

_____

_____

My plan for accomplishing this is to (Include behavior/thought/feeling and

time span) _____

_____

_____

_____

How will you and I know I have succeeded? _____

_____

My reward will be   _____

Ways in which I could potentially sabotage this contract are: _____

_____

_____

_____

I will not use the above to sabotage myself

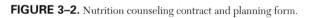

_____

Signature

FIGURE 3–2. Nutrition counseling contract and planning form.

Short Term Goal *I will lose 2 pounds this week*

My commitment is to

1) Increase exercise to 4x/week, 30 minutes each

2) Decrease fast food meals from 7 to 3 times/week

My plan for accomplishing this is to (Include behavior/thought/feeling and time span) *Continue to walk with husband 2x the nights he is home. Walk alone during day 2x other days. Bring watch so I know 30 minutes. Bring lunch to work (sandwich, fruit, low fat dessert) 3x. Pack it in evenings. Weekend-cook 1x*

How will you and I know I have succeeded? *I will have lost 2 pounds. I will probably feel more energetic.*

My reward will be *A day at the beach without the children.*

Ways in which I could potentially sabotage this contract are: *Ignore this contract, forget my watch, feel too tired to walk, be angry with my husband and not want to walk with him, forget to pack lunch, feel pressure to go out and eat with coworkers.*

I will not use the above to sabotage myself

Jane Smith

Signature

FIGURE 3–3. Completed nutrition counseling contract and planning form.

what has happened that session. This time is most productive when the client does the evaluation of what was accomplished and how she or he feels about what has transpired.

Overall Evaluation. The evaluation of medical nutrition therapy/nutrition counseling over the long run is the change that has occurred in clients' nutrition lifestyles. In addition, there may be an improvement in health, a loss or gain of weight, or some other measurable physiological change. However, for the client and MNT, the most important evaluation is the determination of the extent to which the counseling has changed the quality of life for the client. MNT and counselee together need to discuss this as the counseling experience is brought to culmination.

Feedback should provide a review of the client's achievements in incorporating new nutritional behavior, as well as changes in feelings and coping ability. Each counseling session begins and ends with feedback from the client about his or her weekly activities or about the session that is concluding. When the end of the counseling term is approaching, an evaluation of the counseling relationship and its success in reaching long-term goals should be made. After counseling has ended, further monitoring and support should be planned so that results can continue to be evaluated.

Bringing About Closure. Closure must occur at each counseling session and at the culmination of the counseling relationship. Special attention must be paid to satisfactorily bringing about closure in both the cognitive (knowledge) and affective (attitudes, feelings) aspects of the counseling. Clients can be asked to summarize sessions or review commitments. MNTs may occasionally need to interject thoughts, but too much summarizing by a MNT may not help clients to bring about closure. When the client has reached the goal that was originally planned, further counseling is the prerogative of the client. If the MNT has seen a client only two or three times and the work has gone well, both participants will find the termination of counseling satisfying and comfortable. However, most medical nutrition therapy is not truly effective in a few sessions. This is particularly true in situations in which significant lifestyle changes are necessary. Closure is difficult when the MNT feels that the goals have not really been attained. She or he may find the need to take on an advocacy role in requesting more sessions. If this does not work out, then the MNT and client need to bring closure knowing that the best result has not occurred.

Generally, there should be a mutual agreement to discontinue the counseling, or a new agreement should be made between the client and MNT. Goals may not have been met and the MNT may feel uncomfortable dismissing the client. In addition, there may be a warm feeling between the MNT and the client, and both will feel the loss of the relationship. In some instances, termination of counseling sessions may create some anxiety, particularly on the part of clients who have depended on the MNT for support. It is important to provide some advance preparation for the termination. Talking it over and making plans for the future can help, as can increasing the time period between counseling sessions. However, it is also important, once the decision to end counseling has taken place, that the MNT work through the separation and culminate the relationship so that the client can become independent. This does not mean that you should not have the opportunity to follow-up with the client on occasion, to see how things are going, or that she or he cannot contact you for occasional support. Often, phone calls are made to the client to help in the transition of the termination.

There may be cases in which the termination of counseling sessions comes about because the client needs or desires more intense psychological counseling. In such situations, it is important for the MNT to deal with his or her limitations in such a way that both MNT and client recognize the move as one of success rather than of failure.

An important aspect of concluding relationships with patients discharged from a hospital is a referral to an MNT in the community. Clients can be referred to an outpatient department, a dietetic practitioner in private practice, or other community settings. Few, if any, patients make significant nutrition lifestyle changes after a few days in the hospital, so referral after a short hospital stay is important. For most people who require changes that are basic to their lifestyles, 3 months is probably a minimum length of time for nutrition counseling, and 6 months should not be considered too long a time. Weight management and recovery from eating disorders can often take years to accomplish.

Termination of counseling should follow these guidelines (Cormier & Cormier, 1979):

1. Point out the client's achievements and independence.
2. Share your positive feelings about the client and relationship.
3. Plan for a follow-up at a future date.

"Leave your door open" should the client decide to reinitiate counseling in the future.

In summary, Box 3–8 lists nutrition counseling criteria and examples for Stage VI and Figure 3–4 is a nutrition counseling worksheet that can be used to guide you through these stages.

Box 3–8

Nutrition Counseling Criteria and Examples: Stage VI

STAGE VI: EVALUATE PROGRESS

Signals Ending of Session

"We're almost finished for today."
"Before we end . . ."

Summarizes Session

"Do you have any questions?"
"Please summarize for me the main points we discussed."

Gets Feedback That the Client Is Satisfied with the Session and Contract

"I think you have accomplished a great deal today. How do you feel about this?"
"Are you comfortable with the goals you have set for yourself?"

Makes Agreement with Client About Follow-Up

"I will be in to see you again next Monday afternoon at 2:00. In the meantime, if any
        questions or problems arise, you can reach me at _____ between the hours
        of _____ and _____ ."
"Our appointment for next week is _____ ."

Stage I

Counselor introduces him/herself:_____ Date of Birth:_____

Counselor asks client name:_____

Counselor or client states purpose of visit:_____

_____

Overview of session is given:_____

Background information:_____

    Appetite:_____

    Allergies:_____

    Who cooks, shops:_____

    Eating concerns:_____

    Cultural/religious restrictions:_____

    Exercise:_____

    Recent life changes:_____

    Financial concerns:_____

    Medical history:_____

    Lab data:_____

    Height:_____ Present weight:_____ Usual weight:_____

    Time span of gain/loss:_____

24 hour recall or diet history:

Food   **Amount**   **Circumstances** (where, with
                                                         whom, feelings, stress, etc.)

FIGURE 3–4. Nutrition counseling worksheet.

Illustration continued on following page

Stage II

Problems expressed by client: _____

_____

Feelings about it: _____

Physical/emotional/social aspects of the problem: _____

_____

Problems perceived by MNT: _____

_____

Long-term goals: _____

Short-term goals: _____

Nutrition instruction_____

Stage III

Alternatives: (brainstorming)

_____

_____

_____

_____

Stage IV

Alternative solutions should be reasonable, ownable, and appropriate __

_____

Select one or two alternatives_____

_____

Counselor affirms the client's ability to make changes_____

_____

FIGURE 3–4 *Continued*

Include coping mechanisms_____

_____

Stage V

Contract filled out.   _____ Yes   _____ No

If answer is no, give reason _____

_____

Stage VI

Summary of session_____

_____

Plan for follow-up_____

_____

Referrals_____

_____

FIGURE 3–4 *Continued*

Summary

The role of the MNT is to help people make changes in nutritional behavior that will enhance their lifestyles. An eclectic model for fulfilling a counseling role draws from many available theories of human psychology and counseling.

The problem-solving method includes the processes of building a foundation of rapport, defining problems, selecting alternative solutions, reaching a commitment to action, and evaluating progress. This approach is particularly well suited to medical nutrition therapy.

At the conclusion of counseling, both the client and the counselor should feel comfortable that the client can move on. The counselor has the responsibility to remain available should clients wish to return, or to refer them to other professionals if appropriate.

People differ according to their personality structures in their responses to facilitating techniques. Personality differences are not dependent on the type of medical recommendation a client might have had prescribed or the disease entity present. Personality is a combination of genetic makeup, the environment in which the individual grew up, and the present situation.

Suggestions for Further Learning

1. Using the worksheets provided in Figure 3–4 as a guide, begin to practice counseling. You may want to practice on friends or family first if you have had no previous experience in counseling.

2. Next, counsel a person and record the session on an audio or videotape. Observe the processes and compare them to the ones outlined in this chapter.

3. If you practice in an inpatient setting, identify the aspects of this model than can be employed in short-term interactions, then use them in practice.

CITED REFERENCES

Berne E: *Principles of Group Treatment*. New York: Grove Press, 1966.

Brammer L: *The Helping Relationship: Process and Skills*. Englewood Cliffs, NJ: Prentice-Hall, 1985.

Cormier W, Cormier S: *Interviewing Strategies for Helpers: A Guide to Assessment, Treatment and Evaluation*. Monterey, CA: Brooks/Cole, 1979.

Gilliland BE, James RK, Bowman JT: *Theories and Strategies in Counseling and Psychotherapy*. Englewood Cliffs, NJ: Prentice-Hall, 1989.

Helm KK, Klawitter B: *Nutrition Therapy: Advanced Counseling Skills*. Lake Dallas, TX: Helm Seminars, 1995.

Mason M, Wenberg BG, Welsh PK, et al: *The Dynamics of Clinical Dietetics*. New York: John Wiley and Sons, 1977.

Rogers CR: *On Becoming a Person, Sentry Edition 60*. Boston: Houghton Mifflin, 1961.

Schwartz NE: Communicating nutrition and dietetic issues: Balancing diverse perspectives. *J Am Diet Assoc*. 1996;96(11):1137–1139.

Snetselaar LG: *Nutrition Counseling Skills: Assessment, Treatment and Evaluation*. 2nd ed. Rockville, MD: Aspen Publishers, 1989.

Stuart MR, Simko MD: A technique for incorporating psychological principles into nutrition counseling of clients. *Top Clin Nutr*. 1991;6(4):23–39.

ADDITIONAL REFERENCES

Nutrition Counselor: Strategies for Results (videotape). Philadelphia, PA: ARA Services, 1991.

Commission on Dietetic Registration for The American Dietetic Association: *Self-Assessment Series for Dietetics Professionals. Nutrition Counseling Module*. Chicago, IL: American Dietetic Association, 1992.

CHAPTER 4

Nutrition Counseling Strategies

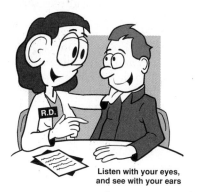

Listen with your eyes, and see with your ears

GOALS

The major goals of this chapter are (1) to explore several client-centered strategies to promote behavior change, (2) to improve the reader's process of listening, and (3) to provide suggestions for counseling techniques in the verbal and nonverbal aspects of communication.

Learning Objectives

At the end of this chapter the reader will be able to:

1. Define listening as both an art and a science.
2. Describe the three basic skills of listening and the barriers to their effectiveness.
3. Explain how proxemics and paralanguage are used as tools for listening to nonverbal messages.
4. Describe mirroring and matching and the benefit of these techniques in a counseling setting.
5. Give examples of each type of verbal response (including humor) described in this chapter.
6. Explain the techniques of confrontation.
7. Identify components of cognitive modeling, relaxation training, and biofeedback.
8. Enumerate the advantages and the disadvantages of group counseling.
9. Discuss issues that influence the empowerment of clients.
10. Begin to practice and become comfortable with the strategies presented in this chapter.

Key Terms

▶ **Listening:** a strategy of communication that involves all of the senses and is the cornerstone for a problem-solving counseling relationship.

▶ **Confrontation:** to "bring to the front" or to discuss problems, concerns, and issues that may be barriers to a healthy nutrition lifestyle.

▶ **Empowerment:** the ability to facilitate a client's recognition and consequent mobilization of his or her inner powers to achieve a healthy nutrition lifestyle.

▶ **Nonverbal Communication:** transmission of meaning through various displays of body language, often unconscious; describes every aspect of communication but the actual words.

More effective nutrition counseling occurs when the disciplines of counseling psychology and nutrition are integrated in the counseling relationship (Isselmann et al, 1993). Strategies for intervening in clients' lives include methods used to establish a relationship, develop problem-solving skills, and motivate clients to change. The strategies described in this chapter have been selected because they fit well into a problem-solving counseling approach and have been used effectively to help people change their nutrition behavior. No one strategy will work with every client. Effective MNTs have many strategies from which they select the ones best suited for each client. The strategies discussed in this chapter simply provide a basis upon which the reader must build a repertoire of intervention strategies. The more approaches with which one is familiar and comfortable, the more creative, spontaneous, and flexible interactions with clients will be.

Counseling interventions have the potential to hurt clients as well as to help them change. Counseling strategies should not be used lightly or as gimmicks. The strong influence an MNT can have on a client's feelings and behaviors must be used in the best interests of the client. In addition, a psychological specialist or therapist should be retained for consultation in understanding clients and evaluating client situations or when there is need to refer a client for psychological counseling.

One study compared counseling skills between two student groups, one group given didactic and simulation experience and the other given experience in health-care settings without formal training (Vickery et al, 1995). The first group encouraged client participation and assessed the client's commitment to change, whereas the second group typically asked "Will you be able to do this?" or "Do you have any questions?" after giving instructions and often did not recognize or acknowledge concerns or feelings expressed by the clients. This chapter discusses several strategies that have been successfully used by MNTs to recognize and address the wide range of issues expressed by clients.

LISTENING

Listening is the most important strategy in counseling because it can serve as a guide to effective problem-solving. It is the prerequisite of all other skills, including empathy, concrete responses, and other relationship skills (Gilliland et al, 1989). Listening enables the discovery of the unique characteristics of each client and guides the selection of interventions. When the MNT is truly listening, more subtle aspects of communication become apparent. Emotions and attitudes that are not expressed directly may be detected in a tone of voice, a pitch or speed of speech, the blink of an eye. The adage "see with your ears, hear with your eyes" can help in the detection of such nonverbal cues. Listening is hard work, but it can be learned by "training, practice, watching a model, and reading" (Gilliland et al, 1989).

Many people engage in what they call "listening," but it is really nonlistening. Real listening is "getting the message," whereas nonlistening is rejecting the message by distorting it or negating it in some way. Listening is a difficult skill to develop for most people because they have long established nonlistening attitudes and habits and must unlearn them. Some degree of introspection is necessary. This can be uncomfortable for the MNT. However, learning to listen is worth the effort.

The result of really listening ("getting the message") from clients will, with incredible frequency, guide you to the most effective interventions. They become spontaneous responses to the client and the situation, more than textbook-learned responses.

To understand clients and select effective responses to clients, it is necessary to interpret communication accurately. One must be aware of the client's world view, ways of solving problems, goals, and lifestyle. The ability to make ongoing assessments of what is happening with clients depends on listening skill more than any other factor. For instance, a better assessment of the success of a weight control program is gained by listening to what the client says than by seeing the weight appear on the scale. The scale does not tell how the client is fitting weight control into his or her lifestyle. Similarly, fine plans can be made for changes that will sound good and never be incorporated by a client if only scientific information about nutrition is used and psychosocial aspects of the nutrition lifestyle are not "heard."

Descriptions of Listening

To begin learning to listen, think about what listening entails. It is both the physiological perception of communication by all the senses (hearing, sight, taste, touch, smell) and the comprehension of the meaning of the communication. Perceiving and comprehending what another is trying to say has been described as both a science and an art.

Listening can be defined as a scientific process. Interpersonal listening is the process whereby the human ear receives sound stimuli produced by other people and through a series of steps interprets the sound stimuli in the brain and remembers them. Birdwhistell (1970) presented the most comprehensive work in this area.

Barbara (1958), in a classic book on listening, described it as an art:

> For listening to be effective as an art, we must be active participants in its whole process. This means not only working just through our ears. It also means responding holistically with our full hearing capacity and our inner perceptions. It entails being fully attentive and awake, alert at every minute to screen out inner prejudices, condemnations or preconceived notions. It means being active in thought and feeling and with one's eyes and ears to avoid inertia. It means being open and receptive to others. It demands of us an enhanced vitality, an aliveness, and a firm desire to commune with others. With all this in hand, we shall grow healthily as human beings, able to influence others with meaning. So we shall arrive at a sustained level of mutual and truthful communication.

Brammer (1985) described listening as an active skill including not only listening with the ears to words and with the eyes to language, but also a total perceptiveness. This kind of listening enables one to answer the questions, "What is going on in this person right now and in this life space?" and "How can I respond in a way that will facilitate problem solving?"

In *Born to Win*, James and Jongeward (1971; p. 48) describe listening not only as the receipt of communication but also as a powerful way of sending a message: "one of the finest strokes one person can give another." This reflects a basic need of most people to have other people listen to them. The effects of fully listening to clients can be astounding. Clients develop high levels of trust for an MNT who listens to them and are influenced to be more open in listening to the MNT in return.

These descriptions indicate the complexity of listening. Both the physical senses and one's attitude are part of the development of three essential aspects of listening: *openness, concentration,* and *comprehension* (Curry-Bartley, 1986).

Openness

Openness is a willingness to receive communication and to allow others to influence one's perception of the world. It means letting oneself receive stimuli from the outside that can influence an ever-changing sense of reality. It involves deliberate effort to receive messages when the incoming message conflicts with preconceived attitudes and beliefs. Hearing ideas that fit easily into one's attitudes and beliefs requires little deliberate effort to be open.

Openness includes both physical and psychological openness. Physical position enhances the perception of messages. A relaxed body position leaves energy for focusing on the client, while a tense body and closed position require both physical and emotional energy for maintenance. Energy that is being used to keep a body tense is energy not available for listening. The upper body and facial muscles are probably the most important ones in regulating listening. Arms held in an open position and jaws, neck, and shoulder muscles relaxed make shutting out messages difficult. Often, attitudes that are blocks to listening can be overcome simply by a conscious effort to position the body openly. The level of openness has a direct effect on the ability to concentrate on the communication at hand.

For instance, if one is worried about a personal problem, the body may be tense and the face may be in a scowl. One will be preoccupied and not listening. A conscious effort to relax, put the problem aside for the moment, and make the body physically open opens the mind to the client, allowing his or her communication into the thought process.

Listening is requisite to empathy, the ability to enter the speaker's world as if it were the listener's own. As much as possible, the MNT must set aside her or his own world view to accept the client. Openness is particularly associated with a willingness to discern messages in an intuitive manner, making the leap beyond logic to perceive subtle nuances detected subconsciously (Curry-Bartley, 1986). This is the art of listening.

Concentration

Concentration is the ability to focus energy on the immediate situation, the here and now. It is an act of will to focus on one point by shutting out everything else. Athletes recognize that high levels of performance require them to concentrate on immediate efforts and to shut out everything else—all fears, irrational thoughts, and distractions in the environment (Curry-Bartley, 1987). The same applies to counseling. Thinking about anything except the immediate situation is irrelevant, for the most part, during a counseling session. Irrelevant thoughts include internal dialogue about what should or should not be instead of what is, worry about peripheral stimuli, or rehearsal of what to say when the speaker stops talking. Concentrating on what the client is saying will prevent preoccupation.

CASE EXAMPLE ·

An MNT became aware of the following internal dialogue while she was counseling a client. "I know I shouldn't scold her for wanting to keep eating salty foods, but I should tell her to stop it because it's really so bad for her, but I shouldn't tell her what to do, and I should have all the answers. Well, I really don't know what I should do and now I don't even know what she's saying!!"

The MNT immediately asked the client to repeat what she had said and concentrated on listening before responding.

· ·

Skill in concentration requires the acceptance of one's feelings and at the same time control of their expression. When an MNT's feelings arise in a counseling situation, they can be self-acknowledged and a decision made as to whether they should be expressed immediately or later, so that concentration can continue to be focused on the client. For instance, a young female dietitian feels a rising irritation when a client refers to her as a "sweet young thing," because she considers the remark insulting. The following case example illustrates this.

CASE EXAMPLE ·

M N T: "Good morning, Mr. Dooley. I am a medical nutrition therapist, here to talk with you about nutrition."

C L I E N T: "Well, good morning you sweet young thing. I'm sure your mere presence will improve my diet."

M N T: (thoughts) Boy, I can feel the irritation when this guy calls me a "sweet young thing." Oh, well, I'll deal with that later.

M N T: (response) "What has your doctor told you about making changes in your food intake that can help address your heart problem?"

· ·

Comprehension

Comprehension is the ability to attach meaning to communication. Concentration on the here and now and openness to communication interact to increase perception and therefore increase the data available for comprehension (Curry-Bartley, 1986). Other factors in comprehension are the tools of interpretation such as a large vocabulary and awareness of the meaning of the client's nonverbal behaviors.

The MNT's frame of reference through which communication is filtered is also a factor. Expanding the frame of reference entails inspection of many cultural biases, which are discussed in Chapter 7, Cross-Cultural Counseling.

Language. Language is an important tool of interpretation. A large vocabulary helps the listener understand what is being said. A vocabulary of the colloquial language of clients is also important. For instance, recognizing unique "Spanglish" words used by Hispanics in their local setting will aid in understanding what they are saying. Hearing other language factors such as lilt, pitch, speed of speech, and inflection may be even more important in interpreting meaning. For instance, fast speech may suggest anxiety. Understanding the theme of what is being said, rather than just the words, is necessary for accurate comprehension (Arnold & Boggs, 1995).

Nonverbal Signs. Nonverbal signs are the most difficult to interpret because they may relay subtle messages that bring truth to communication that the speaker, consciously or unconsciously, may prefer to hide. In addition, nonverbal behavior is culture-bound and if the listener is not aware of particular cultural meanings, miscommunication may result. A good example of this is eye contact. The degree of eye contact among different cultures varies greatly. For instance, there are differences in the ways eye contact is used as a sign of respect. In the United States, direct eye contact is generally thought of as positive (Purtilo & Haddad, 1996). In some other cultures, lowering the eyes is a sign of respect. When the client is from another culture, the MNT needs to adjust interpretation of eye contact.

Congruence of nonverbal and verbal messages also affects meaning.

CASE EXAMPLE ·

M N T: "What is your reaction to the need to lower your salt intake?"

C L I E N T: (fists clenched, big smile on face) "No problem." (too brightly said) The MNT notes the incongruence between clenched fists and smile and too brightly said words. He or she has the choice of ignoring the evidence of feelings or addressing them. The overall situation will determine the direction to take. Confrontation choices include: "What do the clenched fists mean?" and "Would it be a good guess that the 'No problem' statement is to avoid some distress you are experiencing?"

· ·

Frame of Reference. An MNT's frame of reference inevitably distorts messages to a certain extent because of the unique human experience of each person (Purtilo & Haddad, 1996). New information must relate to that which is already known, and since each of us knows a unique bundle of things, each of us hears communication uniquely. Attitudes, beliefs, values, education, self-image, and sensory interaction all affect what is perceived. This cannot be avoided, but these factors can be recognized and skills can be developed to enlarge the frame of reference.

Frame of reference is a function of willingness to be open to others and is a skill that is honed with experience.

Practice. Practice in openness, concentration, and comprehension increases skill in listening, which in turn helps develop effective responses to clients. Practice holding the body open, practice focusing on the speaker, and make it a practice to look up words whose meanings are not clear. Watch nonverbal signs and discuss their meanings with other students or professionals.

Barriers to Listening

Barriers to listening include attitudes such as defensiveness, failure to accept emotional messages, preoccupation, selective listening as described by Mills (1974), and intense feelings. When any of these factors are operating, an individual is usually rehearsing a response that will reduce tension, and consequently the client's message is not fully comprehended.

Defensiveness

Defensiveness creates bodily tension, a rise in feeling, and thoughts directed toward planning rebuttals or questions rather than listening. Rebuttals generally are designed to promote and protect the listener's own irrational thinking. An example of a defensive inner dialogue instead of listening follows:

CASE EXAMPLE ·

CLIENT: "I'm not sure that Dr. Smith knows what he's talking about." (attended by signals of anger)

MNT: (internal dialogue about what she "ought" to say) I don't think Dr. Smith knows what he's talking about either, but if I admit that, he might not send me any more clients, or this client might sue him and then he'd tell other doctors and then they wouldn't send clients to me. I'd better defend Dr. Smith.

MNT: (response to client) "I'm sure Dr. Smith does know what he's talking about." (attended by signals of defensiveness)

· ·

One can also use the other's speaking time to be thinking about a response that will hide the fact that "I don't know everything."

Ignoring Emotional Messages

Another barrier to listening is placing overemphasis on words and intellectual data and ignoring emotional content. In medical nutrition therapy this can result in acquiring a well-documented database regarding nutritional behavior but completely overlooking the problems in changing food habits.

CASE EXAMPLE ·

CLIENT: "The doctor said he wanted me to gain at least 10 pounds."

MNT: "Yes, that's why he wanted you to come see me. I can help you with that. Let's get a diet history first. What do you have to eat in the morning?"

CLIENT: "I have some cereal and coffee . . . It's just that since my wife died last year I don't feel like eating too much."

MNT: "Yes, well . . . Can you tell me how much and what kind of milk you put on your cereal?"

· ·

In this example the MNT was so intent on gathering information she did not (or chose not to) hear that at least part of the client's eating problems stems from being upset over the loss of his wife. He needs to talk about this issue or he would not have interrupted his initial statement.

Placing too much emphasis on data may also be used to mask the MNT's discomfort with feelings. In *How to Listen, How to Be Heard,* Banville (1978; p. xi) points out that "some of the difficulty we have in listening and relating to others is due to the fact that we tend to limit the number of feelings we permit ourselves to experience." Carl Rogers (1961) considered the major barrier to interpersonal communication to be the evaluation of emotionally charged statements. For instance, if you are uncomfortable with anger, you may not notice anger being expressed or you may get scared and stop listening.

Preoccupation

When a person allows life events outside the here and now to intrude and occupy his or her thinking, listening stops. Thinking about the client in judgmental terms also prevents listening. The MNT may become preoccupied with what she is hearing inside her head instead of paying attention to the client. For instance, if the MNT is thinking about how the client should not have brought her children to the session, or that the wife should not be doing the talking, the MNT will probably miss the message being sent by the client. Worry about peripheral stimuli can include such things as responding to a telephone ringing or the smell of coffee or thinking about other things you must or want to do. Especially in institutional settings, an MNT may have concerns related to productivity that can hinder concentration. For an inexperienced MNT, rehearsal of responses, rather than listening, can be a real hazard. He may think he must know all the answers because he is, after all, the expert.

Mills' Nonlistening Types

Three main types of nonlistening identified by Mills include defensive listening, based on an irrational need to defend oneself; authoritarian listening, based on the belief that the other person has more knowledge and therefore must be believed;

and selective listening, hearing people who are more important and not listening to people who are less important (Mills, 1974). Authoritative and selective listening are really two sides of the same coin. The listener gives credence to social status or intellectual status rather than the message.

Feelings

Feelings can also interfere with listening. Frequently, they are a bigger problem than thoughts. Repressed or oppressed feelings and discomfort about listening to others express feelings may break concentration.

Following are two examples of MNT-client dialogue, one in which the person not talking listened, and one in which the person not talking was a nonlistener.

CASE EXAMPLE ·

MNT: "You say you now weigh 140 pounds and you want to get down to 132 pounds?"

CLIENT: "Right."

MNT: "Have you weighed 132 before?"

CLIENT: "Yes, I've weighed 127 pounds, but I literally had to starve. I can't weigh 127 and eat normally. I really am hungry when I do it. It's a number in my head. When I lose weight I don't always lose it where I want to. I lose it in my upper body so . . . (long pause)."

MNT: "You have this fixed number in your head that you think you should weigh, yet when you lose weight you still aren't satisfied because you don't lose it where you want to?"

CLIENT: "Right!"

· ·

In this example, the MNT heard the concerns behind the words and was able to help the client articulate them.

CASE EXAMPLE ·

CLIENT: "What bothers me is that I'm afraid I'm going to eat all the time. I know what to eat."

MNT: "The thing for you to do is to imagine how you felt when you weighed 25 pounds less—how much easier it was for you to get around. Can you picture that for yourself?"

CLIENT: (very faintly) "I guess."

· ·

In this situation, the MNT ignored the expression of fear and also the statement that the client knew what to eat. Either could have been explored to help the client overcome blocks to change. The dietitian's response sounds like a repetition of what she "should" say and is not related to what the client said. The client response reveals passivity and perhaps recognition that the MNT was not listening. The client sounds "put down."

NONVERBAL COMMUNICATION

Nonverbal communication has not received the scientific attention it deserves in light of its significance in expressing the true meaning of communication. This may be due partly to the self-awareness necessary to understand nonverbal communication and the self-revelation required to carefully study it scientifically. Therefore, nonverbal communication is more art than science. It has implications in both listening to and responding to clients. Functions of nonverbal communication include augmenting meaning beyond the ability of words, negating the meaning of the words, releasing emotional tension through face and body, communicating the status of the relationship among the participants in the communication, and maintaining the rules of communication (Littlejohn, 1983).

An example of augmenting meaning would be slamming a fist on the table to emphasize words of anger. On the other hand, shaking the head "no" while saying "yes" tends to negate the spoken words. The face produces the most nonverbal messages, revealing emotions that augment and support or deny words. Good listeners "hear" clearly what they see and respond accordingly. In addition, nonverbal gestures serve to communicate relative status among people, such as dominance and submissiveness. This in turn leads to signals that regulate who speaks when, who can interrupt and who cannot, and so on.

The advent of television has focused more attention on nonverbal communication because televised nonverbal messages are conscious and orchestrated. Studying commercials can be a way of learning a great deal about "getting the message," which is the real intent of communication.

General agreement exists that nonverbal communication transmits the true meaning of communication. Words can be manipulated and figures made to lie, but censoring body language is almost impossible, except by very skilled actors. Consequently, listening to nonverbal communication, rudimentary as it is, can help you understand the client, and straightforward responses that result in consistency between your verbal and nonverbal message will increase your competence. Two areas of study, *proxemics* and *paralanguage,* have developed useful tools for understanding nonverbal messages.

Proxemics

Proxemics, founded by Charles Hall, concentrates on the study of use of space, specifically interpersonal space in communication. Hall perceived space usage as "specialized elaborations of culture." He delineated eight factors that may have an effect on communications, which have been summarized below (Littlejohn, 1983).

1. *Posture-sex factors:* This includes the sex of the participant and the basic position (standing, sitting, lying down, standing straight, slouching knees, crossed legs, arms, etc).
2. *Sociofugal-sociopetal axis:* The word *sociofugal* means discouragement of interaction; *sociopetal* means the encouragement of interaction. *Axis* refers to the angle of the shoulders relative to the other person. The speakers may be facing each other, may be back to back, or may be positioned toward any other angle in the radius.
3. *Kinesthetic factors:* This refers to the closeness in terms of touchability. Individuals may be in physical contact or within close distance; they may be outside body contact distance; or they may be positioned anywhere in between. This factor also includes the positioning of body parts as well as which parts are touching.
4. *Touching behavior:* People may be involved in any of the following tactile relations: caressing and holding, feeling, prolonged hold, pressing against, spot touching, accidental brushing, or no contact.
5. *Visual code:* This category includes the manner of eye contact ranging from direct (eye-to-eye) to no contact.
6. *Thermal code:* This element involves the perceived heat or energy from the other communicator.
7. *Olfactory code:* This factor includes the kind and degree of odor perceived in the conversation.
8. *Voice loudness:* The loudness of speech relates directly to interpersonal space.

Examples are difficult to provide because they are culture-bound. Observing the client's use of speech and speech symbols, as opposed to trying to force one's own style on the client, will increase perception of the client's true message.

Paralanguage

Another guide to listening to clients is watching for cues to their paralanguage. Paralanguage is the use of vocal sounds other than words to augment words. Paralinguistic cues are divided into four types:

1. *Voice qualities:* pitch, range, quality of articulation (forceful or relaxed), and rhythm.
2. *Vocal characteristics:* laughing, crying, yelling, yawning, spitting, belching.
3. *Vocal qualifiers:* the attitude and/or emphasis with which words and phrases are uttered. For example, the statement, "I ate the whole thing" has different meanings depending on which word in the statement is emphasized.
4. *Vocal segregates:* rhythmic factors that contribute to the flow of speech, such as "um" and "ah," pauses, and other interruptions. These are often used to keep the conversation going (Littlejohn, 1983).

When listening to these nonverbal parts of communication the MNT can pick up much of the emotional content of the client message and determine appropriate listening responses. Mirroring and matching techniques are explored at length in the next section on verbal communication. However, a discussion of the client's nonverbal behaviors that can be mirrored and matched is included there as well. Interpretation should be tentative. Remaining open to alternative meanings in different cultures will create the flexibility needed to listen well to people of different cultures. With experience, you will learn to know the different meanings of nonverbal communication among different clients. A more in-depth study of counseling clients from different cultures can be found in Chapter 7, Cross-Cultural Counseling.

VERBAL COMMUNICATION

As mentioned in the section on comprehension, understanding the meaning of words is important for the MNT. A large vocabulary will help. In addition, there are times when it is not as important for the MNT to understand the meaning of a word or statement as it is for the client to understand. So do not worry if not every single word is understood. It is also a good idea to ask for clarification of meaning if you really need to know more about the meaning of the words a client uses. Misinterpretation is possible in any intervention in which the MNT uses a word different from one the client uses.

Word Usage

Clients reveal clues about their thoughts in their use of certain types of words, especially personal pronouns and verbs. Gestalt therapists have been leaders in teaching us how to listen for clues to meaning in the use of words (Corey, 1991). For instance, the use of "it," "you," or "one" instead of "I"—as in "You know it really makes you mad when you have to give up salt in the diet"—suggests that the client may be hesitant to take responsibility for his or her anger. However, sometimes these words are used simply as a habit, a form of speaking people acquire over time. There often is no conscious thought about choice of words. "I feel really mad about having to give up salt in my diet" suggests responsibility of having normal anger about needing to restrain one's diet. Usually, helping clients to see this distinction and to see the power that lies in the words that are used helps them to feel more internal power or empowerment.

Other words that are important are the use of "will not" and "cannot." For instance, "I cannot stay on my diet" usually means "I will not stay on my diet," since it is rare that it is physically impossible for a person to stay on a diet. Generally speaking, the "cannot" suggests either unwillingness or lack of a sense of power. Asking a client to restate a sentence using the more personal word or more powerful word can help him or her move toward a solution for the problem. Other words to listen for include "try," "will," and "maybe." For example, there is a distinct difference in the meaning of these statements: "I will try to cut down on my fat intake this week," "Maybe I'll cut down on my fat intake," and "I will cut down on my fat intake this week." The last is the most powerful statement of the three.

Responses to clients are both verbal and nonverbal. The following strategies for responding assume that before responding you have listened (Arnold & Boggs, 1995). Table 4–1 illustrates appropriate verbal responses. These were originally targeted toward nurses but are necessary for MNTs as well.

TABLE 4–1

Guidelines for Effective Verbal Expressions

1. Keep messages clear, concrete, honest, and to the point.
2. Match content and delivery with each client's developmental and educational level, experiential frame of reference, and learning readiness.
3. Define unfamiliar terms and concepts.
4. Put ideas in a logical sequence of related material.
5. Relate new ideas to familiar ones when presenting new information.
6. Repeat key ideas.
7. Keep language as simple as possible; use vocabulary familiar to the client.
8. Focus only on essential elements; present one idea at a time.
9. Reinforce key ideas with vocal emphasis and pauses.
10. Use as many sensory communication channels as possible for key ideas.
11. Make sure that nonverbal behaviors support verbal messages.
12. Seek feedback to validate accurate reception of information.

From Arnold E, Boggs K: *Interpersonal Relationships: Professional Communication Skills for Nurses.* 2nd ed. Philadelphia: WB Saunders, 1995.

Mirroring and Matching

Mirroring and matching is a strategy that will increase receptivity and listening skills. It is a way of making intuition more available for use in selecting interventions (Bandler & Grinder, 1979). It will also minimize semantic differences and help establish rapport with clients. It is a strategy that has been used successfully by business and sales personnel for years. They seem to know instinctively to mirror the nonverbal behaviors of customers and adjust (match) their word usage to increase their success in the sale or interaction. Mirroring and matching is calculated to make the customer feel a kinship to the seller. An obvious example is the difference in success between a salesperson from New York City who continued to wear New York style clothing while trying to sell farm equipment to overall-clad farmers, and another New Yorker who chose to wear overalls. The point was that people trust someone like themselves more than someone different (LaFrance, 1982).

The authors of this text made observations, with videotaped evidence, that students who were very successful revealed the trait of mirroring and matching. They would follow behaviors of their clients in practice sessions, mirroring them. For instance, when a "client" cocked his or her head, the student therapist's head would soon be cocked in a mirror image. In a similar manner, students would pick up on the words of the "client" and match them in response. Trust between the "therapist" and "client" would be rapid and the two could get down to business quickly. Skill development was enhanced by viewing tapes in class and analyzing interactions.

To develop skill in mirroring and matching, the first step is to focus listening to become more keenly aware of the client's manner of communication. It is simpler to begin by listening carefully to the client's words and matching his or her words and manner of speaking in responses. When confidence in this aspect is gained, focusing on nonverbal behavior can begin. Take note of body movements, such as crossing or uncrossing the legs, the tilt of the head, and the manner of eye contact,

TABLE 4–2

Words Used That Reflect the Three Representational Systems		
Visual (Seeing)	**Auditory (Hearing)**	**Kinesthetic (Feeling)**
"imagine"	"I hear"	"feel"
"look"	"It sounds like"	"sense"
"I see what the problem is"	"heard"	"grasp"
"picture this"	"rings a bell"	"I can handle that"
"show me"	"I hear what you are saying"	
"focus"		

then mirror that behavior. Patterns of eye contact, for instance, can be a stumbling block to good rapport. Rules for eye contact are different in various societies, and are often a bone of contention between people of differing cultures. In some cultures, rules require that people look each other in the eye when speaking; in others, looking down or away is the rule. Many of the mistakes of individuals from high-eye-contact cultures who interact with people from low-eye-contact cultures are made because they perceived a look down or away as insulting. (For instance, consider the admonishment "Look at me when I'm talking to you.")

Mirroring and matching is a powerful strategy and the benefits are great. The client thinks "I've been heard!" and "my message was received exactly as I sent it!" The client usually feels energized. No interpretation or analyzing is necessary.

Representational Systems

Effective mirroring and matching can be further explained through identification of a client's representational system. This refers to the concept that people actually think from one of three main orientations (or representational systems). When engaged in conversation, "internally, [persons] will be either (1) generating visual images, (2) having feelings or talking to themselves or (3) hearing sounds" (Bandler & Grinder, 1979). It is possible to identify which system is used by the words the client uses. For example, the words "imagine," "look," "I see what the problem is," "picture this," "show," and "focus" belong to a visual representational system. The words "hear," "sounds like," "heard," "rings a bell," and "I hear what you're saying" are examples of the auditory point of view. Clients who base their thoughts kinesthetically use words like "feel," "sense," "grasp," and "handle." Table 4–2 summarizes these words matched with their representational systems (Bandler & Grinder, 1979).

To gain good rapport, listen to the words being said and adjust behavior, using the same kind of words the other person is using. For example, the following dialogue shows a difference in the representational systems of the client and the MNT:

CASE EXAMPLE ·

CLIENT: "Well, I could see it for a long time now how, you know, I was really looking good and being successful and losing the weight, and then suddenly, I just looked around and it wasn't there anymore. Can you see that?"

M N T: "Well, I'm beginning to get a sense of the kind of thing you were feeling."

C L I E N T: "It's just that what I'm trying to show you is my picture of the situation."

M N T: "I feel this is important, go on."

C L I E N T: "Well, what I'd really like is your point of view."

M N T: "I sense that perhaps you might want to avoid those feelings by asking me my opinion."

C L I E N T: "I don't see that this is getting me anywhere."

. . . .

Obviously, the client came from a visual representational system and the MNT was more feeling or kinesthetically oriented. The conversation was not going in a problem-solving direction, and rapport was threatened.

Information about representational systems is also available nonverbally. People make movements with their eyes that will indicate which system is being used. Neurolinguistic programmers, who belong to one school of psychological thought, theorize that visually oriented people look up and to their left or right. In other words, they are making pictures internally. Cues to an auditory representational system are eye movement to the left or right side directly. Kinesthetic feelings are represented by eye movement down and to the left (Fig. 4–1).

These representational systems described by neurolinguistic programmers can be used by the MNT in accurately and effectively mirroring the client. These verbal and nonverbal systems can easily be identified in one's communication partner. It is amazing how often people really do look to the side and then say, "Yes, that does ring a bell," or look up and respond, "Yes, I can really see that now!"

Mirroring especially needs to be handled carefully. Selecting which behaviors to mirror is vital because careless use of this method can make people feel as if they are being mocked. People who begin learning and using this method often report that the recognition of their power over the client is at first a little scary. It is

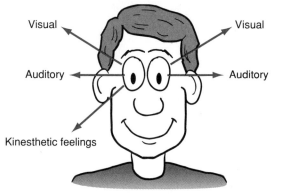

FIGURE 4–1. Neurolinguistic programming visual accessing cues for a normal, right-handed person. Redrawn from Bandler R, Grinder J: *Frogs into Princes: Neurolinguistic Programming.* Moab, UT: Real People Press, 1979.

important to remember that this powerful strategy can be misused. An MNT's use of mirroring must always be in the client's best interest. Mirroring and matching is especially useful in cross-cultural counseling because it reduces the information needed prior to counseling to show sensitivity to clients from diverse cultures.

Because so many nonverbal responses are based on attitudes and are unconscious, the most effective way of making one's nonverbal responses clear is to truly accept the client. However, it is often true that working on techniques to listen well will result in forming favorable attitudes toward clients anyway, so the task is not formidable.

Types of Verbal Responses

There are a number of facilitating responses that are useful in affirming or confronting clients and facilitating change. Each person will feel more comfortable about some than about others, and those with which each person is comfortable are the ones most likely to be used. MNTs need to be comfortable with their interventions; however, this is not the main criterion for selecting them. Often, effective listening responses are not those to which we are accustomed in everyday life. Developing skill includes trying techniques that are uncomfortable and learning to be more comfortable with them. Each counselor needs to attempt new responses, especially if the ones being used do not seem to motivate clients. Observe interventions and evaluate them to see which interventions work and which ones do not and change strategies accordingly.

Affirmation

The basis of the counseling relationship (the empowerment of clients) is affirmation of the intrinsic value and problem-solving ability of clients and, in the case of medical nutrition therapy, affirmation of clients' ability to incorporate specific nutrition behavior into their lifestyles. A client's self-esteem is improved by the positive relationships fostered through affirmation and implication that the client and his or her problems are important to another person (Stuart & Simko, 1991).

The affirmation of clients is the basis of continuing rapport. Many and repetitive affirming responses are needed throughout the counseling sessions. These responses tend to improve client self-concept, and as a result increase clients' ability to see new options for coping with nutrition problems. Some examples of affirmation follow:

1. Refer to clients by courtesy title and last name until some other mutually agreed-on salutation has been determined. This shows respect.
2. Ask for clarification when you don't understand with a question such as "Did I hear . . . ?"
3. Follow a confrontation by pointing out a positive aspect about the client.
4. Verify clients' rights to feel.
5. Consistently communicate trust and respect for the client.
6. Be self-assertive when you have ideas or feelings to express.
7. Use nonverbal responses signifying trust and respect for clients, such as silence when both the MNT and client need to process some communication.

Affirmation of clients may seem very easy at first. However, continuing interaction with a single client is likely to bring awareness of the patience and dedication needed to repeatedly affirm client worth and ability. Frustration may occur because non–problem-solving behaviors and underlying negative thoughts and feelings may continue to be expressed by a client over time. Remember that clients' problems have taken a long time to develop and may take a long time to be solved. The result of consistent affirmation will be realized when feedback from clients provides evidence of new ways of coping. Clients will confirm, in their own words, belief in themselves and report successful behaviors and more positive thoughts and feelings in their daily lives.

Confrontation

Confrontation in the counseling situation is a process of developing an awareness of behaviors, thoughts, and feelings that have been unnoticed or denied by clients (Othmer & Othmer, 1994). It is designed to identify hindrances to change and is not the adversarial process that it may be in other contexts.

Confrontation requires a dialogue between the MNT and the client that will help the client recognize faulty thinking, inaccurate beliefs, and useless, inappropriate feelings that are barriers to problem-solving. Engen and coauthors (1983) listed four basic areas subject to confrontation: (1) discrepancies between self-perception and others' perceptions of the client, (2) discrepancies between the client's words and behaviors, (3) discrepancies between feelings the client says she or he has and the feelings most people would have in the same or similar situations, and (4) discrepancies between stated beliefs and actual behavior.

Affirmation of the client often serves as a kind of confrontation, because many clients do not consider themselves as capable as others consider them. Discrepancies between words and behaviors may be as simple as bringing to the attention of the client that he said "yes," but shook his head "no" and perhaps he really meant "no." Anger is a feeling that many people dislike having, and so may say they are not angry about something that an observer knows quite well would make anyone angry. Clients may need to be confronted when their actions are not consistent with the goals they have set for nutrition counseling.

CASE EXAMPLE ·

CLIENT: (Reviewing what transpired since last session) "I did quite well keeping my intake to 1500 calories each day until my husband *dragged* me out for dinner."

MNT: "He dragged you?"

CLIENT: "Yes." (angry-sounding)

MNT: "What do you feel about that?"

CLIENT: "Oh, it's okay. He meant well."

MNT: "I think of being dragged as something that could cause anger."

· ·

The inconsistency in this example is between the client's use of a word normally associated with becoming angry and the subsequent denial of feeling, with a statement in defense of the husband. This person may have a belief that she should not feel angry.

The need for confrontation is recognized among therapists regardless of their theoretical leanings and they will confront according to their theoretical beliefs. For instance, behavioral therapists confront behaviors. Cognitive therapists confront dysfunctional thinking patterns. From the viewpoint of transactional analysis, illusions are confronted such as prejudice or magical thinking or the use of ego states. Gestalt therapists confront lack of awareness and help clients become aware of thoughts and feelings hindering spontaneous responses in the here and now.

Strategies of confrontation or affirmation are used when client responses indicate that a decision to change is not firm or when clients have been unable to follow through on a commitment. Careful listening will reveal subtle nuances in client responses that indicate the firmness of decisions. For instance, four of the five following responses to "What are you going to do?" indicate a less-than-firm decision.

- ▌ "I am going to try to leave the salt shaker in the cupboard this week." (Use of the word "try" is likely a prediction of failure.)
- ▌ "I am not going to eat as much salt this week." (Very indefinite, since "as much salt" cannot be measured.)
- ▌ "I wish I could leave salt off my food this week." (A wishy-washy decision.)
- ▌ "I want to leave the salt shaker in the cupboard this week." (Wanting is something like wishing, not deciding.)
- ▌ "I am going to eat foods that are naturally unsalted this week." (A to-the-point, measurable, positive action statement.)

Nonverbal behaviors must be watched even more closely than verbalizations for signals of commitment or lack of it. The face and the voice are especially revealing. For example, when the client frowns or does not make eye contact when she says she is sure she can accomplish her goals, or when a client's voice is barely audible while saying his decision is firm, it is indicative of lack of commitment.

When clients make statements indicating low self-esteem, confrontation should be followed by affirmation of client abilities. Clients need consistent reinforcement of their problem-solving capabilities and self-worth to combat self-deprecating internal dialogue patterns that have contributed to ineffective problem-solving in the past. In this problem-solving counseling approach, a wide range of confrontational techniques available to the MNT will increase flexibility.

Skilled MNTs know what problems are the most common in changing eating behaviors. They also perceive accurately the specific problems of a given client and have a wide repertoire of interventions and responses on which to draw in facilitating awareness and change. Unique to nutrition counseling is the need to confront misconceptions about nutrition. Misconceptions about nutrition include faulty ideas about the magical properties of food, food composition, and relationships between food and disease.

Too much confrontation will frighten clients and increase anxiety. Too little confrontation will sabotage efforts to meet goals. Awareness of one's faults and facing sensitive subjects are difficult for clients. They need a steady flow of communication to affirm their value and problem-solving abilities to keep them motivated as their inadequacies are addressed.

The following guidelines are useful in confrontation:

- Push ahead whenever you get the chance and retreat when you meet client resistance.
- Encourage clients to feel whatever they feel, without taking responsibility for client feelings.
- Become aware of your own psychological needs. Do not confront clients to meet your needs.

The goal of confrontation and affirmation techniques is to motivate the client toward a commitment to change. These techniques facilitate each stage of problem-solving and create a climate that leads finally to a commitment to behavioral changes. For example, in Stage II, "Define Problems Multidimensionally," confronting may foster a deeper understanding of the client's problem. In Stage III, "Select Alternative Solutions," both confrontation and affirmation can support the client's imagination in brainstorming. The same is true in Stage IV, "Planning for Change." Confronting strategies also help identify discrepancies that are blocking problem-solving and can help retreat to a previous stage. Stage V, "Commitment to Action," may be the stage in which confrontation is the most vital. A client may express a commitment that is not felt and subsequently fail to keep it if the MNT lets her "off the hook" of confrontation, so to speak. Confrontation does carry the risk of upsetting the client; but it also presents a greater possibility of making real progress toward dietary changes rather than holding back.

Types of Verbal Responses

Every response that the MNT makes to clients is an opportunity to strengthen the client-MNT connection or break it (Arnold & Boggs, 1995). Each one should be made with purpose. Verbal responses can be classified as probing, clarifying, reflecting/reiteration, interpreting, and paraphrasing.

Probing

Probing is questions or statements presented with the purpose of obtaining additional information. It is important to phrase the questions so that clients sense that answers will be accepted without being judged (Arnold & Boggs, 1995). Give no clue as to the expected answer. For instance, it is better to ask, "How much of it did you eat?" than "Did you eat all of it?" The second phrasing could be interpreted as judgmental and does not encourage expansion by the client. Questions that can be answered "yes" or "no" generally frustrate counseling effectiveness, unless quick, simple answers are what is needed. Both open-ended and close-ended questions should be used appropriately, although open-ended ones are usually more productive (Arnold & Boggs, 1995). Probing strategies may also be used to encourage expression of feelings by a client. When a client tells about a frustrating situation, a probing response would be "How do you feel about that?"

Clarifying

There are several reasons for using clarifying responses. One may wish to clarify the meaning of client statements that were expressed in a confused way, to help identify values, or to confront discrepancies. There are many uses of clarifying statements that both confront and affirm. For example, "Could you clarify that for me? You just said what seemed like two conflicting things" (a confrontation), or "Yes, I hear that your recovery is top priority now, that's good" (an affirmation).

Reflecting and Reiteration

These are responses used to elicit elaboration on something the client has said. They are exact repetitions of what was said, and their purpose is to focus on a particular aspect of what the client has said so that it can be made apparent and be more fully expressed. Reflection is particularly valuable in precipitating confrontations. Reflections do not require interpretation by the MNT and they offer the opportunity for the client to hear what she or he has said. For example, "You just said, 'I just can't seem to stop eating,' am I right?"

Interpreting

This is similar to reflecting, but what the client said is put into the MNT's own words, or nonverbal behaviors are interpreted: "You are kicking your foot. Are you angry?" Interpretations of a client's statements or behavior must always be offered tentatively, and different avenues of investigation will be followed depending on the response of the client (Dyer & Vriend, 1988). Interpretations carry the risk that they may not be accurate.

Paraphrasing

This response is a statement that includes the major ideas in the client's statement as well as a verbalization of emotional nonverbal behavior. It is an extension of reflecting and interpreting responses and may come from either the MNT or the client (Dyer & Vriend, 1988). It is a benchmark of progress when clients assertively make these summarization statements.

After each intervention, listen carefully to a client's responses. They will indicate acceptance, "Yes, that's right," rejection, "No, that's not what I mean," or denial, "No, that's not an issue at all." Press on with acceptance and withhold further intervention when rejection or denial occurs.

When using any intervention, the more the client's words are used, the less likely one will be to misinterpret him or her or get into an argument over semantics. Arguing with a client is a digression from problem-solving.

Humor

Recent research has indicated that a good sense of humor moderates the detrimental impact of negative events and enhances the positive elements in life (Kuiper et al, 1995). Humor can be a useful technique in nutrition counseling as a direct way of establishing rapport and as a confrontational technique. A funny anecdote or other spontaneous humor told in the beginning of a new encounter with a client can help break the ice and create a bond. Humor can also be used indirectly as a way of addressing issues and laughing at issues, concerns, and the human condition. However, because of its indirectness and the influence culture and personal background have on humor, care must be taken or humor will become counterproductive (Purtilo & Haddad, 1996). The MNT needs to clearly delineate between laughing *with* someone and laughing *at* someone. Jokes and cartoons need to be carefully thought out as to purpose before being introduced.

Humor is used to ridicule our own or others' ignorance, to cope with stress that is overwhelming (Silberman, 1987; Nezu et al, 1988), to say difficult things indirectly, to relieve anxiety or fear, or as a response to incongruities. In addition, cartoons and jokes rely on some type of half riddle that must be solved by the listener, and most riddles require "inside" information. "Inside" information requires understanding of the cultural context of the joke or cartoon. Care must be taken that humor does not discount clients (Gilliland et al, 1989).

One's sense of humor is what determines which of the uses of humor is funny to him or her. A person's sense of humor is related both to his or her cultural background and to the immediate situation. When feelings are intense one's sense of humor is generally diminished. People who are concerned about being approved of may not respond well to humor. It is often important for the MNT to appreciate the client's sense of humor, yet take it as a serious expression. The following poem written by a patient is humorous, yet expresses negative emotions, hostility, and anger. It is serious.

Poem to a Dietitian

I wrote a letter today to Dorothy Dix
Telling her how you got me in this fix
A thousand calories I'm supposed to get
Why you can't count that far I bet.
One bird egg less any toast
Would be a few calories at the most
Some cracked corn without sugar to make it sweet
Now there's a combination that's hard to beat
And, white fluid called milk, less any cream
I'll see that drink tonight when I dream
That coffee it sure was black
It almost blew my stack.
So, Dorothy Dix will cream, I know
And I hope to get some food to show.

Laughter is not the same as humor or sense of humor. People laugh at things that are not funny as well as those that are. Laughter at something that is not funny or is tragic is sometimes described as *gallows humor* (James & Jongeward, 1978). Sometimes laughter is a sign of arrogance or nervousness or is a technique to cover up an emotion that the person is hesitant to express directly. When using humor, the MNT needs to be particularly careful that none of the negative uses of humor mentioned here creep into his or her communication patterns. The following dialogue demonstrates an appropriate use of humor. The client is being counseled for obesity:

CASE EXAMPLE ·

MNT: "Tell me about what you eat for dessert."

CLIENT: (fidgeting) "I'm a dessert lover. Ha! Ha!" (gallows laugh)

MNT: "Me too! Ha! Ha!"

CLIENT: "That's my main problem. Ha! Ha!"

MNT: (Silent pause)

CLIENT: "I guess desserts really are a major problem for me." (no laughter)

· ·

In this interchange, the original laughter in which both client and MNT produced a gallows laugh served to create a bond between them. However, it was essential that the repetition by the client not receive a light-hearted response because it would create an ulterior communication of some type, suggesting that the MNT was ridiculing the client or conspiring with him to avoid the very problem of desserts. The further response by the client indicated that the interchange guided him toward a partial acceptance ("I guess") of the problem. In their subsequent dialogue, the two addressed the issue of desserts effectively.

COGNITIVE MODELING AND THOUGHT STOPPING

Cognitive modeling and thought stopping is a strategy appropriate for the problem-solving approach to medical nutrition therapy. In this method, clients are provided an opportunity to see, hear, and compare behaviors and thought patterns that are non–problem-solving (Cormier & Cormier, 1979). The MNT can work with the client to articulate problem-solving thoughts instead of non–problem-solving thoughts. Appropriate positive thoughts are identified and can be used in place of negative thinking. Clients are taught to stop thinking negatively and substitute the positive thoughts worked out in the counseling session. For instance, if a person has trouble preparing food without eating some, she may think something like "I can't stop myself from eating while I cook." This thought could be replaced with thoughts such as "I can cook without eating."

In medical nutrition therapy, cognitive modeling and thought-stopping techniques must include articulation of appropriate nutrition knowledge (no magical thinking or misinformation) as well as thoughts that support the capability and self-worth of the client.

Role-Playing and the Empty Chair Technique

Two similar techniques that can be used in cognitive modeling are role-playing and the empty chair technique. In role-playing, two or more people (this can be the counselor and client or, in group counseling, two group members) act out a situation that is a problem for the client. A desirable way of dealing with a situation can be enacted, giving the client practice. In the empty chair technique, the client plays all the roles (Corey, 1991). This technique is derived from the Gestalt school of psychology and is used to probe clients intensively, often dealing with feelings (Gilliland et al, 1989). Using techniques to probe feelings deeply should be left to individuals well trained in psychology. Nevertheless, in a modified version, such a technique is useful in helping clients become aware of anxiety in certain situations, do some self-modeling, and practice such things as assertiveness. Assertiveness is discussed in detail in Chapter 11, Professional Considerations. The following case example illustrates the use of the empty chair technique.

CASE EXAMPLE ·

To prepare for this technique, the client needs to be asked if she is willing to act out or practice what she would like to say in a given situation. The situation may either be an interaction with the client and another person (cognitive modeling) or it can be internal dialogue (thought stopping). Two chairs are set up facing each other, and it is explained to the client that she is to move from chair to chair and play all the roles.

The following dialogue chronicles an internal dialogue.

M N T: "Please sit in this chair and say the thoughts you have when you begin to eat foods that you really don't want to eat."

C L I E N T: "OK. Well, it won't hurt just this one time. No one really will know."

M N T: "Now, go over and sit in the other chair and say out loud what you think of the statement just made."

C L I E N T: (moving to the other chair) "Clara, you know better than that. You know that people will know. You say that all the time, just as an excuse to eat. By the time you've finished saying that you've ruined your diet anyway."

M N T: "Now go back over to the other chair, and tell yourself in the other chair your reaction to the thoughts."

C L I E N T: (moves to other chair) "It is very scolding. I felt mad hearing it."

M N T: "Would you go back to the other chair and say something kinder to yourself about the excuses you think of to justify your behavior?"

C L I E N T: (moves to other chair) "Clara, in the long run you are going to be happier if you stop thinking of those excuses for your behavior."

M N T: "Come on back over here."

C L I E N T: (moves) "I like that much better. When I start to make up excuses, I'll just stop. I'll just say to myself, 'Clara, stop, you're going to be happier keeping your commitment.' I can say it to myself several times if I don't listen the first time."

· ·

Relaxation Training

Inappropriate eating often occurs in situations in which clients feel tense. When such tenseness is the focus of needed change, one approach is relaxation training. Clients can develop the ability to relax through the following process.

1. Becoming aware of situations in which they are tense.
2. Becoming aware of the processes by which they tense themselves.
3. Practicing relaxing by taking three or four deep breaths and then attending closely to regular breathing while at the same time tensing and releasing muscles in all parts of the body, especially those that become tense during inappropriate eating situations.
4. Imagining themselves in the uncomfortable situations and practicing relaxing.

Clients are generally warned that they will feel some tingling sensations or heaviness when they first begin to practice relaxation. Relaxation techniques work best if learned first in situations in which tension is moderate before being attempted in situations in which the client has high levels of tenseness (Warpeha & Harris, 1993).

Biofeedback

Biofeedback is a technique that provides visual information regarding unconscious biological activities in the body. Mechanical devices are used to monitor changes in body temperature and neurological activity to assist people in becoming aware of the biological effects of stress (Warpeha & Harris, 1993).

Although the term is relatively new, the use of biofeedback in weight control has been in use for a long time. A scale can be a powerful tool in weight control and provides some evidence of the biological effect of eating behavior. It has been learned, however, that there are times when emphasis should be focused not on weight itself, but other biological factors, such as changes in stress levels resulting from behavioral changes. Immediate feedback regarding body temperature or neurological changes may be more effective than changes in weight. Biofeedback can be used in conjunction with other relaxation techniques to change habitual reactions to stress.

GROUP COUNSELING

Group counseling is a strategy in which several people come together with the therapist at one time. There are styles in which the therapist serves as a group leader, and members cannot confront one another. This process is individual counseling in a group setting (Berne, 1966). Another style is one in which the counselor allows clients to confront one another as in a discussion group. The danger in this style lies in the possibility that group members will confront each other in nonproductive ways. A great amount of research has established group counseling as an effective approach to change. Much of group therapy has been recognized as common sense (Gilliland et al, 1989). Groups can range from educational groups to problem-solving groups to psychotherapy groups. Family counseling is also a form of group counseling (Corey, 1991).

The advantages of groups include the following:

▋ A group provides feedback between participants.
▋ Members can give each other support and a sense of belonging.
▋ People can test the practicality of their ideas.
▋ People can test reality and recognize faulty thinking.
▋ Groups encourage and support commitment.
▋ Individuals discover that their problems are not unique and are solvable.

The disadvantages of a group include:

▋ Some members may not feel free to be frank and open.
▋ Counselors must be acute listeners who can remain aware of what is going on with several people at a time.
▋ Counselors must be able to prevent undesirable negative interactions between clients.
▋ Coercion of weaker group members can occur if the counselor is weak.
▋ Strong members of a group may attempt to take over the group.

In medical nutrition therapy, groups that come together are most likely to be educational groups rather than actual counseling groups. Educational groups have the primary purpose of imparting information to group members. This is a legitimate function for groups, but it is very different from counseling groups. Counseling groups are not for everyone. Putting a person into a group who is not prepared can set that person up for failure (Edelwich & Brodsky, 1992). Strong, satisfying support systems for people who have similar medical problems, such as diabetes, heart disease, cancer, and metabolic diseases, can result from group activity. Children can benefit a great deal by coming together with other children with similar problems. The group leader needs to be clear as to the purpose of the group. Is it for educational purposes? Is it for counseling, in which more emotional aspects of change are to occur? Group members may become fearful or resentful if they do not understand what will happen in the group.

Groups develop a culture all of their own with each person assuming a particular role in the group (Arnold & Boggs, 1995). Group dynamics must be carefully planned and handled by an MNT who is a group leader. Figure 4–2 describes factors that affect group dynamics.

The setting for groups must be appropriate. There should be ample space, privacy, and adequate physical surroundings. The group should be limited to the number of people the counselor can acutely observe at one time. Four is often a good number. Eight is usually the limit (Ohlsen et al, 1988). When there are more than eight in a group, it is difficult to handle as a counseling group, and better results will be achieved if the group is handled as a nutrition education class.

It is suggested that novice MNTs use groups for educational purposes. As the MNT becomes more practiced, it could prove productive for him or her to study group communication, complete training for group counseling work, or become a partner with a psychological therapist.

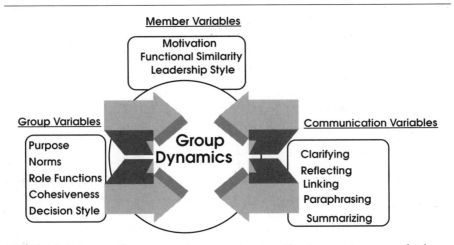

FIGURE 4–2. Factors affecting group dynamics. (From Arnold E, Boggs K: *Interpersonal Relationships: Professional Communication Skills for Nurses.* 2nd ed. Philadelphia: WB Saunders, 1995.)

NUTRITION EDUCATION

Nutrition education of clients is an important aspect of medical nutrition therapy. It is also the simplest aspect. The MNT needs to tailor nutrition education to each client's needs in individual counseling. In group counseling, overall goals need to be developed, even though they may not always meet every need of every client. A strategy of counseling, above and beyond the accuracy of information, is the approach to providing the information. When nutrition information is presented in a logical manner, it is usually more acceptable to clients. "If, then" statements are frequently helpful in applying knowledge. For example, "If you like to eat eggs every morning, then you can still stay within a desirable cholesterol intake if you cut down on some of these other foods high in cholesterol. Let's work together to see how this can be done." Or "A high sodium intake may contribute to the swelling that is bothering you."

The use of "should," "ought," "do this," "don't do that" implies that a client has limited mental capacity and must do what she or he is told to do, be compliant, and follow a prescription. Resistance is very likely to occur (James & Jongeward, 1978).

EMPOWERMENT

Empowerment is the act of investing an individual with authority or enabling him or her to use power as an individual. A dietetic practitioner may be empowered to practice nutrition counseling on both counts when she or he has met a credentialing standard and has also developed assertiveness and a personal sense of power. In nutrition counseling, this power is in turn focused on empowering clients to develop healthy nutrition lifestyles and solve related problems. Although not the direct intent, the empowerment of clients in nutrition-related areas may have the happy result of empowerment in many other aspects of their lives as well.

Power

Power has two general meanings: the physical energy to work, and motivation to do, to think, to feel, and to solve the problems of life. Each of these types of power relies on some source of kinetic energy before power is exerted. The nutrients in food are the source of physical energy. Pinpointing sources of psychological power is much more difficult.

Culture

Culture has a significant influence on perceptions of the source of power, and the values of a particular culture direct the way in which power is used. In general, some cultures teach that power is within, others that it is outside the individual. This has become identified as *locus of control* in psychological terms. Sensitivity to a client's perception of power and values will help turn potential power into action. Appealing to the appropriate power motivates and directs the use of personal power. Clients' statements provide clues as to their perceptions. For instance, when a client says, "God willing, I can overcome this problem," he is giving a clue that he perceives an external source of power. On the other hand, "I know my strength is within me," indicates an internal source of empowerment.

A sense of personal power has been shown to enhance problem-solving in health behaviors as well as in other areas of life (Rody, 1988). Cultures differ in the ways people are taught to exert power, but results are similar. A sense of personal power relates to the dominance and submission expectations of a society. People in submissive positions tend to use indirect modes of exerting power; those who are dominant use direct methods (Cowan et al, 1995). The style of expressing power needs to be appropriate for the client's culture.

Knowledge

In addition to cultural values, knowledge contributes to perceptions of power. Knowledge about nutrition includes nutrition facts, skills in obtaining food, facts about health, and disease-specific information. The proliferation of knowledge, much of it incorrect in the United States, adds a dimension to the knowledge aspects of nutrition counseling; strategies are needed for evaluating the quality of clients' nutrition information. Nutrition education for the client will be effective when motivation has been brought to focus on problem solving. The client's perceived knowledge must also be addressed as part of the solution to his or her problems.

Food Meanings

The complexity of nonbiological meanings of food often confounds the scientific basis for a healthy nutrition lifestyle, and these meanings have a powerful influence on clients' decisions. These were discussed at length in Chapter 2, The Meanings of Food.

Empowerment Tools

Empowerment is the overall goal of the counseling strategies that have been outlined in this chapter. Each strategy provides an opportunity to combine the MNT's power with the client's power to establish a healthy nutrition lifestyle and facilitate problem-solving skills. This produces a synergistic effect: counselor and counselee joining together as a problem-solving team.

The MNT needs to be *flexible and alert,* ready to use whatever the client perceives as a source of power. The MNT needs to be ready to shift gears, interacting with leads coming from the client, working to empower each individual client differently. Working with someone else's motivational sources is a challenging task. The strategy of mirroring and matching is clearly a powerful tool in an effort to be responsive to clients. Empowerment tools include the following:

- Counseling strategies to develop self-confidence and a personal sense of power
- Nutrition/disease education
- Empathy
- Sensitivity
- Flexibility
- Acute observation of client's sense of power

TABLE 4–3

A Comparison of Traditional and Empowering Educational Models in the Treatment of Diabetes

Traditional Medical Model	Empowering Person-Centered Model
1. Diabetes is a physical illness.	1. Diabetes is a biopsychosocial illness.
2. Relationship of provider and patient is authoritarian, based on provider expertise.	2. Relationship of provider and patient is democratic and based on shared expertise.
3. Problems and learning needs are usually identified by professional.	3. Problems and learning needs are usually identified by patient.
4. Professional is viewed as problem solver and caregiver; ie, professional is responsible for diagnosis, treatment, and outcome.	4. Patient is viewed as problem-solver and caregiver; ie, professional acts as a resource and both share responsibility for treatment and outcome.
5. Goal is compliance with recommendations. Behavioral strategies are used to increase compliance with recommended treatment. A lack of compliance is viewed as a failure of patient and provider.	5. Goal is to enable patients to make informed choices. Behavioral strategies are used to help patients change behaviors of their choosing. A lack of goal achievement is viewed as feedback and used to modify goals and strategies.
6. Behavior changes are externally motivated.	6. Behavior changes are internally motivated.
7. Patient is powerless, professional is powerful.	7. Patient and professional are powerful.

From Funnell MM, Anderson RM, Arnold MS, et al: Empowerment: An idea whose time has come in diabetes education. *Diabetes Educ.* 1991;17(1):37–41.

Table 4–3 details a comparison of traditional and empowering educational models in the treatment of diabetes (Funnell et al, 1991).

Power Struggles

Unfortunately, client and counselor may each use power to produce a power struggle rather than to solve problems. Power struggles are attempts to force (or resist) the imposition of one person's value system on another person. Such struggles stem from lack of self-confidence, lack of trust, and other personal and cultural beliefs about what the "truth" is or "how things should be done." Because the MNT must be the more powerful person in the counseling session, and the one trained in empowerment, it is her or his responsibility to conduct counseling so that power struggles are avoided.

The basis of power struggles may be dogmatism on the part of an MNT who has a missionary zeal for her or his particular interpretation of a healthy nutrition lifestyle. Or it may be a belief on the counselor's part that she or he is responsible for finding the correct solution to everyone's problems. Such beliefs are not uncommon among people who go into the helping professions. Part of the preparation for effective counseling is addressing one's own dogma. This is not to suggest that there are never times to challenge client belief systems. Challenges that are empathic and sensitive can be very effective. When resistance is met, the wise MNT retreats, perhaps to address the issue another time when the client may be more receptive.

Empowerment Models

A model for empowering clients was presented by Funnell and coauthors (1991). The authors described empowerment as a way of helping people gain mastery over their affairs through a system of care "in which patients are viewed as equal and active partners in the treatment program."

Key concepts include:

- Emphasis on the whole person
- Emphasis on personal strengths, rather than deficits
- Patient selection of learning needs
- Setting shared or negotiated goals
- Transference of leadership and decision-making to the client
- Client generation of problems and solutions
- Analysis of failures as problems rather than as personal deficits
- Discovery and enhancement of internal motivation toward health
- Emphasis on client-developed support systems

This article emphasizes that an empowered professional is an essential part of implementing their model. Funnell and coauthors quote T. A. White, who described empowerment as a five-step process:

1. Healing yourself and your relationships with others
2. Becoming responsible for yourself and your life
3. Becoming empowered

4. Creating a vision of your life as you want it
5. Committing to action by establishing priorities, goal setting, and goal getting.

A self-empowerment model has been developed by Kirk (1994). According to this model, the first step in empowerment is awareness of choice. Belief in the ability to choose changes the meaning assigned to people and events and leads to behavioral change. Other people do not have to be obeyed and events are not inevitable.

These models were both designed for people with specific health problems, but they are useful in any circumstance in which nutrition counseling is sought. There are several ways of challenging beliefs. The empty chair method will help an individual become aware of his or her belief system. Questioning the logic of belief systems is another method of confrontation.

CASE EXAMPLE ·

C L I E N T: "I can't tell John 'no' when he insists that I join him in eating dessert." (This statement implies a lack of choice in dealing with John. In fact, the client has a choice.)
    The MNT has at least two choices of response.

M N T: 1. "You really can't tell John 'no' (powerlessness) or you won't tell John 'no' (accepting responsibility for actions)?"

        2. "What would happen if you said 'no' to John?" (This response challenges the client to become aware of irrational fears [and occasionally rational fears] she has of the consequences of saying "no" to John.)

· ·

INTERPERSONAL SKILLS

Interpersonal skills bind the processes together and facilitate effective problem-solving. Following is a summary of general interpersonal skills to use and a few behaviors to avoid.

Maintain Eye Contact
Look at client when speaking and when listening, mirroring the client in a respectful way. Do not signal disinterest or preoccupation by gazing around. Focus attention on visuals when applicable, as in "This is a copy of the Food Guide Pyramid, let's look at it together." Be aware of client's degree of comfortable eye contact and respond appropriately. For example, if you notice that Mrs. X is gazing around the room and appears uncomfortable in maintaining eye contact, focus eyes more frequently on materials, visuals, and so on.

Keep Voice Level Appropriate
Be expressive and enthusiastic. Avoid extreme loudness, inaudibleness, or monotone voice.

Demonstrate Confidence

Say something like "I'm sure I can help you devise a plan that can fit into your lifestyle."

Demonstrate Empathy

Use tactile communication when appropriate, such as a touch or a pat on the hand or arm. Use facial expression, tone of voice, and bodily gestures to display empathy. Allow time for client expression, feedback, and response.

Be Nonjudgmental

If a client says, "I had three ice cream sundaes yesterday," respond with something like, "What was your experience of that?"

Talk Sparingly

Give information in a short, concise way. Do not interrupt. Do not take up a lot of time talking or lecturing. Do not give excessive unsolicited information.

Confront Effectively

For example, if a patient rejects his or her food by not eating from the tray or throwing the food on the floor, respond with something like, "I can see that you are upset about something. Do you want to talk about it?"

Provide Adequate Positive Reinforcement

Say things to the client like "This is fine," "That is a good idea," and "Sounds like you are on your way!"

Use Appropriate Physical Distance

Upon initial contact with client, assess his or her need for personal space and position yourself accordingly. If the client jumps or is alarmed upon your entrance, keep a reasonable distance. For example, if the client is on the bed, sit on a chair at the foot of the bed. As the interview progresses and openness is exhibited by the client, you might ask if you can pull your chair a bit closer to hear better or to show visuals.

Ask for and Give Clarification When Needed

Give the client appropriate verbal feedback. Repeat what the client has said to verify facts. Answer questions effectively. Ask for clarification. For example, if the client says, "I eat a box of cookies for breakfast," ask, "About how many cookies is that?" Ask client to repeat, using phrases like "Do you mean . . . ?" and "Did you say . . . ?"

Use Open-Ended Questions Effectively

For example, use questions like "What did you eat when you first got up?", "What did you put in your coffee?", "When in the day is it the hardest for you to avoid food you don't want to eat?", and "How do you feel about that?"

Use Close-Ended Questions Effectively

Ask the client specific questions depending on need, as in, "Do you have any food allergies?" and "Do you think this alternative is realistic for you?"

Maintain an Objective State of Mind Throughout the Session

If a person with diabetes eats sweets excessively, maintain a nonjudgmental attitude. Ask something like, "How do you think this will affect your condition?"

Check Out Incongruent Behaviors or Statements (Verbal Response Versus Body Language)

If you see that a client is responding positively verbally and manifesting negative body signs, confront this discrepancy by asking, for example, "What are you feeling right now?"

Ask One Question at a Time and Wait for an Answer

The habit of not waiting for an answer to a question is common. People ask a second question because they think the first was not good enough. Do not interrupt the client but allow her or him to talk. Interject appropriately to signify listening. For example, "uh-huh" and "yes" indicate that you are following the conversation of the client. Be comfortable with silence. Do not put words in clients' mouths. Schedule adequate time for the interview.

Make Referrals as Appropriate

Depending on the area of concern, refer clients to another professional such as a dentist, physician, occupational or physical therapist, speech therapist, or psychologist, or to social services such as Meals on Wheels or the food stamp program.

Summary

Common to all counseling strategies is the expectation that changes will occur in small steps. The idea that a person would be instructed on a diet regimen and then spontaneously incorporate the entire diet into his or her lifestyle is unrealistic for most people. For instance, a prescription for a 1 g sodium diet for an individual normally ingesting a 4 g sodium diet would be accomplished in stages, reducing sodium intake systematically by setting small intermediate goals on the way to the final goal of a 1 g sodium intake.

Each of the strategies mentioned in this chapter can facilitate changes in nutrition lifestyle. The task of the MNT is to practice different strategies to become flexible in their use. Flexibility leads to skill in selecting interventions based on listening to clients. Learning additional strategies beyond those addressed here will add to an MNT's skill.

It is important for the MNT to accept the challenge of probing factors underlying food choices and to develop the courage to intervene. External support for the client is highly important in the client's ability to become aware of the barriers he or she may have erected to avoid changing.

It is important to remain fully aware of the centrality of food to the human being and its power as a motivator. Food is a primary reinforcer of behavior as well as a symbol of love and belonging. It is deeply entwined with one's self image. Listening to clients will make it clear to the MNT what meanings food has for each client.

For most people, counseling strategies are simply the tools that help to enhance the personal relationship that will develop between MNT and client. That unique relationship is the most important factor in successful counseling.

Self-awareness is a primary tool of effective MNTs. Psychological messages sent to a client relay to him or her what you really feel in spite of anything you say. The greater the congruence between your own behavior and your inner feelings, the more the client will recognize your true strength and the more your relationship will become one of problem-solving.

Suggestions for Further Learning

1. Listen to people you know communicate and observe their listening patterns.

2. Watch news interviews and listen to radio interviews.

3. Tape conversations with friends and replay them to listen to your own communication patterns.

4. Videotape or audiotape an actual counseling interaction and analyze it to determine which techniques you used and if they were effective. It will also afford you the opportunity to listen to the client again. Did you hear or see anything differently this time? Any other strategies that could be employed?

CITED REFERENCES

Arnold E, Boggs K: *Interpersonal Relationships: Professional Communication Skills for Nurses.* 2nd ed. Philadelphia: WB Saunders, 1995.

Bandler R, Grinder J: *Frogs into Princes: Neurolinguistic Programming.* Moab, UT: Real People Press, 1979.

Banville TG: *How to Listen—How to Be Heard.* Chicago: Nelson-Hall, 1978.

Barbara DA: *The Art of Listening.* Springfield, IL: Charles C Thomas, 1958.

Berne E: *Principles of Group Treatment.* New York: Grove Press, 1966.

Birdwhistell R: *Kinesics and Context: Essays on Body Motion and Communication.* Philadelphia: University of Pennsylvania Press, 1970.

Brammer LM: *The Helping Relationship: Process and Skills.* Englewood Cliffs, NJ: Prentice-Hall, 1985.

Corey G (ed): *Theory and Practice of Counseling and Psychotherapy.* 3rd ed. Pacific Grove, CA: Brooks/Cole Publishing Co, 1991.

Cormier WH, Cormier LS: *Interviewing Strategies for Helpers: A Guide to Assessment, Treatment, and Evaluation.* Monterey, CA: Brooks/Cole Publishing Company, 1979.

Cowan G, Bommersbach M, Curtis SR: Codependency, loss of self, and power. *Psych Women Q.* 1995;19:221–236.

Curry-Bartley K: The art and science of listening. *Top Clin Nutr.* 1986;1:14–24.

Curry-Bartley K: *Dietetic Practitioner Skills: Nutrition Education, Counseling, and Business Management.* New York: Macmillan, 1987.

Dyer WW, Vriend J: *Counseling Techniques That Work.* Alexandria, VA: The American Association for Counseling and Development, 1988.

Edelwich J, Brodsky A: *Group Counseling for the Resistant Client.* New York: Lexington Books, 1992.

Engen HB, Iaiello-Vailas L, Smith K: Confrontation: A new dimension in nutrition counseling. *J Am Diet Assoc.* 1983;83:34–37.

Funnell MM, Anderson RM, Arnold MS, et al: Empowerment: An idea whose time has come in diabetes education. *Diabetes Educ.* 1991;17(1):37–41.

Gilliland BE, James RK, Bowman JT: *Theories and Strategies in Counseling and Psychotherapy.* Englewood Cliffs, NJ: Prentice-Hall, 1989.

Isselmann MC, Deubner LS, Hartman M: A nutrition counseling workshop: Integrating psychology into nutrition practice. *J Am Diet Assoc.* 1993;93(3):324–326.

James M, Jongeward D: *Transactional Analysis with Gestalt Experiments.* Reading, MA: Addison-Wesley Publishing Co, 1977.

Kirk CC: *Taming the Diet Dragon.* St. Paul, MN: Llewellyn Publications, 1994.

Kuiper NA, McKenzie SD, Belanger KA. Cognitive appraisals and individual differences in sense of humor: Motivational and affective implications. *Person Individ Diff.* 1995;19(3):359–372.

LaFrance M: Posturing and mirroring and rapport in interaction rhythms: *In* Davis M (ed). *Periodicity in Communicative Behavior.* New York: Human Science Press, 1982.

Littlejohn SW: *Theories of Communication.* 2nd ed. Belmont, CA: Wadsworth, Inc, 1983.

Mills EP: *Listening: Key to Communication.* New York: Petrocelli Books, 1974.

Nezu AM, Nezu CM, Blisset SE: Sense of humor as a moderator of the relation between stressful events and psychological distress: A prospective analysis. *J Personal Soc Psych.* 1988;54(3):520–525.

Ohlsen MM, Horne AM, Lawe CF: *Group Counseling.* 3rd ed. New York: Holt, Rinehart and Winston, 1988.

Othmer E, Othmer SC: *The Clinical Interview Using DSM-IV.* Vol. 1: *Fundamentals.* Washington, DC: American Psychiatric Press, 1994.

Purtilo R, Haddad A: *Health Professional and Patient Interaction.* 5th ed. Philadelphia: WB Saunders, 1996.

Rody N: Empowerment as organizational policy in nutrition intervention programs: A case study from the Pacific Islands. *J Nutr Educ.* 1988;20(3):133–141.

Rogers CR: *On Becoming a Person, Sentry Edition 60.* Boston: Houghton Mifflin Co, 1961.

Silberman IN: Humor and health: An epidemiological study. *Am Behav Sci.* 1987;30(1):100–112.

Stuart MK, Simko MD. A technique for incorporating psychological principles into the nutrition counseling of clients. *Top Clin Nutr.* 1991;6(4):32–39.

Vickery CE, Cotugna N, Hodges P: Comparing counseling skills of dietetic students: A model for skill enhancement. *J Am Diet Assoc.* 1995;95(8):912–913.

Warpeha A, Harris J: Combining traditional and nontraditional approaches to nutrition counseling. *J Am Diet Assoc.* 1993;93(7):797–800.

ADDITIONAL REFERENCES

The Art of Listening (videotape). Lake Zurich, IL: The Learning Seed, 1993.

Bernieri F, Rosenthal R: Interpersonal coordination: Behavior matching and interactional synchrony. In *Fundamentals of Nonverbal Behavior.* Cambridge, MA: Cambridge University Press, 1991.

Blanchard K: Two types of power. *Business Credit.* 1988;Dec:12.

Blumenfeld E, Alpern L: *The Smile Connection.* Englewood Cliffs, NJ: Prentice-Hall, 1986.

Body Language: An Introduction to Non-Verbal Communication (videotape). Lake Zurich, IL: The Learning Seed, 1993.

Del Bueno DJ: How well do you use power? *Am J Nurs.* 1987;87(11):1495–1498.

Flipse R: *Learning Through Laughter.* Chicago, IL: The American Dietetic Association, 1990.

Gretz KF, Drozdeck SR: *Empowering Innovative People.* Chicago: Probus Publishing Company, 1994.

Jackson SW: The listening healer in the history of psychological healing. *Am J Psych.* 1992;149(12):1623–1632.

Pascarell P, Dibianca V, Gioja L: The power of being responsible. *Industry Week.* 1988;Dec. 5:41–50.

Robbins A: *Unlimited Power.* New York: Fawcett Columbine, 1986.

Schlundt DG, Rea MR, et al: Situational obstacles to dietary adherence for adults with diabetes. *J Am Diet Assoc.* 1994.

Self-Assessment Series for Dietetics Professionals: Nutrition Counseling Module. Commission on Dietetic Registration for The American Dietetic Association, 1992.

CHAPTER 5

Selected Perspectives of Psychology and Counseling

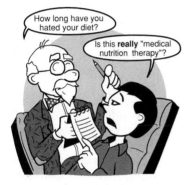

How long have you hated your diet?

Is this **really** "medical nutrition therapy"?

GOALS

The goals of this chapter are (1) to review aspects of psychological theories that have application in the field of dietetics and nutrition, (2) to discuss their implications in nutrition counseling, (3) to provide case examples of how the theory can help explain clients and guide interventions, and (4) to increase the reader's flexibility in counseling approaches.

Learning Objectives

At the end of this chapter the reader will be able to:

1. Identify major concepts from theories presented.

2. Relate various theoretical perspectives to counseling strategies.

3. Apply theoretical concepts to case examples and practice.

4. Develop a broader understanding of human psychology, especially as it applies to nutrition counseling.

5. Develop the ability to respond to clients, as opposed to adhering to one theoretical model.

Key Terms

▶ Action-Oriented Theory (Behaviorist Theory): psychological perspectives that focus on problem-solving and specific changes in behavior, cognition, or feelings.

▶ Counseling Approaches: strategies considered to be effective in facilitating change.

▶ Insight-Oriented Theory (Humanist Theory): psychological perspectives that focus on client awareness and personal growth.

▶ Learning: processes by which people gain knowledge and insight and make changes.

▶ Personality: qualities of a person, based on a theoretical proposition.

▶ Theoretical Tenets: major beliefs, assumptions, and research findings of a particular theory or perspective.

▶ Theory: a possible explanation for, or reasons behind, what happens in the world; a useful theory helps to guide practice.

Humankind finds it much more difficult to study the self than the outside world. Studying ourselves is much too painful. Analysis of humans has often been stymied by influential people. Intellectuals of the past who did study people and came up with theories about us were quite vulnerable to the politics of the time. A prime example is Socrates, who was put to death because he put forth ideas about humankind that were not popular in the society of his time. Even today people who study sociology, psychology, and anthropology are sometimes ridiculed and maligned, especially if they have new ideas that are not provable by experimental methodology such as that used in physics, chemistry, or biology. It is also much harder to study domains such as psychology, because of concern about human rights. People cannot be manipulated in laboratory situations in the same way that innate substances or animals are. Consequently, psychological theories range from those that are more formalized, with some experimental work to support them, to those that are more philosophical in nature, based on experiences of learned scholars who developed theories or models of human psychological function. Some scholars do not accept any current psychological theory as a true theory, but rather as a perspective about the workings of the mind. No single comprehensive human psychology theory has surfaced, but several have been shown to be partially explanatory of human nature (Shilling, 1984).

Summarizing basic concepts of theoretical perspectives, some of which are still in early developmental stages, is a challenge. Some authors present very speculative material as if it were completely proven. Others present material that is confusing and difficult to understand, even though the theory seems to have value. Some of these ideas are presented here anyway, with the caveat that some of the viewpoints presented will change in the future as theorists experiment and learn more about human psychology. Particularly in cognitive psychology, the newest approach to human psychology, theories and models are diverse and often vague. Models of therapy occasionally appear to be very loosely connected to basic concepts of cognitive psychology. This does not diminish the fact that they have applicability to effective dietetics and nutrition practice.

THEORY EVALUATION

Several criteria can be applied to evaluating theories. In general, criteria fall under the following categories:

■ Does the theory explain phenomena sufficiently?
■ Does the theory serve to predict outcomes of counseling sufficiently?
■ Does application of the theory help control events sufficiently?

When the answer is more "yes" than "no" to these questions, the theory can be considered to "work," even though there may be flaws. A working theory is one that can guide practice. Theorists may argue over these flaws in theories and models; however, practitioners usually use several theories to help understand clients, taking aspects of each theory that seem to fit their personal viewpoints. It is from this point of view that theoretical perspectives have been selected for inclusion in this chapter. Each has something to offer in spite of its incompleteness, and each can guide practice.

THEORY CLASSIFICATION

Traditionally, psychological theories have been identified as behaviorist or humanist. Recently, a classification between action-oriented theories and insight-oriented theories has evolved. We have chosen this later dichotomy for organization of the chapter. It is our belief that the action-oriented theories offer cogent perspectives for interventions in nutrition counseling both because of the problem-solving nature of nutrition interventions and because of the limited psychological education of most medical nutrition therapists. Insight-oriented psychologies have much to offer in developing understanding of clients, ourselves, and personal relationships. Insight-oriented counseling strategies tend to be dramatic and bring strong emotions to the surface. No one should use insight-oriented techniques without the educational background that will enable them to work comfortably in the presence of the expression of strong emotions.

The order of presentation in this chapter is, for the most part, chronological, since earlier theories influenced theories developed later. Humanist theories and insight-oriented therapy tended to dominate the early part of the 20th century, whereas behavioral theories and action-oriented therapy have dominated the latter part of the century. Cognitive psychology is in an early stage of development. There seems to be a relatively large number (20 to 30) of theoretical perspectives that call themselves cognitive theories.

Insight-oriented perspectives include psychoanalysis, gestalt, person-centered therapy, and transactional analysis (TA). TA seems to be a bridge between insight- and action-oriented approaches. Action-oriented theories include behavior modification, several cognitive theories, and a transtheoretical theory of change. At the end of the chapter, there is a discussion of the psychology of eating and drinking, a perspective that holds much promise for understanding nutrition behavior. These perspectives emphasize biological theories of human food consumption. All of the perspectives described sufficiently meet criteria for a working theory (Shilling, 1984; Gilliland et al, 1989) and have been shown to work in the practice of nutrition counseling.

The reader is urged to become acquainted with each of the ideas presented here and to use the knowledge in a cumulative manner to aid in enhancing success in medical nutrition therapy. Some theories are more empirically based than others. The reason most often cited in success or failure of counseling modalities is actually the effect of the interpersonal relationship between counselor and client more than a counseling modality, which is a reminder that theories are still limited.

Insight-Oriented Perspectives

Although the seeds of modern theories of psychology sprang from ancient philosophers, Sigmund Freud's landmark work in the late 19th and early 20th centuries was the first work based on scientific thinking. He established the field of *psychoanalysis,* and even though there have been some new concepts developed, the impact of his theories continues to affect psychological thinkers. His youngest daughter, Anna, followed in his footsteps, making significant contributions to psychoanalytical theory on her own. Later psychologies have developed as result or in response to psychoanalysis. Carl Jung, the first of Freud's students to modify psychoanalysis, saw people in a more positive light than Freud. Erik Erikson, a psycholanalytically trained psychologist, produced a positive cogent theory of human growth and development. Jean Piaget provided a theory of cognitive growth and development. Abraham Maslow, among the first to be described as a humanist, originated a theory of human motivation based on the need for self-fulfillment. These last three theories are more fully discussed in Chapter 6, Nutrition Counseling Over the Life Cycle. Others of the humanist persuasion include Frederick and Laura Perls, (gestalt therapy), Eric Berne (TA), and Carl Rogers (person-centered therapy), each of whom described theories of humanist psychology that are still accepted as useful today. They emphasize experiential approaches and therapy that is person-centered and focused on the here and now, awareness, insight, and internal motivations.

Action-Oriented Perspectives

Behaviorist psychology is based on principles of stimulus-response (S-R) theories of learning and motivation. Original thinkers in behaviorist psychology include Watson, Thurmond, and Skinner, who probably did more than anyone to foster its growth. Their viewpoints emphasized the importance of behavior and the reinforcement of desired behavior. As behaviorism evolved, there was a tendency among some theorists to focus very strictly on behavior and behavioral outcomes of therapy. This made it easy to conduct research, but limited full understanding because thinking and feeling were discounted.

Cognitive psychology is a field that has embraced both insight and action perspectives, although individual theoreticians tend to focus on one or the other. In the future, cognitive psychologists may discover more comprehensive theories of human psychology and intervention strategies. No one prominent leader in cognitive psychology has emerged so far. The field is loosely held together with the common thread of belief that thinking can cause feeling and that human brains are analogous to computers. Included in cognitive psychology are perspectives such as social learning theory, neurolinguistics, rational emotive therapies, and numerous others.

There are some major differences between traditional humanist and behaviorist perceptions of human functioning, as illustrated in Table 5–1.

A STUDY APPROACH

As an ongoing exercise throughout this chapter, the reader is asked to refer to the following case example. As the various theories are read, make notes regarding how each theory would (1) interpret and explain the client and the situation described, and (2) guide the MNT in planning interventions. When you have completed the chapter, review all you have written and determine how each theory helped you understand the client and plan intervention strategies. You will probably find that each provides a bit of information that can help plan an intervention strategy, and that all of them together still leave room for your own insights and input. This case will be revisited at the end of the chapter to illustrate each theory in summary.

TABLE 5-1

Comparison of Humanist and Behaviorist Psychology	
Humanist: Insight-Oriented Therapy	**Behaviorist: Action-Oriented Therapy**
People learn through cognitive structures, unique learning, brain structures, and chemistry.	People learn by stimulus-response processes.
Personality is important in understanding people. Personality is not static but is relatively stable.	Personality is not definable, nor important.
Motivation is internal, based on values and self-concepts and self-actualization drives.	Motivation is external, through reinforcement of behavior. There is little free choice.
Therapy is insight-oriented, often dramatic, client-centered. Awareness is essential.	Therapy is action-oriented, often therapist-directed. Behavioral change is essential.

CASE EXAMPLE ·

John Lightfoot, age 52, has been sent to the outpatient department of a local hospital in the aftermath of a myocardial infarction. He is of normal weight. Nutritional needs include a low-sodium, low-fat intake. He is married and is the father of one grown daughter. He lives with his wife of 30 years. He has been working as a lumberjack. The counselor has been working through stage II, problem identification.

M N T: "What do you see as a major problem?"

C L I E N T: "I can't give up salt. Maybe I could just exercise. When I was working I got plenty of exercise. I don't like gyms. Eating salt won't kill me, will it? Oh well, who would care anyway. After this heart attack, maybe I should just die, anyway. My wife fixes my foods. Why don't you talk to her? Oh, I guess you'll have to talk to me for the moment. What are you going to tell me I should do?"

· ·

INSIGHT-ORIENTED THEORIES

Psychoanalytical Concepts

Psychoanalysis is both a theory of personality and a treatment methodology. As a theory of personality, it focuses largely on the unconscious. Freud's theories of the topography of the mind and his descriptions of the structure of personality remain in common usage, albeit with little understanding by the average person who may use psychoanalytical terms flippantly. It is worthwhile to describe psychoanalysis briefly because of the historical background.

Personality

Freud's topography of the mind includes the conscience (*superego*), the instincts (*id*), and the reality (*ego*). These are thought to be not absolute categories, but a continuum. His structural model of personality, consisting of the id, the ego, and the superego is still popular today. The id is the entity in which human instincts reside and where the life force is found, both the will to live and the will to die. The id, which searches for pleasure, is that part of the personality that exists at birth. Soon the ego, that part of individuals that perceives and thinks objectively, and the superego, or conscience, begin to form. Freud conceived the personality as an energy system, always changing depending on the part of the personality that is energized. The process of civilizing a child is to divert energy from the id to the ego and superego (Nye, 1981). If this diversion is socially acceptable, the id is *sublimated.* Sublimation means the expression of socially unacceptable impulses in constructive, socially acceptable forms, often unconsciously. Freud believed that abnormal mental reactions are caused by the repression of desires, rather than sublimation of desires, consciously rejected but subconsciously retained. He believed that no behavior is accidental but is caused by the driving force within each individual. In his practice, he searched for causes of behavior in the subconscious. He would investigate the possible causes for dreaming, hallucinating, forgetting, selective remembering, personal choices, the repetition of the same behaviors over and over, hostility, slips of the tongue, and so on (Corey, 1991). Slips of the tongue, even today, are called Freudian slips, referring to the implied revelation of a subconscious drive when one misspeaks.

Freud's analysis of food in the life of humans would reflect the following. The infant is born with only the id, the pleasure-seeking aspect of personality. The separation from the womb, a place of pleasure, soon brings frustration of need fulfillment, one need being hunger. The response of the id to this frustration creates tension and a demand for release of tension (screaming) in an unfocused way. Feeding reduces the tension, and pleasure results. As the conscious ego develops normally, the child recognizes cause and effect. She or he develops goal-directed behavior, and screaming becomes goal-directed. The ego, the basic conscious aspect of personality, observes and processes reality and produces goal-directed behavior. The superego is the conscience, an internal judge and jury. In this example, the superego would be that part of the personality in which cultural expectations of appropriate food customs would accumulate.

If the representatives of society who influence an infant are too harsh and rigid, the child's ego may be retarded and the superego will be harsh and rigid. Productive energy will not be as available for sublimation because it will be consumed with internal conflict. However, the superego can also be a source of reward, and when the superego is more rewarding than punishing, the individual will have a good self-concept and be able to love and work.

A healthy personality has a strong ego in control and is able to handle reasonably well the demands of reality. Anxiety, a warning to the ego that danger lurks, is minimal and is accepted as a normal part of life. Defense mechanisms are developed by the ego to protect the person from anxiety. Defense mechanisms are falsifications of actual conditions and are assumed to operate unconsciously. Extreme defense building will become psychosis, a situation in which reality is denied altogether, such as in schizophrenia.

Therapeutic Approach

Basically, psychoanalytical therapy is dialogue between client and therapist searching for motivations in the unconscious. Awareness is the goal of therapy. Treatment is long-term, focusing on dreams and other indications of subconscious motivations.

Implications for Medical Nutrition Therapy

The value of psychoanalysis to nutrition counseling lies in its historical value. Analysis of personality and the techniques used require lengthy training and lengthy therapy not at the disposal of therapists and counselors who are not specifically trained in psychoanalysis.

Gestalt Theory

Personality

Gestalt personality theory is a field of psychology that emphasizes human interactions rather than static personality. People are viewed as a part of the environment in which they exist, yet distinctly unique, in a constant process of approach and withdrawal with the ever-changing environment. A healthy personality approaches each new situation spontaneously, creating a new reality based on the new experience, then moving on to the next experience. The unique reality created as people approach and withdraw from situations are called "gestalts," from Gestalten, a German word that has no precise English translation. In English the closest idea to a gestalt is a breathy "Aha!" that expresses sudden insight when confusion, anxiety, and tension are suddenly released. A disorganized situation becomes organized and one "sees" the "simple" truth. Gestalt theory, therefore, does not have an absolute description of personality because a person is always different, growing and learning throughout life.

The personality is considered to be the result of the individual differentiating itself from others, yet connected to others, the I/thou concept. The interface between I and thou is a permeable boundary that allows interaction between the individual and the environment. In addition, the personality is always changing as it interacts with the environment (Gilliland et al, 1989). An interchange of great importance in nutrition is the I/food interchange.

CASE EXAMPLE ·

Metabolic forces interact to cause hunger; the individual sensing the need for food searches for it, takes it in, and metabolizes it into himself. He grows and develops healthily when he accurately perceives need, taking in what is truly nourishing and leaving that which is toxic in the environment. Difficulties in sensing food needs and satisfying them are often changed by problems of the I/thou separation with loved ones and with society.

. . . .

When I/food interchanges are unclear, the distinction between nourishing food intake versus toxic food intake is unsatisfactory. Too much, too little, or inappropriate ingestion of food occurs. Overindulgence in alcoholic beverages is an example of a particularly toxic interchange with the environment.

A number of idiomatic phrases in the language illustrate the psychological impact of food and nutrition, such as:

She bit off more than she could chew.
He just swallowed that idea whole.
My gut feeling is . . .
When I took time to digest that, I understood it very well.
When I heard that, I just chewed it up and spit it out.

Learning

According to gestalt theory, learning is the process by which new gestalts (insights) are formed and new realities are created. Useful gestalts are well-organized, regular, simple, stable, and unique to each individual because each individual has unique experiences. As learning proceeds, new gestalts are used by individuals as a guide to action until a better, more complete truth is perceived and a new gestalt is formed. No distinction is made between intellectual and emotional learning processes (Corey, 1991). An example of learning new gestalts is the process through which the reader is going as a student of medical nutrition therapy.

CASE EXAMPLE ·

In previous educational experiences or by watching others conduct nutrition counseling, you may have learned that diet instructions are given by telling people what they should and should not eat in a 20-minute interview. You may have been following the same process that you have seen others perform. As you began to read that effective changes in nutrition lifestyle take place over time, there may have been some discomfort toward ideas and perhaps confusion in your mind. Perhaps you even accept, intellectually, that it probably does take a long time to change food habits. However, you do not really change anything that you do. Then, suddenly, it dawns on you that a 20-minute interview does not really effect very much change. You *feel* it; you change. You suddenly have a new truth on which to base future actions, and you put effort into seeing clients over time. A new gestalt has been formed.

. . . .

Motivation

Motivation for learning is perceived by gestaltists as based on universal and biological needs to organize stimuli into something personally meaningful. Cognitive structures are the neurological structures in the brain that mediate stimuli and make things meaningful and whole. Humans are drawn toward the unknown to make it organized and complete. If a person has everything organized in a satisfactory manner, with no loose ends or unresolved issues, there is no need to learn (Pettinger & Gooding, 1971).

Many complexities are involved in the formation of new gestalts. The following example analyzes a situation commonly faced in medical nutrition therapy from a gestalt point of view.

CASE EXAMPLE ·

Parents brought their obese child for counseling. In the course of discussing the problem the following conflict (poorly defined expectations) was discovered. The parents often demanded that their children clean their plates because it is a "virtue" to finish everything; otherwise the starving children in India could have eaten the food. Not to leave a plate clean would be a "sin." They also exhorted the obese child not to eat too much. This confused communication left the child in a position of always being wrong. A new gestalt regarding how to interact with the child to reduce confusion was an important part of medical nutrition therapy.

· ·

Polarities

Perhaps more than any other theorists the gestaltists have addressed the tendency of people to see options in life as polarities. All versus nothing, black versus white, should versus want viewpoints limit the alternatives for problem-solving. For instance, when food selection vacillates between what one should eat and what one wants to eat, unsatisfactory food habits often occur. The thought process that results in such a situation is an internal dialogue in which a "top-dog" tells the "underdog" what should be done (always eat right) and the "underdog" obeys sometimes and rebels sometimes. A great deal of psychic energy goes into this internal dialogue. Logical thinking about which food intake would really make sense is excluded. The individual struggles between overcontrol of the diet and indulgence. A functional gestalt to guide behavior is not present. When the individual becomes aware, a new gestalt can be formed that will enable the individual to decide on intermediate options such as thinking of a nutrition lifestyle, not a "diet," that includes desired foods and is also consistent with healthy food habits, according to scientific principles. Furthermore, the individual will find it okay to change as new scientific information modifies his understanding of nutrition and modifies his needs for pleasure from food. The individual will no longer be struggling with the top-dog/underdog internal dialogue of what should or should not be in his or her diet.

Therapeutic Approaches

Goals. *Awareness* in the here and now and *maturity* are the goals of gestalt therapy. Each awareness becomes a part of the whole process of clarifying the self. Specific goals are to become aware of a whole array of polarities that one sets up to limit options and to systematically form clearer gestalts.

Unawareness is described as a state in which a person thinks about the past or worries about the future rather then being aware in the present, the here and now. The person frequently reacts not to the situation in the here and now, but to a similar situation in the past, even when the reaction is no longer appropriate. For instance, a woman's mother often told her, "You should always eat food when it is offered because it is polite. Not to do so is to be rude to your hostess, and her feelings will be hurt." Now this woman feels compelled to follow these instructions even though such behavior is a major problem in maintaining a desirable weight. She goes through periods of time when she never accepts offered food and other times when she accepts food and even takes additional helpings. She considers no other options. She feels fragmented, sometimes overcontrolled, sometimes undercontrolled, complying with "Momma" or rebelling. Therapy might address the underlying issue in this case; the need of this woman to be a polite, not rude person. Some new gestalts that would help this woman are "I am not responsible for everyone's feelings"; "I don't always have to be polite"; and "Keeping desirable weight is more important than anyone's feelings."

Awareness is the key to maturity. It is a principle of gestalt theory that awareness is all that is necessary to bring about change. A person who is mature in regard to nutrition lifestyle eats according to an awareness of immediate and long-term goals for health and pleasure. The immediate situation, the here and now, is allowed to determine the food choices. Behavior is spontaneous, fixated on neither the past nor the future. An example of a person who has gained awareness of his extreme underweight and is mature is one who is comfortable with eating enough each day to increase his weight slowly without making himself extremely uncomfortable by trying to eat too much at a time.

Strategies. Gestalt therapy, aimed at developing a mature person—one acutely aware in the here and now, centered, responding spontaneously, allowing behavior to be determined by the situation at hand, forming ever-changing gestalts—is for people who are willing to become self-aware. Counseling techniques focus on searching the past for the original situations that have resulted in disturbing emotions in the present. The empty chair technique, sentence finishing, and dramatic acting out of emotions are common ways of confronting clients and bringing awareness.

Here and Now Orientation. Clients are encouraged to experience themselves in the here and now—the immediate therapy situation. They "work" on awareness rather than "just talk about things." Direct expression of feelings is encouraged. Clients are confronted with their nonfunctional patterns of interdependence. Poor functioning results from such problems as confusion between self and others, ineffective patterns of approach and withdrawal, inability to recognize polarities, and failure to remain aware in the here and now. Problem-solving is supported in gestalt therapy through the development of a self-support system and a sense of self-responsibility that results from direct experience in the therapy session. It is assumed that interpersonal relationships outside therapy sessions parallel interactions in therapy (Nye, 1981).

High priority is given to developing awareness of internal top-dog/underdog dialogue, the "you should" versus "but I want" internal dialogue. The following comment from a client expresses the curtailing of spontaneous behavior because of the anxiety created from the should/want dilemma.

CASE EXAMPLE ·

"I was going to stop having caffeine when I went to the supermarket . . . I was just like a robot . . . I bought the decaffeinated coffee. Then, the next day, I find out I am not pregnant . . . I started like another robot having my caffeine. I know I shouldn't drink caffeine, but I want to."

· ·

In this situation the gestalt therapist would guide the client toward awareness that she can decide in each instance to choose or not choose decaffeinated coffee and eliminate the robot-like behavior.

Language. Attention to language is important. Language is a clue to inner feelings and thoughts. Descriptive words and the manner in which pronouns are used are clues to a person's sense of personal responsibility. The use of "it," "you," or "one" instead of "I" suggests lack of clarity of self. The use of "I" is a clear recognition of self-responsibility, the others subtly deny the self-responsibility. These substitutions for "I" are common because many people are taught not to use "I" boldly and continue to follow these teachings. The following example shows how language is a clue to the acceptance of responsibility for one's own actions.

CASE EXAMPLE ·

"You know, it really makes you mad when you have to give up salt in the diet" does not accept responsibility for the angry feelings in the same way that "I really get mad when I think about having to give up salt in my diet" does. The therapist (to whom the comment was directed) may or may not be mad about giving up salt, and the client may not be aware of his own anger. The second statement has the potential for awareness of and reconciliation of the normal anger felt when poor health dictates dietary changes.

· ·

Another word to listen for as a guide to self-awareness is "can't" when "won't" would be more accurate. For instance, "I can't stay on my diet" suggests powerlessness while "I won't stay on my diet" usually is a more accurate description of the situation. There are few instances when people in this country do not control their own food intake. Usually, no one but the individual puts the food in the mouth, and even a person being fed can refuse to take it in. Force feeding is the only situation in which a person literally cannot have some control over food intake. "Can't" implies powerlessness, while "won't" implies power and control. The MNT would encourage the client to say the sentence, "I won't stay on my diet," as a method of creating an awareness of the feelings precipitated by this strong statement of self-responsibility.

Nonverbal behavior is considered to be even more important than verbal behavior as clues to inner thoughts and feelings. Nonverbal communication is explored by having the client exaggerate the behavior and then verbalize its meaning. Clients are urged to stay in the here and now and be aware of what is occurring within. Each new gestalt is a part of the ongoing development of maturity.

Implications for Medical Nutrition Therapy

Some of the concepts of gestalt psychology can be helpful in understanding clients. Attention to language can facilitate identifying attitudes and beliefs that indicate difficulties in problem-solving. Gestalt ideas, in this respect, fit quite easily with cognitive therapy approaches that focus on the importance of thinking. Although many of the techniques used in gestalt therapy should not be attempted by therapists who are not adequately trained in gestalt therapy, some, such as the empty chair technique used for role-playing, can be effective in modeling and assertiveness training.

Person-Centered Therapy

Personality

Rogers' theory of person-centered therapy focuses on the processes of change rather than on personality, so there is no explicit description of personality in his teachings. The "self" is always searching for self-actualization (Schilling, 1984).

Self-Actualization. Fundamental to person-centered therapy is the tenet that humans have an inherent tendency to strive toward self-actualization. An environment in which an individual receives unconditional positive regard from others results in the development of positive self-regard, enabling the potential for self-actualization to be realized (Meador & Rogers, 1984). *Unconditional positive regard* is love for the very existence of the individual, not dependent on personal characteristics or behavior.

Parental actions that create an environment of unconditional love and a balance of discipline that neither overcontrols nor indulges the child results in positive growth and development. A person who has developed a positive sense of self can handle both positive and negative responses to themselves without losing a positive sense of self. When children are treated with ambivalence or with unconditional negative regard, they develop a sense of low self-esteem, experienced as a nebulous internal anxiety that is difficult to pinpoint (Nye, 1981).

Therapeutic Approaches

Goals. The focus in counseling is on the immediate experience of the client. The process is not problem-centered, goal-centered, or behavior-centered. The goal is to develop a self-actualizing person who has a positive regard for self and others and is genuine and straightforward. Façades can be discarded, and the individual can experience the full impact of the present.

Strategies. Counseling is very nondirective, based on the belief that people are basically trustworthy and able to understand themselves and make changes for themselves in a supportive atmosphere. The counselor merely responds by communicating that the client's message has been received.

The environment necessary for therapy is a warm, permissive atmosphere in which the therapist unconditionally accepts the client (Rogers, 1961). Throughout his writing, Rogers emphasized the concept of unconditional positive regard for clients. These ideas have influenced counselors of every persuasion.

Counselor Characteristics. Person-centered counselors listen to clients with a nonjudgmental attitude and foster client freedom of expression. At first, clients often experience apprehension in light of so much freedom. As therapy progresses, clients begin to take responsibility for themselves and "become" what they can become to the fullest extent permitted by biological endowment (Rogers, 1961).

Some of the most fruitful research on characteristics of successful counselors has been conducted by Rogers and his followers. The following characteristics have been found to be common among successful therapists (Meador & Rogers, 1984).

- Accurate, empathic—describes a counselor who is accurate in sensing meanings and feeling of clients.
- Unconditional positive regard—this means accepting the client without judgment.
- Congruence, genuineness—the ability of the counselor to understand his or her own inner experience and have it translate as honesty to the client.

Implications for Medical Nutrition Therapy

Person-centered therapy is oriented toward clients' self-expressions, not toward specific problem-solving. The nondirective approach is usually too time consuming to be practical in nutrition counseling.

Efforts to achieve characteristics of successful counselors will have a beneficial effect on the success rate of medical nutrition counselors. As clients perceive the therapist as warm and supportive rather than critical, trust will enhance the relationship and increase the receptiveness of clients to learning new nutrition habits.

Transactional Analysis

Transactional analysis, commonly called TA, provides a bridge between insight-oriented theories such as psychoanalysis and gestalt, and person-centered therapy and behavioral (action)–oriented theories. Berne, and others who followed him, proposed a theory of personality structure and interpersonal relationships. The name transactional analysis comes from analysis of interpersonal communication (transactions).

TA describes the components of personality in a way that is understandable by the lay public and minimally trained counselors. There is no other theory of personality in which constructs are presented in simple ways as well as in complex ways and can as quickly provide insight into personality. TA concepts that are particularly useful in medical nutrition therapy include personality structure, life scripts (self-fulfilling prophecies), transactions, and psychological games (how we do not say what we mean). Understanding these factors will help identify strengths and weaknesses in clients as well as one's own self.

Although several theories of personality are valid and useful, none are presented in the literature in a way that is as readily understandable to nonpsychologists as is TA. In TA, personality is described in behavioral terms easily observable in true life. TA concepts provide a rapid way to become more cognizant of personality and are therefore emphasized here.

Personality

Structural Analysis. Freud can be credited with discovering the "persons within"—the id, the ego, and superego, abstract concepts of psychological phenomena. Berne first based his practice of psychiatry on an understanding of these constructs, but as he gained experience he began to identify personality characteristics of a more concrete nature than those described by Freud. He observed that people often change suddenly from one demeanor and set of behaviors to another for no apparent reason, and that some behaviors and expressions of feelings present in adults are not present in children. He also began to notice that while very small children are emotional, not dispassionate and logical, adults may display logical, dispassionate demeanor and suddenly switch to a very emotional demeanor. These emotional displays took two forms, childlike or parent-like. From these observations, Berne named three distinct divisions of personality: Child, Adult, and Parent, each a distinct "ego state" or "system of feelings accompanied by a related set of coherent behavior patterns" (Berne, 1973; p. 23). A natural or free Child ego state is present at birth. The other ego states are developed as the child watches others and mimics them. Berne thus theorized that the ego states present in an adult are components of personality developed by a growing child and gleaned from adults, generally parents or primary caretakers.

Berne described the Child ego state, the only one present at birth, as representing basic human *feelings* such as anger, fear, sorrow, joy and *needs,* such as food, shelter, love, and sexual expression. The Adult ego state was described as producing dispassionate logical thought. The Parent ego state was described as containing the mores and values of society, providing direction and guidance in fulfilling social expectations. A mentally healthy individual has a personality in which all three ego states are present and available at will to respond to events, using the ego state best suited for solving problems and having fun.

Ego states are identified with a capital first letter: Parent or (P), Adult or (A), Child or (C). If these words are written entirely in lowercase, they refer to people, not to ego states. A TA diagram of a balanced personality is shown in Figure 5–1.

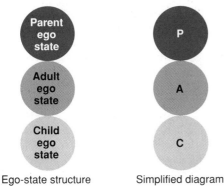

Ego-state structure   Simplified diagram

FIGURE 5–1. Basic balanced (healthy) personality structure: ego states. (From Gurman AS, Messer SB: *Essential Psychotherapies: Theory and Practice.* New York: The Guilford Press, 1995.)

The Child Ego State. The Child ego state is a collection of natural feelings, including sensory perceptions, spontaneous biological urges, uninhibited demands to meet basic human needs, and passionate feelings of anger, fear, joy, and sorrow. The (C) assimilates feelings learned from people who have cared for the child. These are derived feelings such as guilt, learned fear, learned anger, and sentimentality. Both natural and derived feelings influence the child's self-concept, which Berne described as the level of "OKness" felt by a child (Berne, 1973). This Child ego state embodies the part of the personality developed before an individual has the capacity to think logically. Therefore, most of the thinking in the (C) is emotional, irrational, and magical. For instance, thinking that a celebration will be ruined if you do not eat your favorite food, and therefore overindulging, is evidence that you are in the Child ego state because this thinking is irrational. Believing that a particular food or diet regimen will "cure" a disease is also magical thinking. There is no logical basis for thinking that a particular food can cure a disease, except for specific diseases such as those caused by deficiencies. "Wishful thinking" is another way this attitude is described.

TA writings describe the actions and words that are evidence of a Child ego state. The descriptions are based on observations of children. An aware lay person is as capable of developing skill in describing the Child ego state as a trained professional. Just ask, what do children do? What words do they use? What body posture and movements do they show? Even though the individual with whom one is working may have an adult body, if she or he is acting and talking like a child the little boy or girl inside is showing and the person is functioning in the Child ego state.

Some of the following words and phrases are typical (C) behaviors. Children whine, pout, use flirtatious behaviors to win you over, stomp their feet, throw tantrums, jump for joy, shed real tears or crocodile ones, tell you what you want to hear even if it is not true, look up for your approval, ask why, for real or to get attention, believe in Santa Claus, run out in the street because they do not realize the danger of the world, and many other such examples (James & Jongeward, 1978).

Note that some of the examples given seem to express a free spirit whereas others seem to indicate manipulative behaviors. Berne (1973) classified the (C) into two major functional parts, which he named the Free Child (FC) and the Adapted Child (AC). The (FC) is the natural passionate Child—uninhibited, self-centered, and unsocialized. The (FC) is not controlled by outside forces but by the uninhibited demands of the organism and an intuitive (gut feeling) recognition of what is happening in the here and now. Anger, joy, fear, sorrow, and needs for food, shelter, and love are in the (FC).

The (AC), on the other hand, is not in touch with these basic feelings and needs of the individual. This part of the personality has watched others express themselves and manipulate the world and has selected a set of adapted feelings and manipulative behaviors she or he perceived as acceptable in the environment in which she or he grew up. These "derived" feeling and behaviors continue even when they backfire on the individual. In some homes, feelings may be denied altogether. The (AC) figures out what feelings are expected and incorporates them into his or her repertoire. For instance, a little boy may learn that being afraid is not acceptable, so he decides not to have these feelings and to have some other feeling instead, often anger. Conversely, fear or sadness is often more acceptable for girls than anger.

The same is true with behaviors. The (AC) has found that either behaving as a very good boy or girl "works" or being rebellious "works" to exert influence on others. Adaptations frequently mirror stereotypical behaviors of parents, the models of "good and bad." Examples include the woman who has learned that being "afraid" will get others to help her or the man who must always be "strong." Use of the (AC) in food-related behaviors is illustrated by individuals who have eating disorders. It is usually "adapted" feelings and behaviors that become barriers to problem-solving among adults because the individual is not certain about how to change his or her automatic reactions to responses more suitable to the present.

The intuitive part of the personality seemed to Berne to reside in the (FC). He described it as a thought process that was a leap beyond logic; a sense of reality that is able to perceive events happening in the here and now with even more accuracy than logical thought (Berne, 1973). It is the creative and intuitive part of the personality. He named it the "Little Professor." When allowed to function, the "Little Professor" is an excellent aid to problem-solving. It provides the "hunch," the "gut feeling," the extralogical sense of the best course of action.

The Parent Ego State. The Parent (P) is a collection of perceptions of "the adult world" a person learns as a child from the significant others in his or her life and accepts as unquestionable "truth" without logical consideration. These perceptions form a prelogical belief structure of social expectations and values. The internal (P) assimilates outside influences and uses then to make judgments on self and others. The (P) gives "permission" to the (C) to think, feel, and do certain things, and "injunctions" against thinking, feeling, and doing certain other things. An example is the "permission" given by (P) to (C) to cry when emotionally upset that many women learn in childhood. Conversely, many men have learned an "injunction" against crying when upset. The quality of the (P) is influenced by the quality of the permissions and injunctions the caretakers gave to the young child.

Values, as well as feelings and behaviors, of caretakers are also incorporated into the (P). Values, once incorporated into the personality, are used to judge the actions of self and others. The values of the culture in which a child grows up form the matrix of the value system in the (P). For instance, some cultures think a fat baby is a healthy baby. A young mother in today's society may hold this value unconsciously, and will judge her baby's health and the quality of her mothering according to this value. She will experience conflict between her value system which says "fat baby=good mother" and another value system that considers a thinner baby to be healthier—"thin baby=good mother."

In counseling, the mother may be helped to think logically about babies and healthiness and substitute a new value into her (P) that incorporates neither stereotype.

The (P) includes a critical, prejudiced, directive component (CP) and a protective nurturing component (NP), both necessary for a healthy personality. A sufficiently critical (CP) produces a sense of moral responsibility without overriding the nurturing (NP) that serves to love and forgive human frailties (James & Jongeward, 1971). The (P) can be expressed directly through overtly parental behavior or by exerting an influence on the Child ego state. When being expressed directly, the (P) can be recognized by such verbal clues as "Don't eat too much, don't you know that isn't good for you?" (CP) or "I made you a special meal for tonight" (NP). Sometimes, both the critical (CP) and nurturing (NP) can be detected in the same sentence, as in "That was not done the right way, let me help you."

Nonverbal indicators of the (P) include such actions as a pat on the head, a spank on the bottom, a shaking forefinger, or a thumbs-up sign. The influence of the (P) on the (C) is experienced in the (C) as self-love and tenderness or as guilt and self-punishment. For instance, an individual who has an overly strong drive to be perfect, is never satisfied with himself or herself, and thinks degradingly of himself or herself is showing the influence of an overdeveloped (CP). On the other hand, a person who is self-confident and forgiving of his or her mistakes has a well-developed (NP).

The Adult Ego State. In a TA drawing of the personality the Adult (A) is shown between the (C) and the (P). It demonstrates one of the Adult ego state's primary functions, logical mediation between (P) and (C), the two illogical ego states. The (A) produces rational concepts of life and is capable of transforming all types of stimuli into logical information. It is aware of the values and beliefs of the (P), the feelings of the (C), and data from the environment. The (A) can think, analyze, and reconcile the three parts of the personality. It executes spontaneous responses to situations in the here and now (Berne, 1973).

CASE EXAMPLE ·

A young woman, recovering from anorexia nervosa, is learning to use her (A) instead of her rebellious (AC). She is aware of her overcritical (CP) telling her she is fat when she is not, her (C) reacting to the (CP) by refusing to eat, and her (A) understanding the nutrition information that not eating will kill her. She is able to make a healthy decision, which is to eat, the logical thing to do, and at the same time give herself loving thoughts (strokes) for good decision-making.

· ·

A comparison between the (A) and a computer can be made in that they both take in data, organize and analyze them, estimate the probability of various alternative behaviors, and compute answers dispassionately. Unlike a computer, the (A) is also able to "compute" irrational thoughts and feelings. If the irrational part of the personality is repressed and the individual does not think about feeling, the (A) is not fully functioning. A fully functioning (A) is aware of the virtue of feelings and how they can be used to enhance the quality of life.

All ego states are vitally important to a healthy individual. Effective decision-making is possible only when the (A) is in charge and can recognize what the (C) wants, what the (P) thinks "should" be, and what the data indicate.

Integrated Personalities. A healthy or mature individual has a personality structure in which the three ego states are balanced and available spontaneously (see Fig. 5–1). An ego state is activated by the concentration of energy into that part of the personality. The most productive problem-solving use of ego states is energizing the (A) and creative (C)—the "Little Professor"—simultaneously. When both are energized, creative solutions can be found to problems, solutions that are often repressed by the AC and CP. When the (P) is energized, individuals are judgmental, directing, loving, protective, compassionate, critical, or nurturing. If the (A) is not energized also, (P) behaviors are likely to be repetitious parental behaviors copied from early childhood memories of what parents "should" do. These latter behaviors are not problem-solving unless they are also based on knowledge and understanding.

When the (C) is energized, individuals feel and act like children. If the (A) is not energized also, these behaviors are likely to be old reactions to stimuli that are not useful in the adult world. For instance, a woman who manipulated her father by pouting as a child may try that maneuver on a teacher in college and be surprised that it does not work. If she continues to pout to get what she wants, she is in the (AC) responding to the past, remaining unaware of the inappropriateness of her behavior in the present, the here and now.

If only the (A) is energized, behaviors are likely to be "cold-blooded," ignoring emotional needs. The individual will not "feel" his or her feelings, and will be insensitive to the feelings of others. When the (A) is in charge and is aware of the (P) and (C) and the immediate situation, a person has an integrated, functional, problem-solving personality and a high self-concept. In TA terms, he or she is OK.

Unintegrated Personalities. Personalities that are not integrated have an imbalance of ego states or they have confusion and overlapping between them. In some cases, an ego state may be missing completely. Figures 5–2, 5–3, and 5–4 demonstrate several ways in which a personality can be distorted.

Overlapping (contaminated) ego states create prejudicial or magical thinking. In such personalities, the prejudices and values of the (P) or the magical thinking of the (C), or both, are confused with the logical thought of the (A). For instance, when a statement such as, "Women are more emotional than men," is accepted as a fact without research to support it, confusion exists between the (P) and the (A) ego states. A common societal belief may be that women are more emotional than men. Understanding of psychology leads us to know that men and women are both emotional. Magical thinking, a function of the (C), can also be mistaken for logical

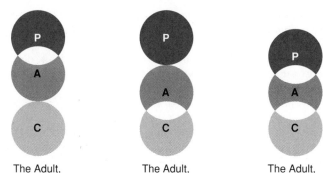

The Adult, contaminated by the Parent

The Adult, contaminated by the Child

The Adult, contaminated by the Parent and Child

FIGURE 5–2. Overlapping (contaminated) ego states. (From Gurman AS, Messer SB: *Essential Psychotherapies: Theory and Practice.* New York: The Guilford Press, 1995.)

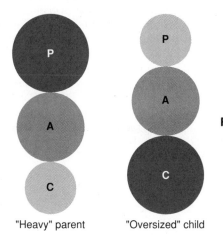

"Heavy" parent   "Oversized" child

FIGURE 5–3. Imbalanced ego states.

FIGURE 5–4. Lax ego states. (From Gurman AS, Messer SB: *Essential Psychotherapies: Theory and Practice.* New York: The Guilford Press, 1995.)

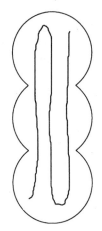

thought (A). Accepting as a fact the idea that a particular food has magical properties, for instance, that a high intake of cabbage will prevent any and all cancers, is an example of (C) contamination of the (A). Perhaps the most frequently encountered (C) contamination of (A) is seen in people who move from diet to diet in a vain hope to find a magical cure for overweight. The (C) hopes to lose weight without making long-term changes in nutrition lifestyle.

In *imbalanced* personalities, some ego states are overdeveloped and others are underdeveloped. When a person is too much in the (CP), she or he may be extremely critical of other people, domineering, and unwilling to listen to any information that is contrary to his or her belief system. Overhelpfulness is a function of an overdeveloped (NP). When a person helps another who can help himself or herself, the person helped does not develop competence. Overhelpfulness is a subtle way of suggesting that others are not really capable of helping themselves, or cannot be trusted to "do things right." People who go into the helping professions may exhibit this personality trait.

A person who is childlike much of the time is described as having an oversized Child (C). She or he often acts like a "good" or a "bad" child, reacting to events in a stereotypical way rather than a thoughtful way. This is particularly annoying when the individual is rebellious, expressing the attitude "You can't make me." A more subtle manifestation of the (C) is the "good little girl" or "good little boy" who always tries to please other people, outwardly complying while secretly rebelling or holding anger that may suddenly be exhibited in a burst of fury toward self or others (see Fig. 5–3).

Lax ego states result in a personality in which a person is unclear about his or her identity. The person will exhibit confusion in thinking and behavior. She may say she feels as if she is falling apart. Such individuals may be candidates for referral to a psychotherapist (Gurman & Messer, 1995).

Identifying Ego States. The energized ego state can be identified by voice, facial expressions, posture, vocabulary, and gestures.

Below are listed some examples of communication patterns from each ego state:

Critical Parent
You should, ought
Do this; don't do this
Stay here.
Look at me when you say that.
Why are you doing that?

These words are likely to be attended by a scolding demeanor. Perhaps the hands will be on the hips, the face frowning, and the speaker will be looking down the nose. The (P) is always superior, and is making an effort to communicate with the (C) ego state.

Nurturing Parent
Let me do that for you.
Let me help you.
I know that hurts.

Don't work so hard.
I'll try to make things better for you.
I love you.

The demeanor likely to be displayed with these behaviors includes looking down the nose, but the face will show concern and seem loving rather than scolding. The speaker may pat the listener as a mother would pat a small child. This (NP) is also addressing the (C) ego state.

Adult

That isn't the way to do it.
This is a good way to do it.
We have a problem to solve.
What do the data tell us about this problem?
How did you feel when that happened?

The behaviors present at the same time include a thoughtful but not scolding look on the face, body held straight, and arms and legs at ease. The eyes are comfortably direct according to the cultural expectations of the participants in the dialogue.

Adapted Child

Why?
I can't!
I won't!
I want it now!
Please. (whining)

The voice of the (C) is likely to be a higher pitch than either (P) or (A), often whiny or petulant-sounding. The eyes may be downcast or looking up for approval. Sometimes there is a stance of defiance, with the hands on the hips like (P), but without the power of the (P).

Free Child

Wow!
Why!
Let's do it!
Boy oh boy oh boy!

These words and similar others are accompanied by the unique innocent look of wonder that children show when they are discovering the world and finding life exciting. With some words, such as "why," one has to listen to inflection and take note of nonverbal behaviors to be able to tell whether the "why" is (AC) or (FC), as will be discussed in the section on transactions. Many subtleties of communication indicate ego states. For instance, sarcasm or whining indicate that the words that in themselves might be coming from the (A) are actually coming from the (P) or (C).

Since we also receive messages in an ego state, the interpretation of communication is affected by the energized ego state. For instance, if we are feeling guilty, a question intended simply to get information may be heard as an accusation. Transactions are discussed in more detail further on in the chapter.

Script Analysis

The TA concept of a script for life is based on the observation that people seem to take on a role and play out a predictable drama as they go through life. They interact with others in such a way that an outsider could watch their behavior and predict the outcome of their lives. Sometimes, this is called the self-fulfilling prophecy. Claude Steiner, a leader in TA script analysis, defined scripts as blueprints for life or dramas based on premature, illogical decisions of the (C) about what life has to offer and how the individual fits into the drama. Two major scripts have been described: "I am a winner" (OK) and "I am a loser" (NOK) (James & Jongeward, 1978). The expectation to win or lose in life serves as a filter through which all future events are perceived. A person filters out communication that does not fit the script as a means of protecting the position in life in which the person has decided he or she belongs (Steiner, 1975).

Berne originally described four life positions taken by an individual based on his or her own sense of OKness and that of others (Berne, 1973).

The winning position
    I'm OK–You're OK
Losing positions:
    I'm not OK–You're OK
    I'm not OK–You're not OK
    I'm OK–You're not OK

Winners are authentically themselves, doing things they like to do, maintaining good self-concepts, living lives consistent with good health, and enjoying satisfactory relationships with other people. Each ego state is available at will for response to inner feelings and thought and for response to the environment, here and now (James & Jongeward, 1978).

Winning is not significantly related to material or social success. It is an inner state of contentment with self and others: I'm OK–You're OK (IOK-YOK). Winners are assertive, straightforward, problem-solving people who at the same time adapt appropriately to their cultural heritage. They feel OK most of the time.

Losers have failed to achieve an integrated personality. They have overlapping or lax ego states or poor development of ego states. They are NOK most of the time. People who feel NOK but think others are OK (INOK-YOK) are likely to be "defined, demolished, bound, or awed by others" (James & Jongeward, 1978; p. 2). Those who find both themselves and others lacking in some way (INOK-YNOK) use tactics in their interpersonal relationships to try make others feel discontent. Blaming others for problems is a common method. A person with an IOK-YNOK script has contempt for other people and rarely seeks counseling of any type.

Most people have a script that has some balance between winning and losing. No one is OK all of the time, but some people seem to make a decision that they are, over all, winners, even though they may occasionally be discontent. They are optimistic. Losers are not NOK all of the time, but they frequently have a feeling of impending doom, even when they are OK. They are pessimistic.

Losers have not made the transition from total infantile dependence on others to independence and thus to the interdependence of an integrated personality. "Big time losers" generally fail to function well in society and may become institutionalized. Mundane losers are often socially successful, but consider themselves NOK in most situations and frequently mask their discontent from all except those closest to them. Clues to specific areas of NOK are apparent in both verbal and nonverbal communication. Conversation sprinkled with phrases such as "if only", "what if," "poor me," and so on, indicate NOKness. Energy is not directed toward problem-solving and the here and now, but rather toward furthering the NOK script, dwelling on the past or worrying about the future (James & Jongeward, 1978).

Winners needing nutrition counseling take information and change their nutrition lifestyle to satisfy their own best interests, with little need for support. Problems in nutrition counseling usually are related to a "loser's" script of some sort. Troubles are proportional to how serious the losing script is. Scripts are very complicated and are subconscious. People have general scripts and also have minor scripts. For instance, a person with a "stupid" script will ignore evidence of his or her intelligence. A person with a "don't grow up" script may excel in school but remain dependent on someone and fail in the world of work. For additional insight into scripts, see *Scripts People Live* by Claude Steiner (1974).

Transactional Analysis

Eric Berne's description of intrapersonal and interpersonal communication reflects the concept that people subconsciously go about "proving" that they are OK or NOK. He used the term "strokes" to describe interactions. Each stroke is a transaction. When people interact, they stroke each other.

Strokes. Berne identified four types of strokes:

- Positive: loving, nurturing
- Negative: critical
- Conditional: based on behavior
- Unconditional: based on existence

Giving and receiving positive strokes supports an OK self-concept, and giving and receiving negative strokes supports a NOK self-concept. Positive, conditional strokes acknowledge desirable behavior, and positive, unconditional strokes acknowledge the inherent value of being alive. Negative conditional strokes are critical of behavior, and negative unconditional strokes discount the inherent value of existence.

CASE EXAMPLE ·

Positive conditional: You did a nice job. Thank you for handling that problem.
Positive unconditional: I love you. Your eyes are beautiful.
Negative conditional: I don't like the way you wrote this letter. Your answer is wrong.
Negative unconditional: I hate you. You make me sick.

· ·

According to TA, all strokes, positive or negative, provide stimulation and awareness of existence. They are the basis of motivation. For infants, an adequate number of strokes are necessary for survival, whether positive or negative. An adequate number of positive strokes are required for normal growth and development and OKness. If positive strokes are unavailable, negative ones will suffice but will lead to a NOK life script (Steiner, 1975). Children tend to grow up OK or NOK based on their early childhood environment. Infants who receive an abundance of positive stroking thrive emotionally and become capable of positive self-stroking and an OK self-concept. The world is an environment of mixed negative and positive strokes. A person who grows up basically OK can withstand negative stroking without losing a sense of OKness. For example, an OK person can have his or her work criticized by another without losing self-esteem.

On the other hand, negative stroking leads to NOKness. A tendency to filter out positive strokes as a means of retaining a poor self-concept develops.

CASE EXAMPLE ·

A college student, while maintaining a 3.5 or even a 4.0 grade point average on a 4-point scale, continued to think of herself as "dumb." The two concepts do not fit together. "Dumb" people do not have 3.5 or 4.0 grade point averages. Upon reflection, that particular student remembered being told often that she was dumb, as in "you dumb kid," an unconditional negative stroke. She had internalized this stroke and developed a NOK self-image related to intelligence.

· ·

In most cultures, the stroke environment tends toward the negative and most people grow up feeling NOK about some aspects of themselves. It is unrealistic to believe there should be a totally positive environment in early childhood. This would not prepare the child for reality. However, children who experience seriously negative environments tend to believe, as adults, that they deserve negative strokes and they reject positive stroking from self and others.

CASE EXAMPLE ·

A dialogue between the Parent ego state and the Child ego state might go something like this when a positive stroke such as the following is given:

HUSBAND: "My, that cake you made looks beautiful and tastes delicious."

WIFE: (internal)

(CP) TO (C): "What does he know? You know you've made better ones and your sister always makes better ones."

(C) TO (P): "You're right, mommy. You know best. I won't accept this stroke, because you say it isn't so."

WIFE: (out loud to husband) "Oh, it's not that great."

This results in rejecting the compliment and serves to give the husband a negative stroke as well.

•   •

Children who are hurried, scolded, teased, excessively punished, or in other ways receive attention that is physically or emotionally damaging are discounted and devalued as human beings. Most unconditional negative stroking is damaging to children, and to adults, for that matter. In medical nutrition therapy, there is little or no need for negative stroking, particularly unconditional negative stroking.

Time Structure. All people need to structure time: time to eat, sleep, play, work, make love, fulfill bodily urges, meditate. Our choices as to where, when, what, how much, and with whom we participate in each of these affect the quality of our lives. They also determine the extent to which problems are solved in meeting our physical and emotional needs. Problem-solving requires changes in time structure, either in outward activities or in thought patterns. Each single change in time structure affects the entire time structure of an individual. For instance, a person dealing with diabetes who has spent a good portion of time eating dessert needs to do something else during the time she or he would otherwise eat desserts. An individual who has bulimia nervosa structures some time with vomiting and purging and therefore needs to fill that time with some other activity. The MNT has to be aware of the possible ramifications of changes in nutrition lifestyle and how they affect the whole time structure of the individual, both physically and psychologically.

Berne (1973) divided time into the following types of psychological activities (getting strokes): withdrawal, rituals, pastimes, work activities, games, and intimacy. *Withdrawal,* which provides the fewest strokes, and *intimacy,* which provides the most, are the least tolerated by most people, while at the same time the most wished for. Most of our time is spent in rituals, pastimes, work, and games. *Rituals* serve the purpose of making events predictable and identifying those like "us" and those who are "outsiders." For instance, food-related rituals regulate what to eat at meals and snacks, foods suitable for us and for others, holiday foods, and so on. Almost all food consumption is ritualized. *Pastimes* and *work* are used to meet other people and find those who will play our psychological games. Many pastimes and work activities also have eating as part of the activity, such as cocktail parties, wedding receptions, coffee breaks, working lunches, and so on. *Psychological games* provide a high level of strokes, prevent intimacy, and further NOKness. They are a serious detriment to problem-solving and will be discussed at length later. *Intimacy* is achieved when people are open and straightforward and have feelings of closeness with one another. To gain intimacy, games must be dropped, and individuals must trust themselves and others significantly.

CASE EXAMPLE ·

A mother-daughter interaction included the mother preparing and leaving food out for her underweight daughter's late-night arrival home from work. The daughter refused to eat the food each night. In medical nutrition therapy, the daughter became aware of her rebelliousness in the interaction, and the NOK feelings for both mother and daughter that resulted. As a result of therapy, the two talked the matter over and both gained positive feelings and a sense of intimacy in place of the negative feelings. The daughter began to eat the food and accepted the love it symbolized.

· ·

Transactions. In the TA view, communication between people is between ego states. An individual energizes the (P), (A), or (C) and communicates through words and body language from the ego state that is in use. In order for communication to progress, each person in the system must respond from the expected ego state. When this happens, transactions are *complementary*.

CASE EXAMPLE ·

A mother coming upon a child about to eat garbage will put energy into the (CP) and yell, "Stop!", hoping to energize the child's (AC) to stop the action about to be taken. If the child stops, looks up and says, "OK, Mommy," this would be a complementary transaction. Both are spontaneous and honest.

· ·

When a person asks a question such as "What time is it?" she or he is usually in the (A). A response from the addressee's (A) is expected, such as "5:14." The transaction is also complementary. If, however, a response such as "What do you care?" occurs, it is obvious that something has gone wrong. The first speaker expected a response from the second speaker's (A), but received one from the (AC). In TA, such a response is called a *crossed transaction,* and communication stops unless one of the people involved changes ego states to resume with complementary transactions. There is something going on in a crossed transaction that does not quite meet the eye. If a person responds to an innocuous question with a sarcastic remark, there is some underlying message being transmitted in an indirect manner. The social message and the psychological message are inconsistent. In TA, this is called an *ulterior transaction,* indicating that the communication is dishonest and has an ulterior motive. Such transactions display a lack of trust among the individuals involved and a lack of assertiveness. Many times, patterns of ulterior transactions indicate the kinds of difficulties people have in solving problems. If, for instance, a parent coming upon an overweight teenager who is starting to eat a large piece of cake yells, "Don't be stupid," instead of something such as "Please don't eat that cake, let's talk about it first," there is a message that the child is stupid, and the communication is about stupidity, not the act of eating the cake. The transaction is ulterior. Most likely the child heard the underlying message and may respond rebelliously by eating the cake, as if to say, "So, OK if I'm stupid. I'll prove it by doing a stupid thing."

Classifying communication into these various types helps the counselor understand clients better. The types of transaction most useful to MNTs are straightforward. They may be complementary or crossed. If a client uses many ulterior transactions, many of the counselor's responses will necessarily be crossed as the client and counselor work through the client's mistrust and lack of OKness until the client realizes that it is safe to be honest.

Ulterior transactions are the basis of manipulative behavior and psychological games (Berne, 1973). They are often complementary in that communication may continue between the game players until one or the other breaks it off. People gain negative strokes from games because they are dishonest and discount the players or the situation. They prohibit effective problem-solving because they detract from the issues and focus on efforts of the players to manipulate one another. Examples of the types of transactions are shown in Figures 5–5, 5–6, and 5–7.

Psychological Games. In common everyday communication, we often talk about psychological games, or "head games," or "laying a trip" on one another. We all know that when one is engaged in psychological games trouble lies ahead, and that the people involved are going to end up losing something, such as a friendship, a job, good health, and sometimes even life itself. Berne (1973) looked at this phenomenon closely in his study of transactions. He noticed that there is a set of ulterior transactions that follows the same pattern, with people repeating the same words, and behaviors with negative feelings always occurring at the end of a set of transactions. He described them as a set of complementary ulterior transactions that are predictable attempts to manipulate the self or others rather than being

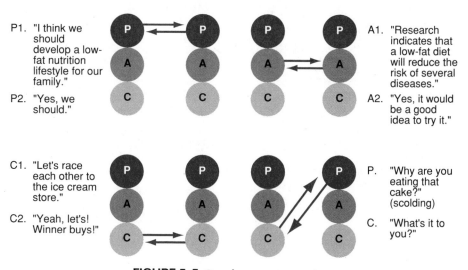

FIGURE 5–5. Complementary transactions.

C. "I'll never be able to follow this diet."

A. "Have you thought about whether you really can't, or you won't follow a different plan for food intake?"

P. "Why are you eating that cake?" (scolding)

A. "Are you scolding me?"

FIGURE 5–6. Crossed transactions.

straightforward and assertive. Real thoughts and feelings are hidden from the self but are usually displayed to others by nonverbal signs or telltale hints in the voice. Thinking is emotional, responding to internal cues from the past rather than to the immediate situation. Listening is also emotional and based on stereotypes rather than on what is actually happening in the present.

Games begin with a transaction that has the psychological intent to put down one or more of the participants in the game. Tension will build between the par-

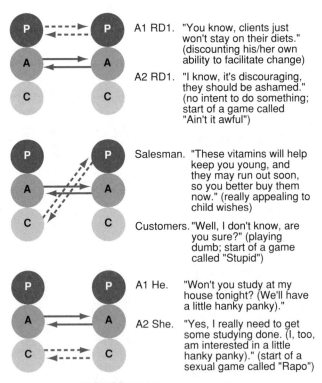

A1 RD1. "You know, clients just won't stay on their diets." (discounting his/her own ability to facilitate change)

A2 RD1. "I know, it's discouraging, they should be ashamed." (no intent to do something; start of a game called "Ain't it awful")

Salesman. "These vitamins will help keep you young, and they may run out soon, so you better buy them now." (really appealing to child wishes)

Customers. "Well, I don't know, are you sure?" (playing dumb; start of a game called "Stupid")

A1 He. "Won't you study at my house tonight? (We'll have a little hanky panky)."

A2 She. "Yes, I really need to get some studying done. (I, too, am interested in a little hanky panky)." (start of a sexual game called "Rapo")

FIGURE 5–7. Ulterior transactions.

ticipants until one wants to end the game and makes a switch. Often the one put down becomes aggressive. Suddenly, participants recognize that they have been "had," and feel bad about themselves and the others in the game. Figure 5–7 shows the general ulterior transaction pattern in psychological games. There are three major roles in games: Victim, Persecutor, and Rescuer. Players will begin games in one role and will switch to another role to end the game.

In TA literature, games have names derived from the way the game is played or the thoughts players have at the end of the game. The first game Berne described was "Yes, but" and it is often played in medical nutrition therapy.

CASE EXAMPLE ·

C L I E N T: "Will you help me work out ways to reduce fat in my diet? I'm confused about how to do this."

M N T: "I'd be happy to help you. Have you thought about using baked meats rather than fried?"

C L I E N T: "Well, yes, but, I really love fried chicken."

M N T: "Oh, maybe you could take the skin off."

C L I E N T: "I've tried that, it tastes terrible!"

· ·

In this game the client started out as the "victim." The "hook" is the statement "I'm confused," which discounts the client's thinking ability. The MNT set out to rescue the client by giving suggestions, possibly in good faith. However, when the client rejected the suggestion, he showed that his "I'm confused" statement was insincere, since he would have accepted the suggestion if he had really wanted help. The MNT was "hooked" and the game is on until one of the players does something to stop it. The client might say, "Boy, you sure don't have many good ideas," switching to the Persecuter position.

The game triangle, also known as the drama triangle, is show in Figure 5–8.

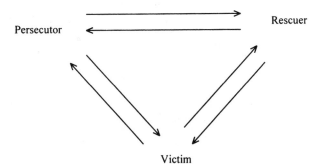

FIGURE 5–8. The drama triangle. (From Gurman AS, Messer SB: *Essential Psychotherapies: Theory and Practice.* New York: The Guilford Press, 1995.)

Games are played unintentionally in everyday life whenever we do not trust ourselves or others to be straightforward. However, confidence men and women use them on purpose. They "con" people into giving them money or other tradable goods under false pretenses. Con artists in the nutrition field cheat victims out of millions of dollars per year. For instance, high-protein compounds are advertised and sold to individuals who want to be good athletes. Advertisements appear to be facts aimed at the (A), but they are really aimed at the wishes of the (C) for magical solutions. Con games are most successful among people who have contamination between the (A) and the (C). Sometimes people continue to believe false advertising for a long time, but when they do realize that there is no magic and they have been conned, they feel foolish or stupid and usually angry at the person who conned them. If they are mad enough they may even sue. The dietetic practitioner may, at times, feel discouraged in the struggle to combat such con games and may even be tempted to use them when it is obvious that those who use games sometimes become rich and often famous.

Therapeutic Approaches

Goals. The goals of TA are to change behavior, thoughts, or feelings and ultimately scripts. It is desirable for clients to become more OK as therapy continues. In most situations, specific goals for therapy are developed between therapist and client. They are often behavioral but may also address thoughts and feelings.

Strategies. TA counselors make use of gestalt techniques to increase client awareness and contracts for planning changes. Counselors teach clients the TA language. The relationship is considered to be one in which client and counselor work together to achieve client goals (Gilliland et al, 1989). Group counseling is common, with much support coming from other group members as they help each other analyze scripts, time structure, and games (Corey, 1991).

Implications for Medical Nutrition Therapy. The concepts of (P), (A), and (C) are easy to explain to clients and an easy way for them to become aware of their thinking patterns and interactions (Gilliland et al, 1989). It can be fun for clients, and it sometimes helps them drop some of their defenses and become more open to learning how they function in non-problem-solving ways and how to change to more productive habits.

Script analysis is best left to a psychological therapist, but the MNT can use knowledge of this concept to recognize script aspects that impinge on a client's nutrition lifestyle. The script a person is playing out to be a loser could include failing in an attempt to incorporate changes in nutrition behavior.

Using the TA concept of games is an excellent tool for helping people understand nonproductive interactions between one's own ego states as well as between individuals. Interactions between counselor and client may reveal the games a person plays and can be used to create awareness in the here and now. Clients can see much more clearly what they are doing by learning to recognize games being played in the counseling situation, the here and now, and taking steps to stop playing them as part of their contracts. (See Chap. 3 for a discussion of contracts and Chap. 4 for a discussion of the empty chair technique.)

Awareness developed by learning about the (P), (A), and (C) and scripts and games contributes to a problem-solving approach in medical nutrition therapy.

ACTION-ORIENTED THEORIES
Behavior Modification

Behavior modification theory is based on stimulus-response explanations for human learning and behavior; the idea of cause and effect in determining human behavior (Gillilland et al, 1989). The earliest behavioral theories focused on organisms responding to stimuli and on a chain reaction in which additional stimuli associated with the original stimulus would result in a behavior even without the original stimulus. The most famous experiments were those by Pavlov using dogs. He first offered food, which resulted in salivation; later he rang a bell simultaneously with the presentation of food. Subsequently, he withheld the food when he rang the bell and noted that the sound of the bell resulted in salivation anyway. This illustrated that responses could be learned through association and behavior could be changed. Watson continued research in this line and developed the basis for learning theory as we know it today. Skinner also made many contributions to behaviorist theory, developing the theory of operant behavior, a theory in which the organism is considered to produce the first stimulus, which receives a response from the environment, starting the S-R chain of learning (Nye, 1981).

Personality

Little attention has been given to personality from the behavior modification viewpoint. There is a tendency to believe that the personality is the result of the stimuli and responses patterns of the person (Nye, 1981).

Operant Behavior Concepts

Skinner's concepts have become the hallmark of behavior modification theory and treatment. Skinner (1974) classified behavior into two types: operant and respondent. *Operant* behavior is behavior with no known stimuli preceding it, while *response* behavior occurs after a stimulus. Skinner considered response behavior to be of little importance. He focused on operant behavior and the consequences of that behavior. The consequences either encouraged repetition of the behavior or discouraged it. Encouragement is defined as a reinforcement (reward). Discouragement is defined as a punishment. To understand behavior modification, the precise definition of *reinforcement* and *punishment* is crucial, both theoretically and in the practical application of the theory in counseling. These words do *not* mean the same thing that they do in everyday language. Specifically, a reinforcement, or reward, is any result of behavior that increases the likelihood that the behavior will reoccur. Punishment is any result of behavior that decreases the probability that the behavior will recur. Effective punishment will completely extinguish behavior. In this definition, the consequences of a behavior do not have to be pleasant to be a reinforcer (Skinner, 1974). For instance, if a child does not get much attention for behaving appropriately but receives a lot of negative attention for misbehavior, the misbehavior is likely to continue because the child gets attention (a reinforcer). This can be applied specifically to teaching a child food habits. Praise for eating wholesome food, such as cereals and vegetables, and ignoring consumption of less wholesome foods, such as candy, can have the consequences of candy becoming much less important to the child.

In cases in which active punishment of a behavior has extinguished it, the behavior is likely to continue as soon as the punishment is stopped (Nye, 1981). It is not uncommon that a child who is scolded for consuming candy will consume it in secret (to avoid the punishment) or will wait until the punishment can no longer be applied and then resume candy eating. Sometimes the wait can be very long, even until adulthood when a person is outside the control of parents. Ignoring behavior has been found to be the best tactic to decrease (extinguish) its occurrence, thus defining ignoring a behavior as a most effective punishment. Skinner believed that people seek unpleasant consequences for a behavior to avoid no response, which is very undesirable. Skinner, like others, disavowed punitive action as an effective means of shaping behavior. Rather, he espoused reinforcing desirable behavior and punishing undesirable behavior by ignoring it.

Skinner accepted no concepts of free choice, believing that behavior is a result of past environmental events and current environmental circumstances, only in the context of an outside stimulus–observable response system. He was interested only in observable behaviors as indicators of all events occurring within the human organism. He did not consider reports of feelings or thoughts as observable (Corey, 1991). Later theorists have begun to include reports of internal "behaviors" as acceptable.

Behavior modification ideas became widespread following publication of Skinner's work. It has become very popular in university and research settings because tracking behavior lends itself to research modalities. It strongly influenced teacher training and counselor training in this country. There has been criticism of behavior therapy for ignoring possibilities of internal control, and the place of feelings in human psychology. Many of the principles of behavior modification have evolved into cognitive psychology and therapy.

Therapeutic Approaches

Goals

The goal of behavior modification therapy is to change behavior. The scientific method is important in determining success of therapy. Client's current problems are the focus of interventions to change behavior. Treatment goals are set out concretely and usually in time-limited statements. Changes are documented and goals are revised according to evolving needs.

Strategies

Putting the behavior modification ideas into practice is not as easily accomplished as explaining its principles. Precise knowledge of the exact "operant" behavior is difficult to determine, as is the precise behavior that it is desirable to reinforce. For example, several behaviors are related to consuming food, such as purchasing, storing food, and food preparation. For one person, the difficulty is in purchasing behavior, for another storage, and for another food preparation. Selecting behaviors to support or ignore requires discovery of the significant behavior and discovery of the reinforcer.

The complexity of reinforcers and punishers not only includes the identification of them, but also the timing. Research has shown that immediate reinforcement is much stronger than later reinforcement. In addition, behavioral change has been shown to occur more readily when reinforcers are carefully regulated. Optimally, in early stages of behavior modification treatment, reinforcement of every instance of the desired behavior should be reinforced. Later, reinforcement at regular intervals is instituted, and lastly the desired behavior is randomly reinforced. The idea behind this is that the behavior is supported because of the unknown aspect of just when the reward is coming (Gilliland et al, 1989). Gambling houses apply these principles quite effectively. Another application of planned reinforcement could be the treatment of hospitalized patient with anorexia nervosa.

CASE EXAMPLE ·

In cooperation with a patient with anorexia nervosa, a plan was made as to the food to be eaten at each meal and the reinforcer to use immediately after the desired behavior had occurred. At first, the patient was rewarded after each meal. When she was doing well, the reinforcement schedule was changed to every third meal, and when appropriate the reinforcer began to be applied randomly. The desired behavior continued and was motivated by the patient's hope for the reinforcement at each meal.

· ·

Counseling strategies include contracting, role-playing, assertiveness training, aversion therapy, satiation, token economics, relaxation, systematic desensitization, and self-management. Several of these are discussed in Chapter 4 and in Chapter 11, Professional Aspects, in the section on assertiveness. Therapy tends to be structured, and a significant amount of responsibility is placed on the counselor. These two factors can be useful in bringing focus to counseling. It can also result in missing the real problems when the real problems are in the emotional realm (Corey, 1991).

Implications for Medical Nutrition Therapy

Many aspects of behavior modification can be applied to medical nutrition therapy. Goals in medical nutrition counseling are to change those nutrition behaviors that are observable and concrete. Behavior modification therapy uses many counseling techniques that address overt behavioral change. Techniques are oriented to problem-solving. Some of the techniques, such as aversion training or desensitization, should be used only by therapists who are trained in their use.

Applying the principles of operant behaviorism, in therapy, involves waiting for the desired "operant" behavior to occur and then reinforcing (rewarding) it, thereby motivating the learner to exhibit the behavior again. For instance, the MNT may note, mentally, that a client reported undesirable food habits. She would ignore these reports and wait for a report of a desirable behavior and then praise that behavior. A difficulty presents itself when the family at home does not follow these principles and reinforcers are not consistent. The effectiveness of the model is diminished.

The adult client can work with the MNT to learn self-management using behavior modification concepts. In discussing the issues in changing food habits, client and counselor together can examine the reinforcers and punishers in individual situations and plan ways in which to obtain reinforcers for desirable behavior. There is abundant research supporting the effectiveness of behavior modification therapy in nutrition counseling. (See additional references.)

Cognitive Psychology

Theories of cognitive psychology and therapy are a loose collection of as many as 25 or 30 theoretical perspectives. They present different rationales and types of therapy, such as attentional processes, memory, coping strategies, cognitive appraisal, internal dialogue, irrational beliefs, self-efficacy, and automatic thoughts (Brewin, 1989). Some have been proposed somewhat piecemeal with no overarching concepts. Even the definitions are diverse. For our purposes, we have broadly defined cognitive psychology as the study of how humans process information. What is meant by information is somewhat vaguely described also. Some writers consider only thought to be information; others also consider all stimuli from the environment, as well as emotional input, to be information. In real life, theories that ignore emotion are probably doomed to failure because emotion is a highly important aspect of human life (Eysench & Keane, 1995). For this book, we choose to accept the definition of information in the broad sense of any stimuli accepted by the brain, including thought, emotional information, and sensory information.

Figure 5–9 displays the several disciplines from which cognitive psychology is drawn.

Information Processing Theory

Much of the early work on this theory was conducted by people in the communication field, primarily Bell Laboratories. Consequently, many terms and concepts are from communication theory. Berlo's Communications Model described the way feedback messages are transmitted. Messages are encoded, sent, received, and decoded. High fidelity makes a message clear. Noise obscures the message. The concepts can be translated into cognitive processes: those processes in the brain which function to make meaningful the stimuli (information) received by our senses of taste, smell, touch, sound, and sight (Berlo, 1960).

Information processing deals with a bewildering diversity of phenomena regarding the way individuals perceive, learn, develop language, establish memory and retrieve information, feel, think, form concepts, and behave. There is not yet one cohesive theory, although there are models of such things as cognitive func-

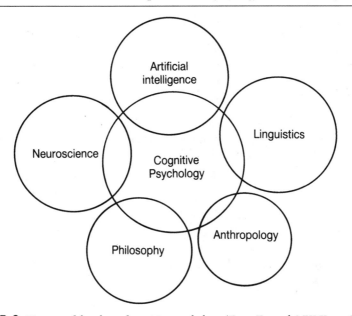

FIGURE 5–9. Diagram of the place of cognitive psychology. (From Eysenck MW, Keane MT: *Cognitive Psychology: A Student's Handbook,* 1995; reprinted by permission of Erlbaum (UK), Taylor & Francis, Hove, UK.)

tion, communication systems, the change process, and problem-solving processes (Gurman & Messer, 1995). The problem-solving process described in detail in Chapter 3 are essentially based on concepts of cognitive psychology.

Basically, theories of cognitive function as information processors compare the brain to the digital computer (Eysenck & Keane, 1995). Psychologists drawn to cognitive psychology from the behavioral sciences tend to be more mechanistic, such as Bandura (1977), whereas those from humanistic psychology, such as Ellis and Harper (1975), make an effort to encompass feelings and emotions as "information" that can be processed by humans. Cybernetics, a field of study that began specifically as a study of industrial systems and their feedback and control mechanisms, also strongly influenced the development of cognitive psychology (Gurman & Messer, 1995).

A Computer Analogy. Generally speaking, the analogy to computer functioning is as follows: (1) sensation (input), (2) short-term memory (RAM), (3) long-term memory (storage), and (4) retrieval (pulling saved information back into RAM) (Littlejohn, 1983). The typist or programmer (an outsider) determines the input into the computer. The person (internal) controls what input is accepted and perceived in the brain by selecting from all possible stimuli. He or she chooses that which is appealing, puts it into short-term memory, checks previous information to see if the new information is compatible, keeps it in long-term memory if it fits, and throws it out (forgets) if it is undesirable. There is also a retrieval system to get something out of long-term memory and back into short-term memory upon demand. This description is, of course, highly simplified. An example of this process applied to nutrition is illustrated by impressions at a cocktail party. In a crowded, noisy room, one must filter out much sensation to attend to significant messages. An individual might filter out the sensations of eating or, if the food tastes good, turn off the sounds of the party and concentrate on the food. In the latter case, stored information might be "cocktail parties have good food," while everything else is forgotten.

Although there are certainly some things to be learned from making an analogy between computers and human minds, it is imperative to remember that there are some critical differences (Guilford, 1987; p. 8).

∎ Computers solve problems given to them; people must identify problems.
∎ Computers solve only one problem at a time; people often face many at a time.
∎ The programs for solving problems are handed to the computer and they are debugged; people must develop their own programs, which probably are full of bugs.
∎ Computers receive a restricted amount of information; people have unrestricted amounts, some of it irrelevant, and may lack relevant information.
∎ The computer will detect inconsistencies, because it cannot deal with them; people overlook many inconsistencies.

In addition, models based on computer processing fail to take into consideration individual differences among people as problem-solvers.

Cognitive Complexity. One important concept not included in the model just described is the idea of cognitive complexity, the complexity in the processes by which people make sense of stimuli. A theory of cognitive complexity originated by Schroder, Driver, and Streufert identifies two elements, (1) what the person knows and (2) how an individual processes thought (Littlejohn, 1983). People vary in the complexity of cognitive systems. People with more simple cognitive systems integrate new information more simply than people who have more complex cognitive systems. For people with complex cognitive systems, new information is integrated with more concepts already known. Meaning will be connected with a wide variety of concepts. For instance, people with more complex cognitive systems will integrate information about someone they meet with less tendency to stereotype than do people with more simple cognitive systems. It appears that cognitive complexity depends somewhat on basic intelligence, but more on how much a person knows about a particular subject. An example of a relatively complex integration of meanings of food is shown in Figure 5–10 (Littlejohn, 1983). It might reflect the integration of the meaning of food that would be common among medical nutrition therapists and probably more complex than some clients' integration of the concepts.

Learning Theory. Learning theorists suggest that the sequential stage model of information processing erroneously assumes that stimuli impinge upon a passive organism. Rather, they propose that it is not the stimulus event, but an individual's in-

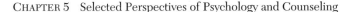

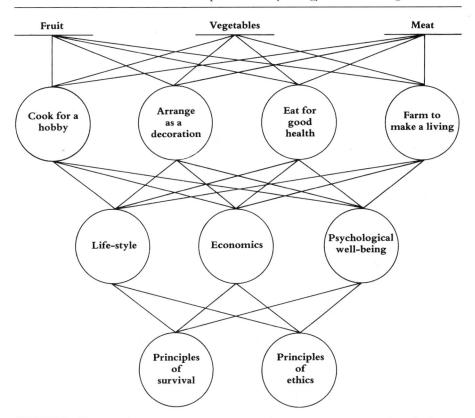

FIGURE 5–10. A moderately complex integration of information processing. (From Littlejohn SW: *Theories of Human Communication.* © Wadsworth Publishing Co, Belmont, CA; 1984.)

terpretation of the stimulus that leads to a response. An individual's past will affect the way in which information is processed. Failure to fully appreciate aspects of an individual's conceptual past is probably the greatest weakness of information processing theories (Eysneck & Keane,1995). In addition, no computer has yet been able to "recall problems, reason, learn and process language with human facility" (Anderson, 1990; p. 2).

Cognitive psychology theory in its current form generally suggests that it is not the stimulus event (information), but an individual's interpretation (cognition) of the event that leads to a response. The cognitive process that results in meaning is learning. To make meaningful is to process information by associating new information with other information in the mind. For instance, for an infant, milk in the mouth is associated with a feeling. Slowly, as the child's brain develops and more information is received, milk becomes associated with words as well as a feeling. The concept has been processed by association and becomes more meaningful. For adults, these associations have become so complex that meaning sometimes becomes confused and convoluted.

In general, it is proposed that the basic drive of humans is to seek information, and that motivation for learning is provided by the need to satisfy curiosity through activity and exploration and to obtain physiological arousal or stimulation. Motivation has not yet been clearly addressed by cognitive psychologists (Gurman & Messer, 1995). There is a tendency among them to consider emotional behavior as resulting from poorly thought out concepts or a lack of information. There may be some merit to this idea, but it must also be considered that emotions are a legitimate response to stimulation of the organism.

This discussion has focused on psychological functioning. Physiological processes have been so little studied that discussion of them is not particularly useful at this stage in their development. Suffice it to say that some people learn best by hearing, others by reading or by talking, and still others by using their hands.

Social Learning Theory

Social learning theory has grown out of behavioral science. It is, at least partly, an attempt to overcome faults in behavior modification psychology caused by the failure to consider multiple factors in the S-R model. In the social learning view, people are not totally driven by inner forces, nor completely dominated by outer forces. Cognitive skills represent an integrated capability among humans to respond to both inner and outer forces (Bandura, 1977).

Social learning theory explains human behavior in terms of the interactions between cognitive, behavioral, and environmental determinants. The concept of interaction "neither casts people into the role of powerless objects controlled by environmental forces nor free agents who can become what they choose" (Bandura, 1977, p. vii).

A major method of learning is observing what others do. In learning theory, therefore, a major method of facilitating learning is to model what is desired. Watching others enables humans to make adjustments. It also may lead to anticipation of the results of stimuli, without actually experiencing the stimuli, known as expectancy learning. This can lead to difficulties when a person has selected poor models for learning. Emotional disturbances such as anxiety may be the result (eg, test anxiety) (Bandura, 1977).

Nutrition lifestyle is usually learned by modeling. Children follow their parents' example, whether or not the example is consistent with the words the children hear.

CASE EXAMPLE ·

A young mother feeding her 10-month-old child cottage cheese remarked, "I hate cottage cheese, but I think it is good for him, so I give it to him." Simultaneously she grimaced and turned her head away as she poked the spoon in the child's mouth. The child spit out the cottage cheese. The mother wondered, "I can't understand why he doesn't seem to like cottage cheese."

· ·

Following is a summary of beliefs and assumptions about people that underlie Bandura's social learning theory (Bandura, 1977):

- Virtually all learning is vicarious.
- Some complex behaviors can be produced only through observing models.
- Capacity to use symbols makes people able to solve problems without having actually to enact all alternative solutions.
- People can produce consequences of their own actions and therefore gain some measure of self-control.
- Humans possess vast potential that can be fashioned by direct and vicarious experience into a variety of forms.

In particular, the concept that people learn vicariously led to the development of observational learning (modeling).

Rational Emotive Therapy

Psychoanalytical therapy began to be seen as an unending discussion of problems rather than provision of solutions. Albert Ellis, schooled in psychoanalysis, became influenced by empirical data from the behaviorists and developed rational emotive therapy (RET) in the 1960s (Ellis, 1984). RET has also been known as rational therapy, semantic therapy, cognitive behavior therapy, and rational behavior training (Gilliland et al, 1989).

Personality. By whatever name it has been called, RET suggests that there is a biological basis for human behavior. Because of the biological nature of human beings, they are predisposed to develop irrational beliefs and create their own emotional responses to life events. Nonverbal cognition has an enormous influence on emotions. In addition, influences are exerted by people's early childhood environments (Ellis, 1984). Only with enormous difficulty can irrational belief systems be changed. Ellis did make some assumptions about human beings that are summarized below (Shilling, 1984):

1. Humans are only human. They can change, but not be transformed. They are mortal.
2. The goal in life for most people is to be relatively happy. Happiness, or hedonism (pleasure), is a valid choice.
3. Human behavior is to some extent determined by strong biological and social forces. People can resist these but only with considerable difficulty.
4. People by and large create their own world.
5. People are born with conflicting tendencies between rationality and irrationality.
6. There is an innate tendency to be influenced by families, those around us, and culture.
7. All normal people think, feel, and act. Thoughts can profoundly effect feelings and behavior, but these can also affect thoughts.
8. Emotional disturbances stem from the individual's response to events.

Musturbating is the term used to describe much of irrational thinking, which is thinking that seems to insist upon focusing on what must be, in an all or nothing perspective (Shilling, 1984). Examples include the following expressed thoughts:

"I must be approved of."
"The world must treat me as I see fit. All people who fail to treat me as I proscribe are idiots."
"I must control my life."

Therapeutic Approaches. Rational emotive therapy is based on a humanistic, educative therapy modality. Strong and very directive and confrontive interventions are advocated. Changing the client's viewpoint is the goal of therapy. Desired viewpoints include (Shilling, 1984):

▌ Belief in self-responsibility
▌ Tolerance of others
▌ Acceptance of self
▌ Attitudes of openness
▌ Ability to make commitments
▌ Acceptance of change

Irrational viewpoints are the basis of emotional disturbances. It is the job of the therapist to dispute irrational beliefs and help clients develop rational thought patterns. Two modes of RET are described, "regular," useful in solving short-term problems, and "elegant," concerned with long-range personal fulfillment. In the short-term versions, immediate problems are addressed. In the long-term versions, the focus is on solving emotional problems, then turning to practical problems (Gilliland et al, 1989).

Such a therapy is dependent on rational thinking on the part of the therapist. This necessitates that the therapist become aware of his or her own crooked thinking. For instance, the thought "The client must do what I think best or I will be considered to be a poor therapist" is irrational, a musturbation. Therapists are expected to undergo therapy themselves as a part of developing competency.

Summary of Cognitive Techniques from Diverse Theories

The common belief among cognitive psychologists and therapists is that negative beliefs, thoughts, attitudes, images, and inner dialogue produce cognitions that influence feelings and concepts of self-efficacy. Changing the cognitions is the method for changing feelings toward the positive side, and developing problem-solving ability. Major techniques include:

▌ Relaxation training and therapy
▌ Systematic desensitization
▌ Mental and emotive imagery
▌ Cognitive modeling
▌ Thought stopping

■ Cognitive restructuring
■ Meditation
■ Self-management
■ Behavioral contracts
■ Biofeedback
■ Neurolinguistic programming

Several of these have been described more fully in Chapter 4. Many of the concepts of cognitive theories are useful in a problem-solving approach to nutrition counseling. It is important to recognize the tendency of some proponents of this system to ignore the important role of attitudes and feelings if the more mechanistic forms of cognitive psychology are used.

Implications for Medical Nutrition Therapy

The two cognitive theories, learning theory and rational emotive therapy, seem to have the most applicability to medical nutrition therapy, as well as being well enough developed that the MNT can easily adapt them to specific situations. A considerable amount of research supports the efficacy of these models in health-related counseling.

Cognitive approaches are practical and have a conceptual framework suitable for problem-solving. The MNT can gain insight into the client's perceptions and faulty beliefs by careful listening. Counseling effectiveness depends on the counselor's ability to confront the faulty thinking and work to change it. The MNT can also help clients become aware of feelings. The choice as to confronting emotions, and the related cognitions, depends on the situation and the therapist's comfort with dealing with emotions.

In medical nutrition therapy, the MNT is most likely to deal with practical problems. An example of an irrational belief that has been expressed in nutrition counseling follows:

CASE EXAMPLE ·

CLIENT: "My life just won't be the same if Aunt Millie doesn't approve of me." (an irrational belief)

MNT: "Is that really true?"

CLIENT: "Well . . ."

MNT: "Think about this statement as being a better thought 'While it would be wonderful if Aunt Millie always approved of me, I can't expect that if I am going to be me. In addition, my fears are irrational. Aunt Millie will probably love me even if she occasionally disapproves of me.'" (a rational belief)

CLIENT: "I guess that's true. My life really wouldn't change that much if she didn't approve of me."

· ·

Another example follows:

CASE EXAMPLE ·

C L I E N T: "I must lose at least 50 pounds. If I don't, people will still think of me as a slob. Besides, I'll just be a failure."

M N T: "What would happen if you lost 49 pounds? Or 40 pounds?" (confronting the musturbation) "Would you really be a failure?"

C L I E N T: "Well . . . I don't know, maybe not."

M N T: "Do you recognize what you do to yourself when you think you 'must' do one specific thing to consider yourself successful?"

C L I E N T: "I never thought of it that way before."

· ·

This case example demonstrates a musturbation, that is, "I must find perfect solutions to my problems."

A Transtheoretical Theory of Change

A theory of how people change, developed by Prochaska and DiClemente (1986), combines several cognitive approaches to understanding clients and planning interventions. It describes four stages of change that interrelate in a dynamic process in which people move linearly from stage to stage over the long run, yet tend to move between stages in a nonlinear fashion in the short run as they go through the processes of change. It is one of the better researched models. Prochaska, DiClemente, and Norcross in a 1992 article in *American Psychologist* describe the stages of change:

Precontemplation: a stage in which individuals are not considering changing in the near future (within the next 6 months). The client just does not see the problem.

Contemplation: a stage in which individuals are considering change in the near future. The client has become aware of the problem, but is not sure she or he wants to change.

Preparation: a stage in which individuals intend to take action within a month and have attempted to take action in the last 6 months, without success. Some small steps toward change may have taken place.

Action: a stage in which individuals actually change their behavior. A considerable amount of commitment is required to make real changes.

Maintenance: a stage in which individuals work to maintain the behavior change and prevent relapse.

Habituation: a stage in which new habits have been formed. For some people, this stage can last for a lifetime.

Most people move in and out of this change model, sometimes relapsing and beginning again at some previous stage. Usually negative feelings regarding failure occur when clients experiences relapses. Research indicates that relapsers do not revolve in an endless circle nor do they tend to relapse into the precontemplative stage. Each stage requires some time for the tasks necessary for working through that stage and preparing for the next stage (Prochaska et al, 1992).

The stages of change model has been used successfully to determine where in the change cycle clients are, and the types of interventions that are most useful for each stage. Mismatching interventions and the stage of change has been found to be a major difficulty in counseling and a reason for early termination of counseling (Prochaska et al, 1986). For instance, insisting on writing out behavioral change contracts with a person in the precontemplative stage is probably counterproductive, perhaps leading to unilateral discontinuation of nutrition counseling by the client.

Implications for Medical Nutrition Therapy

There has been a reasonable amount of discussion and research in the application of the stages of change model to nutrition interventions. Sandoval and coauthors (1994) discussed the application of the stages of change model to nutrition counseling in a family practice setting. Figure 5–11 illustrates the dynamic nature of the model in which habituation (making the new behavior a habit) is included.

The model has a valuable place in nutrition counseling in guiding medical nutrition therapy more effectively. In many instances, medical nutrition therapy and nutrition counseling plans are action-oriented and assume that clients are in the contemplative, preparation, or action stages. Many intervention strategies are designed for taking action and may be inappropriate and therefore unsuccessful (Sandoval et al, 1994). Listening to clients and responding empathetically, and further probing into issues and concerns without pushing for change, is recommended in earlier stages.

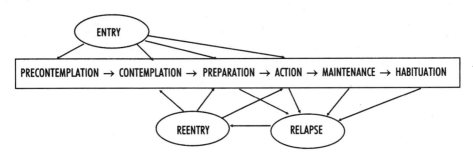

FIGURE 5–11. Stages of change model emphasizing points of entry, relapse, and reentry. (From Sandoval WM, et al: States of change: A model for nutrition counseling. *Top Clin Nutr.* 1994;9[3]:64–69. © 1994, Aspen Publishers, Inc)

TABLE 5 – 2

The Relationship Between Problem-Solving Strategies and Stages of Change Model

Stage	Problem-Solving Strategy

Precontemplation	Building a foundation
	    Establish rapport
	    Limit confrontations
	    Discuss nutrition concepts in an intellectual manner

Contemplation	Problem identification
	    Discuss barriers to change; brainstorm solution possibilities
	    Discuss values, interpersonal relationships, meaning of food
	    Begin to set goals

Preparation	Plan for change
	    Small increments
	    Revisit nutrition education
	    Build feelings of self-efficacy

Action	Commit to change
	    Construct behavioral contracts or other commitment to change
	    Set time limits for specific change activities
	    Encourage and support change

Maintenance/Habituation	Evaluate counseling
	    Plan for follow-up
	    Support empowerment
	    Explore additional coping strategies
	    Let client become more independent but emphasize availability in case of relapse or other needs for continued support.

Putting the stages of change model in juxtaposition with the problem-solving counseling method can help the MNT recognize the readiness of a client to change. Table 5–2 displays the effective relationship between problem-solving strategies and the stages of change model.

There is also value in using the stages of change concepts to document medical nutrition therapy. An assessment of the stage of change from which a client started and of the client's progress through the stages of change provides a better picture of the efficacy of medical nutrition therapy than the achievement of a goal such as compliance or success in reaching some weight goal (Sandoval et al, 1994). These goals assume a client is in the action stage and discount the positive effects of moving clients from the precontemplative stage to the preparation stage, for instance. Documentation of progress through the early stages can provide justification for extended counseling, with a positive prediction for success.

The stages of change model has also been effectively used in tailoring nutrition education messages to fit the stage of change among patients in a primary care setting (Campbell et al, 1994).

PSYCHOLOGICAL THEORIES OF HUNGER AND EATING

Although obtaining food is a major behavioral activity of humans, it has been only in recent years that psychological theories of eating and drinking behaviors have begun to develop. To date, the theories are physiologically oriented, but they do add a useful perspective to psychological theories. In the future, there should be much progress in amalgamating physiological theories with psychological theories in a more comprehensive understanding of why we eat what we do and how to be effective change agents.

Most of the data are the result of animal studies, and caution is urged in extrapolating these to humans. Studies regarding food intake have addressed hunger and thirst, issues of genetic or environmental influences and abnormalities, physiological structures and processes, and psychodynamic processes (Logue, 1986). Increasingly, evidence is pointing to significant biological influences and interventions. There may someday be pills to take to control eating abnormalities. Nevertheless, the current status of knowledge is so rudimentary that psychodynamic theories, themselves still tentative, are the main avenues available for medical nutrition therapy.

Hunger. Theories of hunger and the regulation of how much an organism eats have been varied and inconclusive. The only consistency that seems to occur is suckling among infants. A review of research indicates that regardless of theories of cause, it does appear that over the long run, all animals defend a weight below which they eat more and above which they eat less. Regulation of this "set-point" may be quite different in the short-term as compared to the long-term. *Peripheral theories* postulate that hunger does not involve the central nervous system. This view is particularly popular currently. Stomach distention as a control of food intake has been shown to have an effect, as has the temperature of the environment. *Energy commitment* models have studied both the effect of glucose and fatty acid blood levels. *Central nervous system* theories have focused on the hypothalamus. None have adequately explained hunger. The current tendency is to give more consideration to a peripheral theory of neuronal passageways that regulate initiation and termination of eating. The difficulty with these and other physiological theories has been that the theories have ignored any nonphysiological factors (Logue, 1986).

Brief Review of Concepts

Psychoanalytical theory, while accepting a physiological basis for hunger (both quantity and quality) suggests that hunger even immediately after birth is affected by learning. This early learning, prior to development of linguistic thinking, is so intertwined in physiology that it is inseparable (Logue, 1986). Behavior theorists have not addressed food intake specifically to any significant degree. Some learning theorists have suggested that personality and complex social behavior depend on feeding patterns and how the hunger drive was satisfied in formative years (Lyman, 1989). There is widespread speculation, but no clear picture has evolved. The psychological meanings of food have been addressed more by sociologists and anthropologists than by psychologists (Lyman, 1989). There is abundant opportunity for study in this area.

Human beings do seem to have a genetic preference for sweet-tasting foods and for fats and salt. It should be noted that studies that look at these preferences do not seem designed to manipulate the three elements in the same food. Evidence to date indicates that most food habits are learned and that psychological associations affect the importance of specific foods in a person's life (Lyman, 1989).

A review of studies regarding food and emotions noted that there is confusion between cause and effect. For example, foods preferred in depression, amusement, and friendliness are apparently eaten as a result of feeling, not to cause it (Lyman, 1989). Lyman's general conclusions were:

1. Food preference and emotion relationships are complex.
2. People tend to prefer, but may not always eat, what is best for them.
3. Foods tend to be used to reduce or terminate negative emotions and prolong positive ones.
4. Social interactions affect food intake.

In general, there does seem to be a strong connection between food and emotions and behavior. Below are listed some common themes in the literature. They are more speculative than proven.

1. Preparing food is a way of saying "I love you." Receiving food makes one feel loved because there is a sense of basic needs being met.
2. Some foods, such as candy, are perceived as rewards.
3. Giving up liked foods leaves a sense of deprivation.
4. Giving and taking food are connected with rituals in life and people dislike breaking that connection, so social events become an "excuse" for retaining old habits.
5. Many people "take care of themselves/give love to themselves" by partaking of food to relieve psychological stresses.

There also appears to be an array of psychological reasons that people have difficulty changing food habits. Inability to change food habits may be related to one or more of the following factors:

∎ A tendency to be rebellious
∎ A way of denying the existence of problems
∎ A psychological illness such as anorexia nervous
∎ A general feeling of anxiety and depression
∎ An interpersonal relationship that will be threatened by change

Changes in health behaviors such as lowering cholesterol or losing or gaining weight occur slowly, and many people in our society want immediate results so impatience becomes a barrier to change. It takes the mentality of a long-term investor rather than a trader on Wall Street, who wants his or her profits today, to make long-term changes in food habits.

The literature strongly suggests that factors other than basic knowledge of food and nutrition inhibit behavior change, although inaccurate knowledge may be a barrier to appropriate change. The public is bombarded daily by the media and others with nutrition information of all sorts. In the psychology of food, the effect of food on behavior has been of concern. What has been written about the effect of nutrition on behavior seems well documented only in extremes of weight or in deficiency states (Kanarek & Marks-Kaufman, 1991). However, much information in this area is very speculative, and studies vary in their reliability and validity.

Summary

Each of the perspectives presented in this chapter represents a view of human nature that can help the MNT understand clients and enhance his or her abilities to facilitate problem-solving. Each perspective has limitations due to blurry concepts, lack of research, or failure to address certain aspects of human psychology. Concepts have been selected for inclusion based on their applicability to medical nutrition therapy.

Individual counselors will find that some theoretical viewpoints fit his or her basic beliefs and assumptions better than others. Each reader is encouraged not only

TABLE 5 – 3

Comparison of Theoretical Perspectives on Human Nature on Three Variables			
Perspective	**Personality**	**Learning**	**Therapeutic Approach**

Psychoanalytical	Id/ego/superego
	
	Basic drives are
	  motivators
			Overcome negative aspects
			  of personality
			Analyze the past
			Insight-oriented

Gestalt	Inner control in
	  interaction with
	  the environment
	  both negative
	  and positive
		Holistic through
		  unique
		  cognitive
		  structures
		Forming new
		  gestalts
			Focus on here and now
			Experimental
			Relatively nondirective
			Dramatic
			Insight-oriented

Person-centered	Self-actualizing
	Always changing
	Positive/good
	  inner control
		Through
		  awareness and
		  drive for
		  self-
		  actualization
			Person-centered
			Unconditional regard
			  for client required
			Nondirective
			Insight-oriented

Transactional
  analysis
	Relatively stable
	  but changeable
	Based on
	  life scripts,
	  both negative
	  and positive
			Insight- and problem-
			  solving oriented
			Uses both directive and
			  nondirective
			  strategies
			Dramatic use of gestalt
			  techniques

Behavior
  modification
	Product of
	  stimulus-response
	Outer control
		Operant
		  conditioning
			Problem-solving
			Directive
			Emphasize reinforcement
			  of desired behavior

Cognitive	Rational/irrational
	  thinking and
	  influences
		Cognitive
		  structures
			Socratic/didactic
			Both directive and
			  nondirective

to undertake more in-depth study of these, but also to consider the values in viewpoints that were previously unknown or regarded with skepticism. Current psychological knowledge is still relatively primitive. Intuition and trial and error in medical nutrition therapy is often still the best guide to counseling success.

A comparison of the tenets of each theoretical perspective on the variables of personality, learning, and therapeutic approaches is presented in Table 5–3.

The stages of change model is a theory of how people change. Six stages are identified: (1) precontemplation, (2) contemplation, (3) preparation, (4) action, (5) maintenance, and (6) habituation. Usually people do not go through the changes linearly, but in a dynamic way. Relapse may occur at any stage, and a previous stage will be re-entered.

The psychology of eating and drinking emphasizes the biological nature of food habits. It serves as a reminder that biological strategies may be needed with or without nutrition counseling. There may be more biological limitations to changes people can make in nutrition lifestyle than those of which we are now aware.

Suggestions for Further Learning

1. List and describe the concepts from each of the theories or models in this chapter.

2. Write an analysis from each theoretical perspective of the case study presented at the beginning of the chapter.

3. Make a list of concepts that most parallel your own beliefs about human psychology.

4. In a class discussion, compare the ideas generated in activity # 3.

5. In practice or role-playing, conduct counseling activities and analyze the interactions from the various viewpoints.

6. Read more about the ideas that are of particular interest to you.

Analysis of Case Example
CASE EXAMPLE ·

John Lightfoot, age 52, has been sent to the outpatient department of a local hospital in the aftermath of a myocardial infarction. He is of normal weight. Nutritional needs include a low-sodium, low-fat intake. He is married and is the father of one grown daughter. He lives with his wife of 30 years. He has been working as a lumberjack. The counselor has been working through stage II, problem identification.

M N T: "What do you see as a major problem?"

C L I E N T: "I can't give up salt. Maybe I could just exercise. When I was working I got plenty of exercise. I don't like gyms. Eating salt won't kill me, will it? Oh well, who would care anyway. After this heart attack, maybe I should just die anyway. My wife fixes my foods. Why don't you talk to her? Oh, I guess you'll have to talk to me for the moment. What are you going to tell me I should do?"

· ·

- A psychoanalyst might perceive a conflict in the "id" between the wish to live and the wish to die. This would be explored.
- A gestalt therapist might explain the situation as one in which the client is confused and ambiguous in thinking. Therapy would be directed toward awareness of the situation and the formation of a new and more useful gestalt.
- A Rogerian therapist would not really attempt to explain the client, but would act as a sounding board, so the client could continue talking, become aware, and experience the feelings of the moment.
- A therapist with a background in TA would notice language ("should" and "want"), and ego states, (P) and (C). The "yes, but" game would be confronted.
- A behaviorist would focus on desirable behavior and reinforce the statement about exercising. Therapy would be directed toward exercise goals.
- A cognitive therapist would notice the irrational thought pattern and focus therapy on recognition of the irrational thoughts and ways to change the thoughts, thus modifying the feelings being expressed.

Each of these viewpoints provides explanations that can help a counselor understand the client and develop interventions that will motivate a client to solve the problem being faced. Having a variety of approaches available also enables the nutrition counselor to try different methods, according to the needs of the client.

CITED REFERENCES

Anderson JR: *Cognitive Psychology and Its Implications.* 3rd ed., New York: Freeman and Co, 1990.

Bandura A: *Social Learning Theory.* Englewood Cliffs, NJ: Prentice-Hall, 1977.

Berlo DK: *The Process of Communication: An Introduction to Theory and Practice.* San Francisco: Rinehart Press, 1960.

Berne F: *Games People Play.* New York: Ballantine, 1973.

Corey G (ed): *Theory and Practice of Counseling and Psychotherapy.* 3rd ed. Pacific Grove, CA: Brooks/Cole Publishing Co, 1991.

Ellis A: Rational-emotive therapy. *In* Corsini RJ (ed): *Current Psychotherapies.* 3rd ed. Itasca, IL: FE Peacock Publishers, 1984, p. 196–238.

Ellis A, Harper AH: *A New Guide to Rational.* Englewood Cliffs, NJ: Prentice-Hall, 1975.

Eysenck MW, Keane MT: *Cognitive Psychology: A Student's Handbook.* Hove, UK: Lawrence Erlbaum Associates, Publishers, 1995.

Gilliland BE, James RK, Bowman JT: *Theories and Strategies in Counseling and Psychotherapy.* 2nd ed. Englewood Cliffs, NJ: Prentice-Hall, 1989.

Gurman AS, Messer SB: *Essential Psychotherapies: Theory and Practice.* New York: The Guilford Press, 1995.

James M, Jongeward D: *Born to Win: Transactional Analysis with Gestalt Experiments.* Reading, MA: Addison-Wesley Publishing Co, 1971.

Kanarek RB, Marks-Kaufman R: *Nutrition and Behavior: New Perspectives.* New York: Van Nostrand Reinhold, AVI, 1991.

Littlejohn SW: *Theories of Human Communication.* Belmont, CA: Wadsworth Publishing Co, 1983.

Logue AW: *The Psychology of Eating and Drinking.* New York: WH Freeman and Co, 1986.

Lyman B: *A Psychology of Food.* New York: Van Nostrand Reinhold Co, 1989.

Meador BD, Rogers CR: Person-centered therapy. *In* Corsini RJ (ed): *Current Psychotherapies.* 3rd ed. Itasca, IL: FE Peacock Publishers, 1984, p. 142–195.

Nye RD: *Three Psychologies: Perspectives from Freud, Skinner and Rogers.* 2nd ed. Monterey, CA: Brooks/Cole Publishing Co, 1981.

Pettinger OE, Gooding CT: *Learning Theories in Educational Practice: An Integration of Psychological Theory and Educational Philosophy.* New York: John Wiley & Sons, 1971.

Prochaska JO, DiClemente CC: Toward a comprehensive model of change. *In* Miller WR, Heather N (eds): *Treating Addictive Behaviors: Processes of Change.* New York: Plenum Press, 1986.

Prochaska JO, DiClemente CC, Norcross JC: In search of how people change. *Am Psychol.* 1992; 47(9):1102–1114.

Rogers CR: *On Becoming a Person.* Sentry Edition 60. Boston: Houghton Mifflin, 1961.

Sandoval WM, Heller KE, Wiese WH, Childs DA: Stages of change: A model for nutrition counseling. *Top Clin Nutr.* 1994;9(3):64–69.

Shilling LE: Perspective on counseling theories. Englewood Cliffs, NJ: Prentice-Hall, 1984.

Skinner BF: *About Behaviorism.* New York: Vintage Books, 1976.

Skinner BF: *Beyond Freedom and Dignity.* New York: Bantam, 1971.

Steiner CM: *Scripts People Live: Transactional Analysis of Life Scripts.* New York: Bantam, 1974.

ADDITIONAL REFERENCES

Baldwin RR, Falciglia GA: Application of cognitive behavioral theories to dietary change in clients. *J Am Diet Assoc.* 1995;95(11):1315–1317.

Buckman ES: *The Handbook of Humor: Clinical Applications in Psychotherapy.* Malabar, FL: Kreiger Publishing Co, 1994.

Campbell MK, DeVellis BM, Strecher VJ, et al: Improving dietary behavior: The effectiveness of tailored messages in primary care setting. *Am J Pub Health.* 1994;84(5):783–787.

Corsini RJ: *Current Psychotherapies.* 3rd ed. Itasca, IL: FE Peacock Publishers, 1984.

DeCarvalho RJ: A history of the "Third Force" in psychology. *J Human Psych.* 1990;30(4):22–44.

Kramlinger R, Huberty T: Behaviorism versus humanism. *Training Dev J.* 1990;41–45.

Lowenstein LF: Humanism-existentialism as a basis of psychotherapy. *Int J Ment Health.* 1993;22(3):93–102.

O'Leary A: Self-efficacy and health. *Behav Res Ther.* 1985;23(4):437–451.

Sporny LA, Contento IR: Stages of change in dietary fat reduction: Social psychological correlates. *J Nutr Educ.* 1995;27(4):191–199.

CHAPTER 6

Counseling Across the Life Span

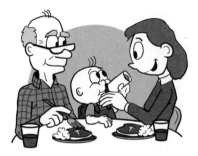

GOALS

The major goals of this chapter are (1) to review current information on human growth and development, (2) to develop concepts of biosocial, cognitive, and psychosocial growth, and (3) to discuss the implications of these subjects for nutrition counseling.

Learning Objectives

At the end of this chapter the reader will be able to:

1. Summarize the theories of human growth and development that are presented.

2. Provide examples of and explain the interactions between biological, social, and psychological growth.

3. Describe the medical nutrition states that are most likely to be a problem at different stages of development.

4. Examine scenarios and suggest counseling strategies.

5. Begin utilizing the understanding of human growth and development in counseling sessions.

Key Terms

▶ **Human Growth and Development:** the processes by which humans change over time and/or the processes by which they remain the same.

▶ **Biosocial Development:** biological growth and change and the social factors that influence them.

▶ **Cognitive Development:** growth in thought processes, perceptual abilities, and language mastery.

▶ **Psychosocial Development:** development of emotions, personality, and interpersonal relationships and the complex social contexts in which they occur.

Awareness of the need to increase interdisciplinary approaches to the study of food and human development has been increasing (Peters & Rappoport, 1988; Angulo, 1988; Sue, 1990). As of this writing, a comprehensive biopsychosocial framework for studying nutrition has

139

yet to be developed (Peters & Rappoport, 1988). Interdisciplinary literature is growing in a somewhat scattered manner that is not well integrated. No theory is proposed in this chapter either, but some practical applications of information are presented that take into account biological, sociological, and psychological factors and their relationships.

The growing effort among health-care professionals to treat patients/clients in a holistic manner has led to attempts to understand the whole person as he or she changes over the life span. Earlier efforts were often addressed singularly toward physical development, social development, or psychological development. However, the importance of genetic endowment on both physical and personality characteristics of an individual is beginning to be viewed as pervasive and entangled with the environmental forces of culture. Nature and nurture seem to be "dancing together," but it is hard to tell who is leading. Currently, the trend is toward investigation of genetic influences in biology, social interactions, and psychology.

Several theories of human growth and development are reviewed briefly in this chapter along with the implications they have for adjusting nutrition counseling techniques to the developmental status of a client. Because most readers of this book have a significant background in biological growth and development, more emphasis is placed on social, cognitive, and psychological aspects and the interactions between them and nutritional needs over the life span. As we continue in an era in which the links between nutrition and stage of life become more evident, it is increasingly important to understand those links. As Kart and Metress (1984; p. 3) wrote, "Aging does *not* occur in a psychosocial vacuum." Health-care professionals have the responsibility to include assessment of nonphysiological factors when assessing and treating (or preventing) nutritional problems.

One aspect of human growth that is very important, psychosexual development, is not emphasized in this chapter because it is not usually directly addressed in nutrition counseling. This is not to say that sexuality is not a factor in some counseling situations, such as in patients with eating disorders. The reader is urged to study further in the area of sexuality when working in situations in which sexuality is an issue.

Although it is recognized that an individual may or may not be in the particular "stage" usually associated with his or her age level, most investigations of human growth and development are conducted using a general framework of chronological age. That stratification is also followed here. The reader is warned that the danger of stereotyping is ever present; if the client does not fit the theoretical model, it is necessary to adjust the theoretical concept, not the client.

THE CONTEXT OF HUMAN GROWTH AND DEVELOPMENT

Much of the literature on human growth and development has been dictated by studies of the dominant culture (Bloom, 1985). This presents certain biases that must be taken into account in practical applications. Nevertheless, there seem to be some general patterns that can help in understanding people from any culture.

Overview of Domains of Growth and Development

The study of human growth and development naturally involves many disciplines—biology, psychology, sociology, medicine, nutrition, economics, genetics, public health, demography, history, literature, and the arts. Because such a broad interdisciplinary subject is difficult to comprehend, it is necessary to divide the subject into smaller domains. Berger described three domains as follows:

> the *biosocial domain,* including brain and body changes and the social influences that guide them; the *cognitive domain,* including thought processes, perceptual abilities, and language mastery, as well as the educational institutions that encourage them; and the *psychosocial domain,* including emotions, personality, and interpersonal relationships, and the complex social contexts in which they occur.
>
> *Berger, 1994; p. 5*

All three of these domains are important to dietetic practitioners. For instance, understanding how to feed a very young child and getting an older child to eat healthily depends on understanding the whole child and the dynamics of the family. Satter described the feeding of young children as an interactive process that is important in the whole development of the child. Not only is the course of early childhood development affected, but also that of later development. Satter (1987; p. 3) says, "Most, if not all adolescent and adult eating disorders, obsessive (and often failed) weight management efforts, and neurotic attitudes and behaviors about eating have their roots in early childhood feeding interactions." Reciprocally, overall patterns throughout life affect our nutrition lifestyles.

THEORIES OF SOCIAL-PSYCHOLOGICAL GROWTH AND DEVELOPMENT

The field of human growth and development is so broad and quickly growing that it is impossible to review all of the theoretical proposals available. Therefore, theories have been selected for the value they have in dietetic practice and how the concepts they present have stood the test of time.

Psychoanalytical Theories

Psychoanalytical theories provided the first scientific approach to human growth and development. The perspective of Freud and his followers interpreted human development in terms of the internal forces that influence a person's development throughout the life span. One of Freud's followers, Erik Erikson, formulated a theory of human growth and development that today continues to provide one of the most comprehensive points of view. In *Childhood and Society,* Erikson (1963) describes the eight stages of human development and the developmental tasks of each stage. Following is a summary of his theory, and descriptions of behavior that define a person as living through a particular stage.

The Eight Stages of Human Development

Erikson described life as continuous growth and development of an individual through a series of developmental crises or tasks (Erikson, 1963). Each developmental task, centered on the individual's interaction with his or her environment, must be resolved satisfactorily before the individual can proceed on to the next stage. It was not his intent to propose a structure for developmental goals, but to describe crucial points in life during which individuals have a potential for self-fulfillment as well as a potential for maladjustment (Bloom, 1985). The way in which an individual meets these crises determines the path of that person's life. Successful resolution leads toward self-fulfillment; failure to resolve developmental tasks leads toward degeneration and despair.

In the achievements of each stage lie the foundations for future triumphs, just as the losses and failures of each period leave us vulnerable to future struggles. At no stage is a challenge fully met, yet at no time is it impossible to address a previous challenge anew with greater success. All the aspects of development are present all the time, and each person addresses the task in his or her unique developmental pattern (Bloom, 1985).

Trust Versus Mistrust. The first challenge of infancy is to trust self and others. In many ways, successful achievement of this task is as much the responsibility of caretakers as of the infant. Those interactions between caretakers and the infant that help make feeding easy and pleasurable, sleep deep and satisfying, and bowels relaxed and smoothly functioning set a course for life toward achievement. When "mother" is consistently available to the child, trust in the "other" in his or her life enables the child to trust himself or herself without "mother" present. The first human social accomplishment is remaining comfortable alone, ready to explore the enveloping world. A rudimentary sense of identity is gained, and the difference between "I" and "thou" recognized. Yet, the inevitability of weaning also produces the prototype for the human sense of abandonment and the resulting helpless rage. The infant's level of trust or mistrust depends on the quality of care. For example, an infant who can depend on being fed is more likely to develop trust in her or his bodily signals for food than one whose caretakers are slow or inconsistent or who force the infant at feeding time (Satter, 1987). Rage will arise among children who experience the latter.

Absence of basic trust is not evidenced in that reasonable moment of reservation that is appropriate to new situations, but is a lack of trust where trust is warranted. It is revealed through statements and behaviors that discount one's own abilities and those of others. For example, both people who refuse to delegate tasks and those who refuse to take on challenges are exhibiting basic mistrust.

Autonomy Versus Shame. Muscular maturation around the age of 2 years sets the stage for learning how to "hold on" and "let go." The child becomes able to grasp and release both voluntary and involuntary muscles. The most dramatic, although not the only, manifestation of this developmental task is learning to control the bladder and bowels. The tactics used in toilet training appear to be a strong influence on physiological function and psychological patterns of holding on and letting go emotionally in later life. In this stage, again, the quality of caretaking is a vital element. Outer control that is consistent, firm, and reassuring is necessary for the satisfactory resolution of shame and the development of autonomy. Protection must be provided for the child against *shame* due to lack of ability to hold on and let go with discretion, and *doubts* about himself or herself when "accidents" occur. Inconsistency and shaming may lead to either overcontrol or rebelliousness in a person. Adult expression of doubt and shame is often in the form of reticence to express thoughts and feelings or lack of creativity in solving problems. When clients make comments such as being ashamed of their food habits or when they exhibit poor ability to say "no" to food offered by others, they are displaying characteristics of shame and doubt rather than autonomy.

Initiative Versus Guilt. When self-control and autonomy develop, the child develops self-confidence in the face of both acceptance and rejection from others. She or he is ready to take the challenge of social interaction in a wider world other than that close to home.

The successfully developing 4-year-old will have plenty of energy to explore the world and take the initiative to "attack" life without undue anxiety. She or he is aggressive just for the sake of being aggressive. The child has entered the struggle in what will be a futile attempt to conquer the world. The differences between fantasy and reality will begin to be recognized. Magic can be seen for what it is and hypocrisies of adults will come to light. Rage at the imperfection of the child's world (especially the parents) must be resolved if it is not to be carried into later life, both overtly and as guilt. Control that protects the child without stifling initiative results in helping the child to learn cooperation as well as competitiveness and to face reality. Much developmental energy is used in resolving disappointments about adhering to social rules. In respect to eating, this means accepting rules about what is and what is not eaten, and on whom responsibility for intake rests.

When initiative is neither supported nor guided and rage is repressed rather than refocused, a prohibition of initiative in self and others and retention of magical beliefs may result. Among adults, magical thinking about food and nutrition may be an example of leftover failure to fully resolve acceptance of the real world.

Industry Versus Inferiority. The normally advanced child is able to sublimate the direct attack on the world and learns to win recognition by socially acceptable means. It is a socially decisive stage; industry involves doing things along with others and acquiring a sense of the division of labor and the work ethic. In all cultures, children at this stage receive some systematic education. A sense of inadequacy and inferiority will develop if a child does not succeed in school or in the technology of society, and she or he may retreat to earlier developmental stages. Failure to make the transition successfully from home to the larger society is the disruption point in many lives. Home has not succeeded in preparing the child for school, and school does not fulfill the promise of early childhood.

Poor food habits and undesirable health conditions seem to plague people who do not resolve the issue of industry versus inferiority. Dietetic practitioners in programs that target segments of society in which individuals have not succeeded socially see many individuals who have become virtually stuck at this level of human development. The nutrition lifestyle of such individuals and their coping strategies may be deficient for themselves and for their future children.

Identity Versus Role Confusion. During adolescence, developmental tasks not completed successfully at earlier stages can be revisited, and in supportive environments there is opportunity to resolve that which was unresolved. The intellect has become strong enough to think about where one fits in this world.

In addition, youth is faced with a physiological revolution. Puberty brings about its own crisis in identity. Basic drives and feelings are intensified as hormonal levels rise. Adolescent experiences encompass acceptance of self as reflected by acceptance by others. Peers are the primary group of influence as the child struggles to become separately identified from his or her parents. It is a time of turmoil for most people. Young people form cliques, get crushes, worship heroes in efforts to see what "selves" are available in attempts to discover who "I" will turn out to be. Although puberty does create turmoil and sexual issues exist, Erikson did not see sexuality as an all encompassing issue, but rather as part of the development of identity, as a person, as a worker, and as a philosophical being.

Intimacy Versus Isolation. The young adult sufficiently confident of his or her own identity is ready to risk a commitment to others. Success at this stage leads to successful partnering even though it may require significant sacrifices and compromises. Role confusion will lead to isolation and self-absorption. Partnerships may result in which both parties protect each other from intimacy. Love is a central issue. Families are usually started during this period.

Generativity Versus Stagnation. Erikson believed generativity to be the uniqueness of humans, their evolution as a teaching and productive being. Generativity is the expansion of intellectual interests and an intuitive investment in biological and social regeneration. A sense of immortality is acquired from influencing the future through child-bearing and instruction of the young. The next generation will be seen as a vehicle for immortality. When faith in the future is absent, a regression results, carrying with it a sense of stagnation and personal impoverishment. Middle-age, then, may become a time for lamenting what was not done, and growing old will be feared.

Ego Integrity Versus Despair. "Only when man [sic] has taken care of things and has adapted himself to the triumphs and disappointments adherent to being the originator of others or the generator of products and ideas—only in him may gradually ripen the fruit of these seven stages" (Erikson, 1963; p. 268). The contrast can be seen between older people who are seen as wise and full of vitality, and those who are crotchety, complaining, and foolish.

People who develop a sense of ego integrity usually have the following characteristics:

A sense of world order and spiritual meaning to life.
Acceptance of one's one and only life cycle, and a new and different love for one's parents.
The ability to find comradeship with others yet readiness to defend one's own lifestyle against all physical and economic threats.
The recognition that one's life cycle is autonomous and that all those with whom one associates are also autonomous.

The cycle is complete when each new generation has a supportive environment in which to face developmental tasks.

Humanistic Theories

Humanistic theories perceive people as being unique among animals in that their development is motivated by a variety of needs to achieve their full potential or *self-actualization.* Notable among the humanists were Abraham Maslow, who proposed the theory of need gratification, and Carl Rogers, who established client-centered therapy.

Maslow's Ideas

In *Motivation and Personality,* Maslow (1970) set forth a hierarchy of needs that motivate human growth and development. He called it a "holistic-dynamic theory." He identified two types of needs—deficiency needs and growth needs. Deficiency, or survival, needs are physiological needs—air, water, food, shelter—and safety needs—stability, security, dependency, structure, protection, belonging, and love. Growth needs are those of esteem and self-actualization. Deficiency needs must be met to a certain extent before individuals can strive toward growth needs. People act to reduce tension by getting rid of deficiency needs, such as hunger and approval by others, and they seek pleasure from growth needs, such as hiking up a mountain alone, learning to give speeches, or establishing a healthy nutrition lifestyle.

Children are more likely to be concerned with physiological needs, such as safety, belonging, and being esteemed by others. Children in a supportive environment may also strive for higher needs through creative activities in art, music, or games. Meeting needs for self-esteem and self-actualization are most often the efforts of adulthood and later adulthood (Maslow, 1970). However, people who have been deprived in one way or another may still be concerned with lower needs. It is only when one need is satisfied that another level of need becomes apparent. For instance, a starving individual will seek something (almost anything) to eat as satisfying his or her need. When food is more available she or he may become more selective in the choice of food and think about the possible dangers of this or that food and whether to share with others. It is only when there is enough food to share that individuals become creative in food preparation. They seek approval and esteem and perhaps seek to satisfy their creative drives. Great achievements can result through the fulfillment of needs for belonging and esteem, as well as self-actualization needs. Once survival needs are satisfied sufficiently, it is not always easy to know by outward behavior what may be motivating the person. For instance, only the individual may know if maintaining a healthy nutrition lifestyle is motivated by a need for approval or by an internal need to take care of one's self.

One perspective on fulfilling higher needs is to view it as a process of repeated choices to meet higher needs rather than meeting safety needs. When a person is generally motivated by growth needs, decisions will most often lead to being more progressive and daring. The person will choose growth over safety in a moderate fashion (Biehler & Snowman, 1982). For instance, when a person takes the risk involved in drastically changing food behaviors, or when she or he decides to start her or his own business, motivation is often the need for self-fulfillment.

Maslow's hierarchy of needs is shown in Figure 6–1.

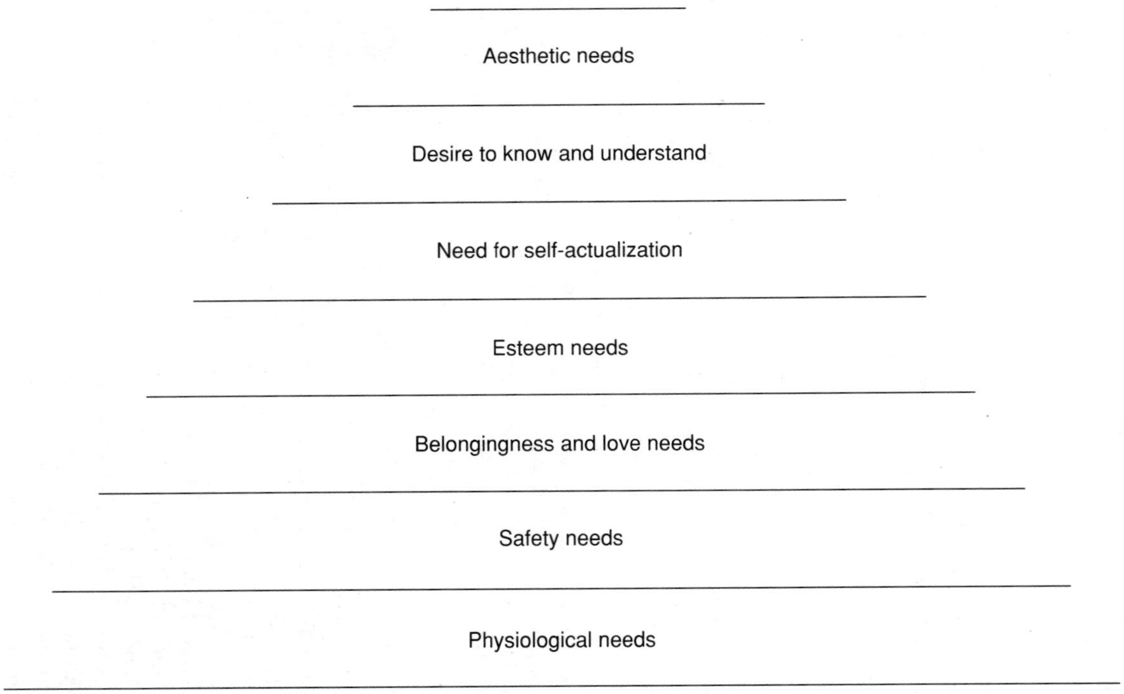

FIGURE 6-1. Maslow's hierarchy of needs. (Redrawn from Maslow AH: A theory of human motivation. *Psych Rev.* 1943;50:370.

Aesthetic needs

Desire to know and understand

Need for self-actualization

Esteem needs

Belongingness and love needs

Safety needs

Physiological needs

Rogers' Ideas

Carl Rogers, the originator of client-centered therapy made his proposal from a practical viewpoint rather than a theoretical one. Probably the most significant contribution that he made to the ideas of growth and development is the concept of unconditional positive regard for clients; the belief that every person has human worth and dignity. He believed that every person has an idea of the way she or he would like to be and that, with the right environment, the person would be able to figure out for himself or herself the direction to take in life (Rogers, 1961). As a therapist, Rogers considered the relationship between himself and the client as the major factor in success of counseling, and he also believed that every relationship a person has can contribute to or stymie growth and development.

Cognitive Theories

Cognitive theories of development are concerned with the structure and processes of thought and the ways in which these processes affect understanding of the world (Anderson, 1990). Two viewpoints have been most influential in developing cognitive theory: Piaget's theory of cognitive development and the information processing theory.

Piaget's Ideas

Sensorimotor Stage. Jean Piaget defined four stages of cognitive development. According to him, the *sensorimotor stage* is one in which the world is known through the senses. Babies experience objects by what they can do to them; suck, touch, squeeze, and so on. They do not yet think with language (Campbell, 1976). For example, the infant experiences sensations from sucking and from having a full or empty stomach that become part of memory.

Preoperational Stage. When children learn that objects exist even when they cannot see them, they begin to think symbolically. This *preoperational stage* is characterized by the development of language and imagination (Campbell, 1976). Children begin to understand points of view other than their own; however, they cannot think logically in a consistent way. In experiments, preschool children respond in ways that indicate that they do not understand that quantities can be conserved in different configurations (Biehler & Snowman 1982). For instance, a 4-year-old would be unlikely to recognize that a 1/2 cup serving of food is a 1/2 cup whether presented in a bowl, on a plate, or in a measuring cup.

Concrete Operational. By the time children begin elementary school, they have refined their logic and can think in concrete terms about their immediate world, the stage that Piaget named *concrete operational.* Children tend to think in terms of concrete experiences. It is a good time to approach scientific concepts with experimentation. Children can think in terms of cause and effect and classification of objects. For example, by 7 or 8 years old, children can experiment with foods by putting them into groups. They understand that a particular food can be classified in more than one way, such as a peach being classified as a fruit, or a yellow food, or a dessert or snack.

Formal Operational. Around the age of 12, children begin to develop the ability to think in abstract terms, which Piaget called *formal operational,* and can begin to think about several alternatives to problem-solving and philosophical ideas (Campbell, 1976). Children develop abilities to generalize and hypothesize. They are able to understand abstract terms such as minerals, vitamins, protein, and so on. This is the best time in the lifespan to teach nutrition science effectively.

Piaget believed that this process is guided by an individual's need to have new experiences reconcile with past experience. When new experiences do not fit well with past understanding, confusion occurs. This is part of the process that eventually results in growth, as a person modifies old ideas and constructs new ones through mental manipulation. Many people find it uncomfortable to be confused and do not realize that it is an inevitable part of learning.

Teenagers have developed the ability to hypothesize as to the consequences of behavior and to test them in their heads. A teenager does not necessarily have to experiment with eating too much and observing weight increases. She or he can figure it out mentally. When teenagers establish poor food habits, factors other than the ability to reason are usually involved.

Piaget's theory has valuable application among children. However, he stopped in young adulthood, assuming that the height of mental development was reached during the teenage years (Anderson, 1994). Yet it is evident that not all adults reach levels of formal operational thinking. Some seem to grow throughout life and to think abstractly in some areas and not in others. For instance, an individual may think abstractly about physics, but not about the implications of nutrition lifestyle (or vice versa).

Piaget's theory has been questioned by several researchers. Kastenbaum (1979) noted that children in the preoperational stages who were given opportunities to focus on similarities and differences in objects learned basic conservation concepts that, according to Piaget, they should not have been able to do. It can be speculated that Piaget did not always give as much credit to factors such as attention span or the social context of learning. In addition, there is now much evidence that thinking qualities continue to change and grow throughout adulthood. Piaget's theory does not account for the wisdom achieved by some people.

Table 6–1 compares Erikson's and Piaget's theories of growth and development.

TABLE 6–1

Comparison of Erikson's and Piaget's Models for Emotional and Cognitive Development

Erikson	Approximate Ages	Piaget
Basic trust vs. mistrust	0–2	Sensorimotor stage
Autonomy vs. shame	2–4	Preoperational stage
Initiative vs. guilt	4–6	Preoperational stage
Industry vs. inferiority	6–10/11	Concrete operational stage
Identity vs. role confusion	11–25	Formal operational stage
Generativity vs. stagnation	Reproductive years	
Ego integrity vs. despair	Older adult years	

Modified from Worthington-Roberts BS, Williams SR: Nutrition Throughout the Life Cycle, 3rd ed. St. Louis: Mosby-Year Book, 1996.

Information Processing Ideas

The invention of the computer has led to new theories of growth and development that are analogous to computer processing. Information theorists have described the process in steps of (1) registering the stimulus, (2) discarding it or storing it for short or long periods, and (3) retrieving it. Additional factors have been described by various authors, but they essentially reflect this basic structure. Learning processes differ between children and adults. The major differences seem to be in the control processes that regulate the flow and analysis of information (Berger, 1994).

The value of this approach over Piaget's ideas is that it considers development throughout adulthood and describes control processes that can improve intellectual skills. For instance, training in memory strategies can help people retain more information, thus improving problem-solving and reasoning skills (Littlejohn, 1983).

Children become increasingly able to learn as they mature because they have learned "what they must do" to accomplish tasks. The maturing of cognitive structures through the years increases the ability of children to screen out distractions and to develop selective attention. Selective attention enables problem-solving and more abstract reasoning.

Implications in Medical Nutrition Therapy

Theoretical concepts in human growth and development can help to explain (1) kinds of developmental problems likely to be encountered, (2) possible causes, and (3) characteristics that are considered to be normal or desirable (Thomas, 1990). The ability to identify the developmental stage of clients serves as a guide to the strategies and techniques most likely to be effective.

Erikson's theory informs us as to psychosocial maturity level and motivational factors. For instance, is an elderly client expressing ego integrity or despair? Is a mother expressing generativity in her child-care activities or the inability to teach a child (stagnation)?

Piaget's ideas provide guidance in instructional activities appropriate for different cognitive stages, what style of language to use, and variations in the use of concrete or more abstract approaches.

Information theory probably is most useful in enhancing the understanding that teaching a person about food and how to make decisions is more effective than trying to produce rules to follow. Many cognitive counseling methods are closely related to information processing theories.

It may be that the most important observations involve inconsistencies in development. For instance, a person may be well into the stage of formal operations (abstract thinking) and emotionally less developed, perhaps even on the autonomy versus shame level, exhibiting good understanding of dietary needs yet rebelling against changing.

A REVIEW OF HUMAN GROWTH AND DEVELOPMENT STAGES

In the following pages, a review of normal (sometimes optimal) human development is reviewed, followed by implications for nutrition counseling. Developmental difficulties and abnormal development are discussed only in regard to problems most likely to be encountered by the MNT.

Birth Through the First Two Years

Biosocial Growth and Development

In the modern birthing environment, many babies are quickly examined upon birth, then given to the mother for cuddling, and then given to the father. The family recognizes the moment as special. The infant is prepared to begin the challenge of growing up. The biological growth of the infant is rapid, physiological states become more regulated, and the infant is more and more responsive to the outside world. Newborn infants both sense and perceive their environment. Normal newborns see, hear, smell, and taste and respond to pressure, motion, temperature, and pain, although they seem to screen out stimuli that are more than a foot away from their eyes (Berger, 1994). The development of motor skills is dramatic.

Potential Medical Nutrition Problems. Nutrition is a vital factor in satisfactory growth and development during this period. Feeding-related concerns, such as colic, spitting up, and nursing bottle syndrome, are common complaints among parents.

The most common biosocial difficulty for children is low birth weight. Low-birth-weight babies are at high risk for many problems. Their first need for survival is getting sufficient oxygen, and their second is digesting enough food. Since the main cause of low-birth-weight babies is malnutrition in the mother, she is often a candidate for nutrition counseling. It is considered by many practitioners that better prenatal care and nutrition counseling would be a more effective approach to saving these babies than post-birth efforts (Pipes & Trahms, 1993).

Inborn errors of metabolism are a second significant problem requiring nutrition counseling. It is vital that children with metabolic problems be fed appropriately as soon as possible and over the long term. Most often, children born with inborn errors of metabolism receive specialized care in the context of a team health-care approach.

When babies are born with medical problems, the potential for appropriate social bonding is decreased. The child may not tolerate much cuddling.

Failure to thrive is diagnosed when an infant (or child) fails to grow at the expected rate over a few months (Pipes & Trahms, 1993). In about 3% of these cases, growth is delayed by environmental factors, including undernutrition, rather than organic causes like neurological problems. The MNT plays a pivotal role in assessment and treatment, whether the failure to thrive is organic or inorganic in nature.

Cystic fibrosis is an inherited disorder of the mucus-producing glands in the pancreas, bile ducts, bronchi, and intestines. The average life expectancy of a person with cystic fibrosis is about 20 years (Zemen, 1991). Nutritional treatment is long-term and is usually collaborative with the physician, nurse, physical therapist, respiratory therapist, and social worker.

From birth, individuals are not exempt from many diseases that require nutrition intervention. Renal disease, cancer, obesity, diabetes, and developmental disabilities are a few of the conditions that can and do afflict infants and the elderly alike.

Cognitive Development

Much diversity and variability of cognitive development has been discovered in the development of sensorimotor skills in infants. Cultural differences have been found to have an important role in the nature and pace of development. The stimulation customs of a culture will influence the pace of development. Children need stimulation and opportunities to use limbs and sense organs. They are in the sensorimotor stage in which communication and thinking are still nonverbal. Much behavior is semi-intentional (trial and error) as children investigate their environment. Universally, by the time the infant has reached about 2 years of age, adults are able to communicate with them using simple language, even though language at this stage is not much like adult language (Lidz, 1976).

Psychosocial Development

The first emotion that can be discerned in the infant is distress. It is expressed emphatically by wailing. The baby soon learns to smile and laugh and engage in social interaction. Between 6 months of age and 1 year, most babies express fear of strangers and anxiety at being separated from the mother. Emotions tend to intensify over this period. The interactions between the child's temperament and the environment begin to shape the personality of the child, and caretakers modify their responses as each learns the other's personality. The development of trust is also crucial in the first year of life. Trusting they will get fed when they signal hunger is fostered by the parent's prompt responses. Tactile stimulation—touching the infant—is important in bonding and establishing trust. Holding an infant while feeding is a primary method for bonding (Williams & Worthington-Roberts, 1996).

Implications for Counseling Parents

Most parents want what is best for their children and are open to guidance from the MNT. However, the developmental stage of the parents will determine their parenting skills. Parents who are able to develop intimacy will care for their child much differently than parents who are emotionally isolated.

Breast-feeding seems to be beneficial for both mother and child and an activity to be encouraged, yet care must be taken not to engender guilt feelings among mothers who have difficulty breast-feeding or do not wish to do so. People who have a "non-perfect" baby need emotional support to deal with the difficulties that arise in taking care of the child, and perhaps with their own feelings of inadequacy for having produced a child who is not perfect. Usually, empathy on the part of the MNT smoothes the way to nutrition education. In many cases, health care for newborns with problems is a team effort and support comes from a variety of sources. When this is the case, the role of the MNT is fairly straightforward. She or he has to both assess the nutritional needs of the child and become aware of the effect of the interaction between parent and child. It is often helpful to observe the feeding process. In some cases, the parents may "over-manage" a sick child and add to the problem (Satter, 1987). The MNT is responsible for providing not only nutrition education but also guidance in feeding the child.

For normal children who have eating problems, the role of the MNT may be more subtle. She or he may recognize that the feeding problem is actually one of interpersonal relationships. Clients may not expect the dietetic practitioner to address interpersonal relationships, and intervention needs to be delicate. In reality, such children do not always receive the attention that would solve the problem (Satter, 1987).

Cultural influences are present even at this early age. The type and time of introduction of foods to the child's diet is culturally based and needs to be considered (Williams & Worthington-Roberts, 1996). For example, some Hispanic Americans give their infants mashed beans with some cooking liquid at age 2 to 4 months.

Whether well or sick, children need the appropriate approaches for developmental age and a maintenance of a positive feeding relationship. For information on specific age-related techniques refer to Satter's *How to Get Your Kid to Eat, But Not Too Much* (1987). For more detailed information see the reference lists at the end of the chapter. The following case example is one in which the mother's motivation resulted in an easy solution.

CASE EXAMPLE ·

Mary is a happy and healthy 6-month-old baby. Her mother was a bit worried about her "overweight," however. At a well-baby check-up at the clinic, the mother related Mary's daily intake of 40 ounces of formula, 8 tablespoons of dry baby cereal, and 4 jars of strained fruit or vegetables. Guidelines for appropriate feeding amounts were given to the mother, along with support and encouragement for other current feeding practices. At a return visit at 1 year of age, Mary's height had caught up to her weight, and she was eating solid foods and drinking milk from a cup.

· ·

Ethical issues may arise in counseling parents of infants when neglect may be present. The MNT may find it necessary to report suspicions of neglect to the appropriate professionals and authorities.

The Preschool Years

Biosocial Growth and Developement

In the preschool years, the brain is maturing much faster than other parts of the body. Children begin to retain a stable image of an object (most importantly parents) when the object is absent from view. Little is known about exactly what is happening in the brain at this time. Patterns of development are related to gender, heredity, and environmental factors. Gross motor skills improve dramatically while fine motor skills remain immature (Anderson, 1990). Physical, cognitive, and social skills are strengthened through play, using toys, planned play routine, imagination, friendships, and other social interactions. A major responsibility of adults is to bond effectively with their offspring and keep children safe during this period of moving out into the world (Bronfenbrenner, 1985). Children's appetites at this stage are relatively smaller than at earlier stages of development, and this may cause concern for parents (Satter, 1987). Activity levels in children increase during the first 2 or 3 years of life, then begin to decrease, resulting in lowered caloric needs.

Potential Medical Nutrition Problems. Children who have been diagnosed with long-term conditions usually mature more slowly than normal children, and normal growth grids and psychosocial measure of growth and development may not be appropriate. Biosocial, cognitive, and psychosocial development are usually affected. However, it must be cautioned that medical problems do not automatically mean there are also problems of mental retardation. A few children contract serious diseases such as cancer, but this is not common. Most illnesses in children in the preschool years are short-term and easily remedied.

Cogntive Development

The cognitive development of children in the preschool years is one of the most delightful experiences for adults. Children are endlessly curious and make surprising connections between concepts. In addition, the inconsistency of their logic and their honesty, imagination, and rigid literal-mindedness combine in many unexpected ways that seem precocious to parents (Anderson, 1990).

Children center on more obvious aspects of the environment in an either/or belief system. For instance, they perceive that they are either "bad" or "good" rather than perceiving that they are children who sometimes act "bad" and sometimes act "good." Usually, distracting a child will change behavior as well as or better than scolding or trying to give long explanations (Lidz, 1976). Children are not likely to understand cause and effect, such as eating too much can cause a stomachache, or not eating enough can cause a stomachache. Among children of this age, concepts of numbers begin to emerge as well as a rudimentary ability to see that there are viewpoints and emotions other than their own. Research by Lev Vygotsky, a Russian psychologist, which actually took place about the same time as Piaget's research, concluded that learning is much more a social activity than a matter of individual discovery. He concluded that guidance, both in quantity and in quality, had a great effect on children's achievements. Language accomplishments are astounding during this period, both in the size of vocabulary learned and the pragmatic aspects of communicating effectively. This is Piaget's preoperational stage (Biehler & Snowman, 1982).

Psychosocial Development

Children become more skilled in social interactions during the preschool years. Through play, they have opportunities to try out roles that they see modeled in adults. For instance, games such as cops and robbers require taking on specific roles of hero, victim, and bad guy. Roles of parent or teacher are also evident as older children "parent" younger children. The response of adults to children playing probably has a major effect on which roles children ultimately choose as part of their identities. Letting children take the initiative sometimes proves difficult for parents (Satter, 1987). This may be a significant problem when children have health problems, such as diabetes. In addition, interactions between parent and child often vary among children in the same family depending on stresses in the family and community and on the personality differences of the children (Berger, 1994).

Implications for Counseling Parents

Many parents exhibit anxiety over what defines normal eating habits during this period. When they seek the help of a MNT, the major focus of counseling often is on anxiety reduction and assessment to be sure that nutritious foods are offered to the child.

Parental influences are strong in this age group. The nutrition knowledge of the parents as well as parental food preferences appear to be important factors in the children's food choices (Williams & Worthington-Roberts, 1996). Parental responses to food jags and transient food dislikes of a preschooler may influence their passing or their becoming permanent food habits. Overcontrolling responses are likely to result in rebellious retention of undesirable food habits. Environment and interactions at meal times also affect quality and quantity of food consumed.

The use of food as a reward usually begins as a child's cognitive capacity increases. "If you finish your peas, you can have dessert" is an example. The long-term effects of the practice of using food as a reward are often negative. Children with special needs continue to need nutrition intervention.

Parents who come for nutrition counseling may need nutrition information, but most often they need help in establishing an effective pattern of responsibility for eating. The parent is responsible for providing appropriate food and environment, the child is responsible for eating. Letting children develop independence in their eating is often difficult for parents. Helping parents learn effective interactions at feeding time is no different than helping them learn any aspect of parenting (Satter, 1987). It is frequently necessary for the nutrition counselor to observe the interaction between parents and children before he or she can know exactly how to guide parents. Getting children to try and like new foods usually is best accomplished by a positive atmosphere and repeated offering of new foods without coercion. Influencing children to like many foods is probably the one best way to help them achieve a healthy nutrition lifestyle. Even at a young age, however, a child's interest in trying new ideas in general will be reflected in attitudes toward trying unfamiliar foods.

In addition to social support, specific disease-related information is very important in enabling parents to cope with the nutritional needs of children with special needs.

CASE EXAMPLE ·

Three-year-old Jimmy was an only child and his parents were concerned that he was not eating enough. Observations by the MNT at mealtime clearly showed a control struggle. Mother and father both talked to him incessantly; coaxing, cajoling, and bribing him to eat. The child whined and cried and did not eat. This frustrated the parents, so they tried harder. The stress level was uncomfortable even to the objective observer. The parents were not aware that it was their responsibility only to provide the food for Jimmy. It was Jimmy's responsibility to eat it or not. The counselor confronted the issue of the tension level with them and worked out a contract with the parents to present the food and then simply allow Jimmy to eat with a minimum of attention. They also planned activities to help themselves endure the anxiety produced by changing their behavior. At first Jimmy continued his undesirable behavior, but as the parents stuck to their new behavior he began to eat better. It took several weeks for them to become comfortable and for Jimmy to respond completely.

• •

The Early School Years

The early school years include approximately ages 7 to 11, the elementary school years. Children are becoming independent, yet they are still very dependent on parents. All cultures engage in formal education of children during this period. It is most likely that this is the youngest age at which an MNT counsels a child directly.

Biosocial Growth and Development

For many children, the years from 7 to 11 are relatively passive and pleasant emotionally. Disease and death are rare. Motor skills develop rapidly and sexual urges seem to be submerged, although differences in development related to gender are becoming more noticeable. It is a time when children test the world to determine where they are going to fit. Hero worship is common.

School-aged children can perform almost any motor skill that does not require too much strength or refined judgment of distance or speed. However, variations in physique and motor and intellectual skills become more apparent. Children who are "different" or who are maturing at a different rate than others, either physically or mentally, may lose confidence and become unhappy.

Children from poorer socioeconomic environments may have more extensive experiences with birth, violence, and death than children in higher socioeconomic groups.

Potential Medical Nutrition Problems. Studies of school-aged children have found that most are adequately nourished (Williams & Worthington-Roberts, 1996). Weight-control problems are among the most common ones that the MNT is apt to encounter. Both peer pressure and adult pressure have an influence on weight control. Difficulties abound for both the underweight and the overweight child. The overweight child may suffer significant rejection by both peers and adults. In contrast, there is so much admiration for thinness that even among abnormally underweight children, images of normal weight are perceived as "being fat." Peak age of onset of insulin-dependent diabetes mellitus is 13 years for boys and 10 years for girls. Iron deficiency anemia and dental caries are also nutrition-related concerns in school-aged children. Many risk factors in cardiovascular disease can be modified by dietary changes at this early stage (Williams & Worthington-Roberts, 1996). Among lower socioeconomic groups, pediatric malnutrition may be a problem that requires nutrition counseling intervention.

Cognitive Development

Piaget's description of cognitive development is generally accepted among psychologists although some believe that cognitive changes do not follow Piaget's timing scheme (Berger, 1994). Logical thought is much improved in the early school years, yet the logic remains concrete and oriented to the present (Campbell, 1976). For instance, an elementary school–aged child will recognize that taking insulin as expected will help him feel better, but does not necessarily internalize that he is protecting himself from complications in later life.

Children enjoy discovering logical relationships, and magical thinking diminishes. Jokes often center on riddles that require processing logical connections. For example, "Why did the chicken cross the playground?" Sandy asked her father. "Why?" asked father. "To get to the other slide!" Sandy delightedly told him.

Information processing theorists have observed an increase in processing capacity and children begin learning how to learn and are able to memorize (Anderson, 1990). More flexibility in language develops. For example, a child may be able to speak in two distinct languages or two dialects of the same language. Children from deprived environments do not seem to grow at the same pace as children who have more supportive environments.

Psychosocial Development

According to Erikson, a sense of competence or incompetence (industry versus inferiority) is the result of this stage of development. Adults still have a strong influence on children, but they are beginning to recognize that there is a larger world and are learning to get along in it. Values other than those of the parent begin to have meaning. Peers begin to be a strong influence on development. Interface with a broader world creates a greater awareness of a child's own shortcomings. Because children spend most of the day in school, life becomes adjusted to more of a routine. They have more access to money, food stores, and vending machines, meaning that less nutrient-dense foods are temptingly available to them. School seems to have the effect of lowering self confidence for many youngsters. They become susceptible to learned helplessness, a belief that they are unable to overcome past poor performance. This may result in giving up attempts to succeed (Berger, 1994).

The stability level in the home influences the problem-solving abilities of children in this stage of development, affecting younger children more seriously than older ones who can understand more of what is happening. Children tend to blame themselves for troubles between their parents and can become disturbed.

Although poverty takes its toll in all three domains, it may be most devastating in the psychosocial domain (Berger, 1994). For instance, one reason for the debilitating effect of poverty during the early school years is that children at that age focus so much on the tangible and notice the differences between those who have material things and those who have not. Rage at being a "have not" can become a major focus, disabling much other growth.

The influence of television, and now computer and video games, adds to a child's sedentary lifestyle, which may result in nutrition problems. It has been estimated that children watch television an average of 22 to 25 hours per week (Williams & Worthington-Roberts, 1996). Television advertising also influences food attitudes and requests for foods. Children are solidifying their nutrition lifestyles at this stage.

Implications for Counseling Parents

One problem that may face the MNT counseling parents is dealing with hyperactivity among their children. Hyperactivity has also been termed attention deficit disorder, hyperkinesis, and learning disabilities or dysfunction. It affects 5 to 10% of school-aged children (Whitney et al, 1990; Williams & Worthington-Roberts, 1996). Most often the child diagnosed with attention deficit disorder simply cannot tolerate sitting for long periods of time without effective and stimulating teaching. There has been speculation that certain additives (salicylates), sugar, and caffeine may be causative factors, although scientific studies have not confirmed these theories (Williams & Worthington-Roberts, 1996). The MNT may take the opportunity to provide some nutrition education to both parent and child (be sure it is fitted to the age level and is stimulating). There often is a need to encourage solutions other than changes in food intake. All too often, trying to solve problems of hyperactivity through diet results in delays of more appropriate treatment, such as drug treatment.

CASE EXAMPLE ·

A young mother related to a nutrition counselor that, after spending many hours a day for several months preparing special foods for her child, she had finally realized that when the child wanted to misbehave or act "crazy," he always obtained a candy bar to eat just prior to the undesirable behavior. In addition, he had become quite aware that he was controlling a great portion of her time. When she quit spending so much time catering to the child and did not let his intake of sugar serve as an excuse for his behavior, episodes of undesirable behavior were dramatically reduced.

· ·

Weight-control problems have become significant in American society, even in this young age group. Increasing exercise may be a more productive way of attacking overweight problems than implementing strict controls on food intake. Parents can be encouraged to exercise with their children, probably to the benefit of both. Success may depend on changing the nutrition lifestyle of entire families. A team approach is usually needed in situations of significant underweight or overweight.

For the underweight, the challenge for the MNT is to help parents mitigate the strong social pressures for thinness.

It is important to consider the many social changes that may impinge on families who have elementary school–aged children. Single parenthood changes dynamics in the family; parents may be overindulgent or overprotective. Allowing children to take the lead in handling their nutrition lifestyle is very important. Parents are not always aware that even though their child may seem passive at this age, poor handling of eating can lead to serious problems with the child in the teenage years (Satter, 1987). When it is apparent that parent-child interactions are negative, or when socioeconomic status and living conditions create high stress levels, other problems in a child's life may need to be solved before problems with eating can be addressed.

McKelvey and coauthors (1989) stated that among children aged 7 to 11 years who had diabetes, those who did well received appropriate guidance and control from parents. Parents with the most knowledge about the disease provided the best guidance and control for their children. Giving too much responsibility to the younger children of this age group was not productive.

A counseling system that combines knowledge specific to the disease and a clear understanding of developmental stages is most likely to be effective. For instance, recognizing that children between 7 and 11 generally test their abilities to "get away with things" is a challenge. Setting limits and yet helping children learn ways to be self-limiting requires significant commitment on the part of parents.

A review of psychological aspects of children with diabetes found that most youngsters are able to cope with their disease, but that children in poorer health and from dysfunctional families coped less well. This may be true of children with other childhood diseases as well (Johnson, 1988). If the MNT suspects family problems, he or she should seek a consultation with a psychotherapist. Collaborative treatment is recommended for continuing care of children with long-term special needs.

Implications for Counseling Children

Some of the same caveats apply to the MNT as to the parents of school-aged children. It is important to let children take a major part in managing their nutrition lifestyles, while heeding the need to set limits so that the child does not face anxiety from being given too much responsibility.

An overbearing approach may anger a child. Even when children seem passive, they may be seething underneath, waiting to reach the age at which they can break free of adult authority. Children between 7 and 11 or 12 years of age like the scientific approach. Let them know the facts without too much reference to the far distant future, then provide the support they need to make their own decisions. Humor can be well-utilized among children of this age group.

Modeling and contracting techniques can be effective with children of this age. They need immediate and repeated reinforcement of desired behavior. Involving the entire family is usually very productive. An unfortunate example of the failure of the family to cooperate with a contract is in the following case example. More total family involvement might have avoided failure.

CASE EXAMPLE ·

In a group therapy situation, a 10-year-old girl, Emma, made and followed through on a contract to follow her regimen for cystic fibrosis for 5 days at home and at school. She contracted for a reward of going shopping with her mother on Saturday, to which her mother agreed. When the day came, however, the mother decided that Emma really should follow her regimen longer before a reward could be given. The result was that the next week Emma refused to make any effort to eat appropriately.

· ·

Sometimes a child needs someone to talk to who will be supportive, because support is not always available at home. By spending a little time working with a child on any problem, an MNT can establish a relationship that will foster the development of a desirable nutrition lifestyle for the child that can be a basis for his or her entire life.

The child who has diabetes continues to need nutrition guidance throughout his or her life. As Satter (1987) says, it is important to remember that the patient is a child with diabetes, not a diabetic who is a child. The disease state should not be controlling the child or the family. This is true for any medical or nutrition problem in children. The child is the focus.

Adolescence

The placid years before adolescence seem somehow analogous to a placid lake that slowly rises behind a dam until there is so much pressure that the dam breaks and a torrent rushes forth, uprooting everything in its path. In a similar fashion, adolescence comes upon a child in a torrent of biosocial, cognitive, and emotional changes. Children grow taller, heavier, and stronger; the peer group becomes all important; the mind turns more toward abstract thought; and the child's body matures into a fully functioning sexual adult body (Bloom, 1985). Socioeconomic status has a significant effect on growth in all three domains at this time. It also affects the length of time that the psychosocial aspects of adolescence continue. Some children begin to earn a living for themselves and perhaps their families. Some young girls become mothers. Both circumstances tend to limit adolescents' potential for growth. Other young people continue to be dependent on their families as they continue in school or look for work, often late into their 20s (Berger, 1994).

Biosocial Growth and Development

Most children experience a spurt of growth during adolescence, both in height and weight. Growth usually begins with the extremities and proceeds toward the torso and head. The nutritional demands of the body usually increase. Most adolescents are vitally concerned with their appearance and may feel considerable anxiety over it. Weight is a problem for many. Girls in particular are apt to be dissatisfied with their weight, even when it is normal. Boys usually are more concerned with height and muscularity. Early-maturing girls and late-maturing boys seem to have the most difficulty with adolescence (Berger, 1994). Boys may have a strong need to depend on the mother and an even stronger need to deny their need.

Potential Medical Nutrition Problems. Issues of weight management are central because of the developing sense of body image. Teenagers struggle with eating disorders, anorexia nervosa, bulimia nervosa, and obesity. Fitness activities and sports competitions further aggravate struggles with weight. Chronic diseases like diabetes and cystic fibrosis are difficult to manage in this developmentally turbulent time. Experimentation in drug and alcohol use, with the potential of substance abuse, could lead to medical nutrition problems. Pregnancy is likely to require a medical nutrition care component whether its course is normal or complicated.

Cognitive Growth and Development

Teenagers become adult-like in their cognitive functioning, reaching Piaget's stage of formal operations, the ability to manipulate abstract ideas mentally. A show of intellectual bravado combined with self-centeredness can lead to conflict if parents and other authorities, such as an MNT, lack understanding of the processes that are occurring. Whereas a younger school-aged child can deal with scientific facts, the teenager is able to think in terms of scientific reasoning—the development of hypothetical situations and alternative solutions to problems. Decision-making begins to include reasoning about the consequences of behavior (Bloom, 1985).

Psychosocial Growth and Development

"Who am I?" and "What am I going to do?" seem to be the questions people are asking and attempting to answer in the adolescent years. When pressures are too great, young people may prematurely foreclose their options, the result being role confusion and residual anger in many cases (Berger, 1994). Adolescence may come to an end much more quickly in a person who is not allowed a longer period of time, through school or other opportunities, to investigate possibilities. Drug use may be a factor in failure to develop at this stage. Pregnancy in teenaged girls is a major detriment to optimal growth and development, as well as being a major social problem in this country. Body image is paramount. Developing an image of the physical self that includes an adult body is an intellectual and emotional challenge that is intertwined with nutritional concerns (Williams & Worthington-Roberts, 1996).

Implications for Medical Nutrition Therapy

The pubescent teenager is likely to be dealing with the development crisis defined by Erikson as identity versus role confusion and to have the operational cognitive abilities described by Piaget. Among some adolescents, belonging to a certain group is a strong motivation; other individuals are motivated by higher-level needs. However, even among people at higher levels of human growth and development, medical problems, especially at their onset, are likely to cause some regression in development. The MNT must be alert to these factors.

Usually, much counseling effort needs to be directed toward encouraging the teenager to want to change before discussion of the actual types of change can take place. Parents often need to be included in nutrition counseling, but their role should be one of support, not intrusion (Williams & Worthington-Roberts, 1996).

Teenaged girls probably have the poorest nutritional habits of any group in this country. Both underweight and overweight are significant problems. Neither is easy to address, and a team approach is usually the most successful. The topic of eating disorders is addressed at length in Chapter 9.

Because adolescents are subject to peer pressure, they may need help in resisting offers of inappropriate food. A study of resistance training for teenagers with respect to offers of alcohol indicated that the individual's attitude toward the social acceptability of a behavior, and a belief in the good effect of a treatment were strong influences on success of the training (Donaldson et al, 1995). Studies of teenagers with bulimia came to similar conclusions (Brown, 1991).

The rebelliousness of adolescence may prove a hazard for patients with diabetes or other diseases that require significant restrictions on food intake. Teenagers may not respond well to contracts and rigid dietary programs, and they should be allowed to lead the way in the approach to their needs. Diabetes educational programs have been among the most progressive in implementing effective techniques in dealing with resistance. For instance, there has been an effort to change some vocabulary used, such as dropping references to "compliance" (Jenkins, 1995). These programs can serve as a model of approach for nutrition therapy for patients in other disease states.

For many parents of children with chronic and serious diseases, it is a challenge to let the child develop his or her independence because of well-founded fears of the dangers the child faces who rebels against his or her body. However, to succeed in later life, the child must develop independence. Parents often need support in dealing with their anxiety as they relinquish control of their children.

Pregnant teenagers bring much emotional baggage and many physical hazards with them. Their nutritional needs are the greatest at a time when it is very difficult to meet them (Guttierrez & King, 1993). Although it is impossible to tell exactly what may have happened to her, a pregnant teenager almost always has suffered significant emotional if not physical assault before coming for nutrition therapy. It is safe to say that pregnant teenagers are at least ambivalent about having a baby, and, in many cases, are quite hostile toward the idea. Motivation is often difficult, and patience is needed along with the Rogerian attitude of unconditional acceptance of the client. Her problems are many and she may need not only knowledge and support for a healthy lifestyle for herself and her child, but also an advocate to help her cope with the realities of her world. A collaborative effort among health-care professionals increases the effectiveness of counseling and treatment. Table 6–2 presents the suggested professionals needed to guide adolescents in issues arising in pregnancy. In fact, the American Dietetic Association issued a position statement (Rees & Worthington-Roberts, 1994) on the nutrition care of pregnant adolescents, stating, "It is the position of the American Dietetic Association that pregnant adolescents have unique biologic, psychosocial, and developmental vulnerabilities placing them at nutrition risk. Throughout their pregnancies, adolescents require nutrition care provided by dietetics professionals in interdisciplinary programs specialized in serving this age group."

TABLE 6–2

Suggested Members of Health-Care Team to Guide Adolescents in Issues Arising in Pregnancy

	Discipline					
Issues	Obste-trician	Adolescent Medical Specialist	Nurse	Nutri-tionist	Social Worker	Psych-ologist
General health and planning of continuous care		X	X	X	X	
Complications of pregnancy	X	X	X	X		
Labor and delivery preparation	X	X	X			
School program					X	X
Economic resources			X		X	
Substance abuse (cessation and education)		X	X	X	X	X
Psychological adjustment and stress	X	X	X	X	X	X
Developmental delay			X		X	X
Infant-care education		X	X	X		
Relinquishment counseling			X		X	X
Nutritional care		X	X	X		
Nutritional care: Education		X	X	X		
Nutritional care: Resource coordination			X	X	X	
Family or marital conflict					X	X

From Worthington-Roberts BS, Williams SR: *Nutrition Throughout the Life Cycle.* 3rd ed. St. Louis: Mosby-Year Book, 1996.

Drug use may bring an adolescent to nutrition counseling because of the resulting malnutrition or renal failure or some other life-threatening condition. At times, young people are facing severe food restrictions. It may be a matter of life and death that they follow the treatment plan. Severe illness can lead people to ambivalence about death (Kubler-Ross, 1975). When working with children who may be dying, it is important that the MNT work with a care team and that she or he take care of her or his own stresses. Children may want to talk about death over time. Because children recognize how uncomfortable this can be, they may sometimes choose a new person in whom to confide. If an MNT has established a good rapport with the young client, she or he may be chosen. It is important to facilitate a climate of openness and let the child (or an adult for that matter) talk. Often, there is no need for any response except empathy.

CASE EXAMPLE ·

A dietitian had been working over several weeks with a 17-year-old male patient on dialysis. At one session, the client seemed agitated and preoccupied for several minutes into the conversation and was not interested in nutrition. The MNT kept bringing up issues that had been discussed previously, thinking that she would land on the problem (without success), when the following occurred:

C L I E N T: (suddenly bursting into tears) "I'm going to die. I thought I was to get a kidney transplant yesterday, and when I went for the match, it didn't match. I don't want to die."

The MNT was not aware the client had been close to getting a transplant, and was a little startled and was silent for a moment before answering.

M N T: "Would you like to talk more about that?"

Following this dialogue, several minutes of conversation about dying and frustration ensued, after which the client was much calmer and the two were able to return to considerations regarding the nutrition needs of the client.

· ·

Early Adulthood

Early adulthood is characterized, in Erikson's theory, as a time of intimacy versus isolation. Most people marry or establish partnerships in early adulthood, and most become parents. Young adults are energetic, fortunately, because it takes a lot of energy to become parents, and to work and play. Overall health is good for the vast majority of people in early adulthood. By and large, their energies are available for social and psychological growth.

Biosocial Growth and Development

Young adults do not grow much taller, but they typically grow stronger and fuller in their bodies. It is the prime of physical life. It is the major stage of life for reproduction, starting a new family, and embarking upon a job or career. A cultural shift occurring over the last few decades has resulted in a greater emphasis being placed on commitment to self and a delay in marriage and family. It appears that people who choose parenthood, either biologically or through adoption, show greater evidence of generativity than those who remain childless (Kotre & Hall, 1990).

Potential Medical Nutrition Problems. Young adulthood is the time of life when the need for nutrition counseling is lowest. Pregnancy, whether associated with normal or abnormal health conditions, may warrant nutrition counseling. Gestational diabetes is the most common medical disorder to complicate pregnancy. Women who are happy that they are going to have a child and have no complications in pregnancy may be the most easily counseled people. They learn what they need to know and proceed with their lives. They may find it easy to eat well because they are motivated by the thoughts of the child soon to be born, and perhaps because they know that the nutrition requirements of pregnancy are time-limited.

People in this stage also seek nutrition advice about disease prevention, especially if there is a strong family history of disease or if there has been a recent illness or death of a family member. Certainly, appropriate intake of energy-producing foods, adequate intake of essential nutrients and fiber, and variety and moderation in the diet have all been shown to be preventive factors for various diseases (Whitney et al, 1990). People who suffer from chronic diseases continue to need the assistance of an MNT, either ongoing or intermittently.

Cognitive Growth and Development

Cognitive activities in this stage focus primarily on career and family functioning. The proposed stages of adult development are described in Table 6–3 and in the following pages (Schaie, 1977–78).

Scholars have realized that thought processes develop in the adult beyond the level defined by Piaget as formal operations. This further stage has been termed *post-formal thought*. The central features are the ability to adapt thought to the subjective, real-life circumstances that arise and the ability to find solutions to problems by assessing the effect of past solutions (Kastenbaum, 1979).

Psychosocial Growth and Development

Berger (1994) identified two major needs of adulthood, the need for affiliation (love) and the need to achieve. The young adult embarks on tasks to fulfill these needs and goes through several periods of re-evaluation and transitions. Social standards have a great influence on mating and marriage. Not infrequently, social expectations and personal expectations are not synchronized. Both work and family environments support or inhibit generativity, and people will grow or stagnate through interactions between themselves and their environment. Research indicates that as people grow and develop in adulthood, Erikson's life stages appear to

TABLE 6–3

Stages of Adult Development	
Stage	**Developmental Process**
Childhood and adolescence	Acquisition—learning unspecialized knowledge and skills
Early adulthood	Achieving—goal-directed learning
Middle adulthood	Responsibility—integrating personal goals with those of family, community, social systems
Late adulthood	Reintegration—a time of wisdom

After Schaie KW: Toward a stage theory of adult cognitive development. *J Aging Hum Dev.* 1977;8(2):129. By permission of Baywood Publishing Company.

Behavioral Expressions of a Sense of Intimacy Versus Isolation: Stage 6	
Characteristic Behaviors of People Who Have a Sense of Intimacy	**Characteristic Behaviors of People Who Have a Sense of Isolation**
1. They have been able to establish a firm sense of their own identity.	1. They have not been able to establish a firm sense of their own identity.
2. They tend to be tolerant and accepting of the differences perceived in other people.	2. They tend not to be particularly tolerant or accepting of differences perceived in other people.
3. They are willing and able to trust others and themselves in the relationships they form.	3. They are not particularly willing to trust either themselves or others in the relationships they form.
4. They are able to form close emotional bonds without fearing the loss of their own identity.	4. They are hesitant to form close emotional bonds because of fear of losing self-identity.
5. They tend to develop cooperative, affiliative relationships with others.	5. They tend to develop competitive relationships with others, making cooperative efforts more difficult.
6. They find satisfaction in their affiliations with others but can comfortably isolate themselves and be alone when they . choose.	6. They tend to prefer more separation from others; they feel uncomfortable when affiliations with others are too close.
7. They are willing and able to commit themselves to relationships that demand sacrifice and compromise.	7. They have difficulty committing to relationships that may demand sacrifice and compromise.
8. They are inclined to perceive relationships as something one gives to.	8. They are inclined to perceive relationships as something one takes from.
9. They tend to perceive sex as a means of both achieving physical closeness and expressing love.	9. They tend to perceive sex as a means of achieving physical satisfaction, but not necessarily expressing love; partner is seen more as an object.
10. They are able to express their caring feelings in a variety of ways and to say the words "I love you" without fear	10. They have difficulty expressing their caring feelings for others and find the words "I love you" hard to verbalize.
Implicit Attitude	**Implicit Attitude**
1. I'm okay and others are, too.	1. I'm okay, but others are not okay.
2. Others can generally be trusted.	2. Others cannot generally be trusted.
3. Life can be difficult, but through mutual interdependence we can make it.	3. Life can be difficult, and people have to learn to take care of themselves.

TABLE 6–4

From Hamacheck DE: Evaluating self-concept and ego development within Erikson's psychosocial framework: A formulation. *J Couns Dev* 1988;66:354–360.

be appropriate for both males and females (Erikson, 1963). The behaviors that are indicative of this stage of psychosocial development, as defined by Erikson, are presented in Table 6–4 (Hamacheck, 1988).

Implications for Medical Nutrition Therapy

Young adults are more likely to seek nutrition counseling for help in parenting than for problems of their own. The MNT should keep in mind that those few patients who have developed chronic or serious disease are dealing with significant losses besides the loss of good health. For instance, they may not be able to move forward in their career and may not have medical coverage. They may be unable to support a growing family. People facing illness at this time of life may have difficulty thinking that nutrition is an important issue. By the same token, healthy people may not recognize that an optimal nutrition lifestyle can diminish their vulnerability to disease later in life.

Many strategies and techniques of counseling work well with young adults. In most instances, the client's cultural background is more significant in selecting the approach to use in counseling than is the stage of life. Cross-cultural counseling is discussed in detail in Chapter 7.

CASE EXAMPLE ·

Mrs. Jones is a 38-year-old woman with a blood cholesterol level of 262 mg/dL. No other health problems exist and she is within a healthy range for weight. The rest of her lipid profile is normal. Her mother died of a stroke several years previously; her maternal grandmother died of a heart attack. Mrs. Jones was sent by her doctor to the MNT with a diagnosis of hypercholesterolemia. She did not understand why the doctor did not just give her medication for her condition. The following dialogue began after a good rapport had been established.

CLIENT: "I am so busy I can't be bothered with changing my diet! I don't know why the doctor didn't just give me some pills. I have a family to feed ." (pause)

MNT: "Perhaps there won't be much to change. In addition, a change that's good for you might also be something the whole family could change. Let's go over the food you eat now and how you go about feeding your family."

A nutrition lifestyle inquiry followed. When it was finished the MNT continued.

MNT: "Now tell me what you have heard about nutrition that could help lower cholesterol."

CLIENT: "Well, I guess lowering fat intake would help."

MNT: "As you think back over what we have talked about, what is one easy thing you could do to decrease fat intake for yourself and perhaps for your whole family?"

CLIENT: "Well, I bet no one would even notice if I changed to low-fat milk instead of whole milk and I could leave off cream and put milk in my coffee. Would that be enough?"

MNT: "That would be a good way to start. Does facing this problem seem less difficult now?"

CLIENT: "Yes."

· ·

Middle Adulthood

There is a tendency among Americans to avoid the term "old" and to fear it. This negativity seems to conflict with scientific evidence that middle adulthood is a stage of much growth and development (Kart, 1994). The age bracket for middle adulthood is quite indistinct. It may be as early as 35 for some, and well into the 60s for others.

Biosocial Growth and Development

Middle adulthood seems to be getting later and later in life for some people. Sheehy (1995), in *New Passages,* advises people to read any descriptions of aging with the thought in mind that if they are now 50, descriptions of 40 will fit them; at 60, they are more like descriptions of 50-year-olds, and so on. For some people, this may mean that they get a new chance at a mid-life crisis. Unfortunately, the circumstances of life make significant differences in the biosocial status of people as they become older. Some people are much older than others in later years. The poor, ethnic minorities, and those with poor habits tend to have poor health and die younger. The homeless, about whom little is known, are the group most vulnerable to poor health. Although genetics and culture have a bearing on health in middle adulthood, socioeconomic status is more influential (Kastenbaum, 1979).

For all people, however, the body begins to deteriorate, and strength and vitality diminish. Chronic disease states begin to appear. Less is known about health problems of women, because traditionally research has focused on male studies, often extrapolating to women (Thomas, 1990). Table 6–5 displays the increments of chronic disease over the adult life span.

There is a cultural shift in attitudes that encourages optimal health habits and disease prevention, or at least delay. People are encouraged to exercise, eat right, drink only small amounts of alcohol, maintain a healthy weight, and not smoke. For many people exercise is one of the most attractive ways to take control over poor health habits (Berger, 1994). Coping effectively with stress seems to enhance health status, although those who are most bothered by life's stressors also seem to be the ones who are least likely to seek help in coping with stress (Aldwin et al, 1996). For both females and males, the sexual-reproductive system slows down. For some, these changes are negative; for others, especially women, greater enjoyment of sexual activities occurs.

Potential Medical Nutrition Problems. The incidence of chronic diseases and the physical deterioration in which nutrition plays a role increase in middle adulthood. Cataracts and arthritis are two age-related changes that have a nutritional link (Whitney et al, 1990).

Cognitive Growth and Development

Longitudinal studies over the last 25 years have led to the conclusion that previous ideas about intellectual deterioration are incorrect. Intelligence may improve throughout middle-age and even into late adulthood. Intellectual competence is multidimensional and multidirectional, characterized by significant differences

TABLE 6–5

The Increments of Chronic Disease

Age	Stage	Atherosclerosis (Hardening of Arteries)	Cancer	Arthritis	Diabetes	Emphysema	Cirrhosis
20	Start	Elevated cholesterol	Carcinogen exposure	Abnormal cartilage staining	Obesity, genetic susceptibility	Smoker	Drinker
30	Discernible	Small lesions on arteriogram	Cellular metaplasia°	Slight joint space narrowing	Abnormal glucose tolerance	Mild airway obstruction	Fatty liver on biopsy
40	Subclinical	Larger lesions on arteriogram	Increasing metaplasia	Bone spurs	Elevated blood glucose	Decrease in surface area and elasticity of lung tissue	Enlarged liver
50	Threshold	Leg pain on exercise	Carcinoma in situ	Mild articular pain	Sugar in urine	Shortness of breath	Upper gastro-intestinal hemorrhage
60	Severe	Angina pectoris	Clinical cancer	Moderate articular pain	Drugs required to lower blood glucose	Recurrent hospitalization	Fluid in the abdomen
70	End	Stroke, heart attack	Cancer spreads from site of origin	Disabled	Blindness; nerve and kidney damage	Intractable oxygen debt	Jaundice; hepatic coma
Prevention or Postponement		No cigarettes; no obesity; exercise	No cigarettes; limit pollution; diet; early detection	No obesity; exercise; minimize stress on any one joint	No obesity; exercise; diet	No cigarettes; exercise; limit pollution	No heavy drinking; diet

°Abnormal replacement of one type of cell by another.
From Berger KS: *The Developing Person Throughout the Life Span*, 3rd ed. New York: Worth Publishers, 1994. Reprinted with permission.

among individuals. There is a practical knowledge that develops from experience as well as philosophical knowledge that some individuals develop (Berger, 1994).

Psychosocial Growth and Development

Shifts in family structure (children leaving home, adult children returning home, no children at home), and changes in the work place can all create a time of crisis for adults in mid-life (Berger, 1994). People begin to realize that time is limited and dreams of youth are not likely to be achieved. Men seem likely to be distressed by mid-life. Women seem to vary more between becoming depressed and feeling liberated. Many women return to work or school during this stage of life (Kotre & Hall, 1990). For some people, work is a source of satisfaction (sometimes an obsession); for others, it is a source of discontent. Certain traits seem to stabilize in mid-life, such as extroversion, agreeableness, conscientiousness, neuroticism, and openness. People seem to improve in personality, that is, "mellow out," and some become wise. This stage was described by Erikson as stage 7, generativity versus stagnation (Table 6–6).

Implications for Medical Nutrition Therapy

Clients in middle adulthood exhibit wide ranges of intellect and education. Messages need to be tailored to each client. The client's vocabulary and use of clichés and nonverbal signs will indicate which strategies to use. The use of medical jargon can exacerbate communication problems. Medical nutrition problems, especially the onset of chronic disease states, are likely to unsettle clients significantly. In addition, conflicting results have been reported on the effect of knowledge on the patient's adjustment to disease. It has been suggested that in some instances, an overemphasis of knowledge not linked to goals is counterproductive. It is suggested that the practitioner provide only information that is goal directed (Eckerling & Kohrs, 1984).

An MNT can expect a significant proportion of clients from this age group. There may be wide-ranging differences in the contexts in which individuals seek advice and counsel from a dietetic practitioner. Clients' goals will range from hoping to delay aging by magic, to very common-sense plans for extending a life of good health, to coping with serious illness and death. Perhaps the most important task is to avoid stereotyping middle-aged adults (as well as older adults) by chronological age (Thomas, 1990). Even people who are themselves in middle and later years may be prone to contributing to stereotypes and ageism (Kart & Metress, 1984). A young MNT needs to keep in mind that she may have some distortion in her view of older people. In addition, she may perceive older clients as parental figures and "countertransference" attitudes toward parents to the client.

Flexibility of approach is important with middle-aged adult clients. A variety of techniques and motivational tactics available to the MNT enable an adjustment to working through problems in a way that best suits the client. In addition, the MNT should have the same teaching materials available at different levels of vocabulary. Culture and gender may be more important variables than actual age in the world view of clients.

TABLE 6 – 6

Behavioral Expressions of a Sense of Generativity Versus Stagnation: Stage 7

Characteristic Behaviors of People Who Have a Sense of Generativity	Characteristic Behaviors of People Who Have a Sense of Stagnation
1. They feel personally concerned about others, their immediate family, which includes future generations, and the nature of the world in which those generations will live.	1. They are concerned primarily with themselves and show little interest in future generations.
2. They reflect varying degrees of involvement with enhancing the welfare of young people and making the world a better place for them to live and work.	2. They have little interest in producing or caring for children of their own.
3. They reflect a parental kind of concern for the children of others.	3. They show little by way of a parental kind of concern for the children of others.
4. They tend to focus more on what they can *give* to others rather than on what they can *get*.	4. They tend to focus more on what they can *get* from others rather than on what they can *give*.
5. They tend to be absorbed in a variety of activities outside of themselves.	5. They tend to be absorbed primarily in themselves and their own needs.
6. They are interested in leading productive lives and in contributing to society.	6. They are not particularly interested in being productive or in contributing to society.
7. They display other-centered values and attitudes.	7. They display self-centered values and attitudes.
8. They are interested in enhancing what is known, even if it means changing the status quo.	8. They are interested in maintaining and preserving what is known in order to conserve the status quo.
9. They feel a strong inclination to develop some unique talent or to express themselves creatively.	9. They do not feel any particular inclination to develop some unique talent or to express themselves creatively.
Implicit Attitude	**Implicit Attitude**
1. What can I give to others?	1. What can I get from others?
2. Risks I would like to take include . . .	2. Risks I would like to avoid include . . .
3. I enjoy being productive and creative.	3. I prefer routine and sameness.

From Hamacheck DE: Evaluating self-concept and ego development within Erikson's psychosocial framework: A formulation. *J Couns Dev* 1988;66:354–360.

Later Adulthood

As the population grows older, there have developed distinctions between the young-old and the old-old. The differences may have some relation to chronological age, but more often it is a distinction of vitality and health. Kastenbaum (1979) stated that there really is no integrated "proven" theory of aging that accounts for biological/social/psychological dimensions. The tendency to be narrow in focus seems more prevalent among those who study biological changes than those who study the social and psychological functioning of the elderly (Kart, 1994).

Biosocial Growth and Development

Contrary to prejudice and stereotype, most old people are happy, healthy, and content, even though physical deterioration is taking place. The brain continues to function well, if more slowly, among healthy people. Aging is not synonymous with disease, but it does make the body more vulnerable to disease (Kart & Metress, 1984; Tischler, 1996). Loss, grief, and mourning are prevalent issues among the elderly. Among the life patterns most resistant to change are nutrition lifestyles, because they are so inextricably linked to so many meanings of life (Peters & Rappoport, 1988). Each individual has a different set of ways in which he or she will change. For instance, one individual may not be willing to drink skim milk instead of whole milk but is willing to eat lowfat cheeses.

Stress seems to be a factor in people's ability to adapt to aging. Those who see life in a positive way are more willing to make lifestyle changes that are likely to forestall illness and result in longer, healthier lives.

In later adulthood, most people are retired and must adapt to a new lifestyle to remain content and develop a sense of meaning as they grow old. The freedom and leisure time can be priceless or it can become a burden. Unfortunately, there is a tendency in the health-care community to consider the problems of the elderly to be inevitable and not worth addressing very seriously (Berger, 1994).

Potential Medical Nutrition Problems. Chronic and sometimes multiple diseases manifest themselves as people age. The occurrence of diabetes, heart disease, gastrointestinal disease, cancer, and hypertension have important nutrition implications. Biological aspects of aging include cellular-level changes and organ-level changes. Physiological changes include neurological developments and coordination of functions. All body systems deteriorate to some degree. Nutrient requirements change for older people. Loss of bone occurs, making osteoporosis the most common bone disorder among older people. Drug and nutrient interactions are very important for the elderly. Because of the incidence of chronic diseases in this age group, they use about 25% of all prescribed drugs (Williams & Worthington-Roberts, 1996).

Cognitive Growth and Development

Thinking processes slow, memory declines (primarily short-term memory), but quality of thought may improve. The sensory register declines, and other indications of deterioration appear in tests and examinations. In the real world, most elderly are not handicapped, although some disease states, such as Alzheimer's disease, have a debilitating effect on cognition. Depression becomes more common, especially among those with one or more chronic illnesses. Still, people tend to become more philosophical. Religion and spiritual ideas may become more important (Fieldhouse, 1995).

Psychosocial Growth and Development

Three theories of psychosocial aging have been developed: activity theory, continuity theory, and disengagement theory. The disengagement theory suggests that there is a mutual withdrawal between society and the elderly. The activity theory holds that people who disengage less are happier. The continuity theory proposes that personality traits stabilize among the elderly, and that the changes that occur with age are less disruptive than those that occur in younger years (Berger, 1994). As people live longer, healthier people remain "young-old" much longer. They continue to enjoy working or find satisfying and productive generative activities in

TABLE 6 – 7

Behavioral Expressions of a Sense of Integrity Versus Despair: Stage 8

Characteristic Behaviors of People Who Have a Sense of Integrity	Characteristic Behaviors of People Who Have a Sense of Despair
1. They reflect many of the positive ego qualities associated with earlier stages, such as trust, autonomy, initiative, industry, and identity.	1. They reflect many of the negative qualities associated with earlier stages, such as mistrust, shame, guilt, inferiority, and identity confusion.
2. They believe that who they are and what they have become are largely the consequences of their own choices.	2. They are inclined to believe that who they are and what they have become is not something over which they have had much control.
3. They accept death as an inevitable part of the life cycle.	3. They show signs of fearing death and do not accept it as part of the life cycle.
4. They are able to admit to themselves and others that, for the most part, they have no one but themselves to blame for whatever troubles or failures they have experienced.	4. They tend to blame others for whatever troubles or failures they have experienced.
5. They are ready and able to defend the dignity of their own lifestyles against all physical and economic threats; that is, they are not easily pushed around.	5. They offer little resistance to physical and economic threats to their lifestyles; that is, they are easily pushed around.
6. They are able to look back on their lives with feelings of pleasure, gratitude, and appreciation.	6. They tend to look back on their lives with feelings of displeasure, regret, and depreciation.
7. They tend to be reasonably happy, optimistic people, satisfied with their lives.	7. They tend to be fairly unhappy, pessimistic people, dissatisfied with their lives.
8. They approach the final stage of their lives with a sense of personal wholeness.	8. They approach the final stage of their lives with a sense of personal fragmentation, an incompleteness.
9. They are able to integrate their past experiences with current realities, and in this way generate a kind of "wisdom:" about how to live one's life and cope successfully.	9. They seem to be stuck at the level of blame and disappointment, which makes it difficult for them to learn from their mistakes.
Implicit Attitudes	**Implicit Attitudes**
1. I have much to be thankful for.	1. I have little to be thankful for.
2. I am in control of my life.	2. I have little control over what happens to me.
3. I accept myself for who I am, and I accept others for who they are.	3. I do not accept myself for who I am, and I wish others could be different.

From Hamacheck DE: Evaluating self-concept and ego development within Erikson's psychosocial framework: A formulation. *J Couns Dev* 1988;66:354–360.

retirement. They seem to tolerate the aging process satisfactorily, even though they sometimes have several medical problems. The death of a spouse or long-term companion becomes a common experience. Men seem to have more physical problems after the death of their partners than women do. When older people are unable to care for themselves, families usually assume the responsibilities—at least in the beginning. With advancing age, minorities, the poor, and women are the most likely to live in institutional settings. The quality of care for the elderly in nursing homes greatly influences the direction they take in Erikson's last stage, integrity versus despair (Table 6–7).

Implications for Medical Nutrition Therapy

The most rapidly growing segment of the US population is the group of people over the age of 65. Within this group, the group of those over 85 years old is growing most rapidly. Dietetic practitioners, legislators, insurers, and service providers must recognize this changing demographic and prepare for the ensuing issues (Chernoff, 1996).

Among the elderly, symbolic meanings of food may be so central to world view that a person may "prefer a food for the views and practices with which it is associated and for which it stands, rather than for its physiological significance" (Angulo, 1988; p. 41). Angulo compared studies from the viewpoints of macrobiotics and nutrition science and came to the opinion that, among the elderly, the world view of the individual determines which view, if either, individuals would select as a belief system about food. People distanced from the mainstream would be most likely to accept the system of belief offered by alternative philosophies. People who share the dominant belief that health and well-being come about through science accept a scientific view, and the elderly who have an ideology of independence reject any programmatic system. These findings suggest strongly that the MNT needs to investigate the client's world view before beginning a traditional nutrition education process (Angulo, 1988). Other factors influencing food selection patterns of older people are listed in Table 6–8.

Nutrition counseling for the elderly may be more productive if its focus is not on specific information about food but on maintaining or establishing a healthy nutrition lifestyle. Many older people have a great deal of information, some of it questionable. Their problems lie in life patterns, attitudes, beliefs, and perhaps economics.

People who live alone may need to be encouraged to participate in social environments and to share eating time with friends and family. Among the poor, strategies for obtaining food may need to be devised. There are many community programs for the feeding of elderly persons that can and should be utilized. Especially with the very old, the dietetic practitioner may need to take on the role of advocate, as well as the role of MNT.

When the client is a frail elderly person, the family member mostly likely to be the caretaker is a woman, usually a daughter or daughter-in-law. As with women caring for the young, women caring for the elderly are usually quite open to nutrition information and suggestions for how to care for their loved ones. Often, caretakers need encouragement and support in allowing independence and autonomy for their elderly relative in much the same manner as parents need encouragement to let children lead the way in eating.

TABLE 6 – 8

Factors Influencing Food Selection Patterns of Older People		
Psychological Factors	**Physiological Factors**	**Socioeconomic Factors**
Social activity	Appetite	Age
Self-esteem	Taste acuity	Sex
Nutrition knowledge	Olfactory acuity	Income
Perceived health benefit	Dental status	Cooking facilities
Loneliness	Prescribed diets	Daily schedule
Bereavement	Chronic disease	Retirement and leisure time
Symbolism of food	Food intolerance	Education
Mental awareness	Health status	Distance to food store
Food likes and dislikes	Physical disability	Availability of transportation
Food beliefs	Physical exercise	Availability of familiar foods
	Use of drugs	
	Vision level	

From, Worthington-Roberts BS, Williams SR: *Nutrition Throughout the Life Cycle.* 3rd ed. St. Louis: Mosby-Year Book, 1996.

CASE EXAMPLE ·

Over the years roles change between parent and child. The following conversation was a guide to the nutrition counseling that followed.

DAUGHTER: (speaking to her mother, a nursing home resident) "Mom, you always told us to eat our veggies because they were good for us. Eat your vegetables, they're good for you."

MOTHER: "Humph! I'm 86 years old, I must have done something right."

DAUGHTER: (to MNT who happened to be in the room): "Don't you agree that mother ought to eat her vegetables?" (an attempt to get the MNT on her side)

MNT: (to daughter) "Let me ask you a question about that. What was your reaction when your mother told you to eat your vegetables?"

DAUGHTER: "Umm—I didn't like it much, I guess. OK, Mom, I guess you have done something right in 86 years."

Probably what the daughter (and the mother in past years) really means is "I love you and want to take care of you." If the daughter does not exhibit defensiveness, the issue could be explored. Perhaps foods "Mom" would eat could be determined and communication between daughter and mother could be improved. If the daughter is defensive, the MNT will have the satisfaction of knowing that she avoided being a scapegoat in a conflict between the two.

· ·

Nutrition Support. Understanding psychological aspects of nutrition support is necessary. For example, if a patient is being fed enterally or parenterally, the act of eating accompanied by the physical sensations of tasting, chewing, and swallowing food will be missing. Feelings of insecurity, anxiety, and loss of control may occur. If the patient is able, have him or her participate in scheduling the intravenous or tube feedings to help retain a sense of control (Bayer et al, 1983). Empathy and understanding are important in establishing rapport between the patient and the dietetic practitioner. This will pave the way for the MNT when the patient is again able to eat and may need nutrition counseling.

The Post-Surgical Patient. A post-surgical patient may consider the timing good for a weight loss program since he or she may not feel much like eating anyway. The MNT may need to provide information about the nutritional needs for healing, and the effect of bowel activity, pain, medication, infection, and the emotions of the post-surgical period on the patient's nutritional status. In addition, the MNT must be alert to the effect of other therapies that may result in pain or fatigue, which will interfere with eating.

For older patients whose partner, friends, and acquaintances may have already died, the will to live may be low. There is probably no one on the staff better qualified than the MNT to provide effective support for such patients, even if not one word about nutrition science is needed. The MNT is in the unique position of being able to provide both tempting food and psychological support to encourage the will to live.

The Dying Patient. When nutrition counseling is requested for the dying it is most often an effort to help survivors feel as if they are doing something for the person they hate to lose. It is also important to remember that when a person dies from a long illness, or even from the slow deterioration of physical faculties, the family will become worn out and may feel quite ambivalent about the death of the person. Death and dying are discussed at length in Chapter 8, Emotional Factors.

CASE EXAMPLE ·

Herbert is a 78-year-old man who lives alone in an adult apartment building where there is no food service. His only income is $480.00 a month from Social Security. He lacks the money to buy the foods he has been told to eat. Herbert has trouble chewing because his dentures do not fit . He has a cataract in his right eye, congestive heart failure, and dyspnea. He is taking various medications. He also has a history of depression and has negative feelings about medical treatment ever since his wife died. He is losing weight and has been referred to the MNT consultant by his HMO. When the MNT visits him in his apartment, he tells her all of these problems and it is easy for her to see that before anything much can be done about his food habits, there is a need for someone to help him find assistance within the health-care system. He needs an advocate, and she chooses to help him obtain dental care and other services. When the time comes to directly attack the nutrition problems, both the MNT and the HMO supervisor, who was pleased that the MNT was willing to solve problems a little outside her "job," proceeded with excellent rapport, which in itself became a motivating factor for Herbert.

Summary

It is not possible to effectively understand an individual without having some data on all the aspects of human growth and development—biosocial, cognitive, and psychosocial. Yet, this subject is so broad, it is not possible to study it without looking at each domain separately. Several theories of human growth and development have been proposed. Two that have stood the test of time are those of Erikson and Piaget. In recent years, and in the milieu of people living longer, new theories of development are beginning to emerge. Among them, theories of human development are being proposed by cognitive psychologists. Strategies of medical nutrition therapy and flexibility of style that takes into account the client's stage of growth and development can facilitate change. For both the very young and the very old, caregivers are responsible for providing a healthy nutrition lifestyle for those for whom they care. By the time a child is in school, some direct nutrition counseling will be beneficial. However, until a person has reached early adulthood, it is probably more productive to include parents and perhaps entire families in nutrition counseling.

As people reach middle and later adulthood they vary greatly in their stage of development. Those who have lived in less advantaged environments are more likely to become ill and die younger. Among those who live longer, retirement years may become a joy or a burden. The oldest population consists mostly of women, and most people over the age of 85 can expect to spend time in a long-term-care facility. A significant proportion of the elderly can benefit from nutrition counseling.

Suggestions for Further Learning

1. Read more in-depth reports about an age group that is of particular interest to you.

2. Interview people you know from different age groups and compare your experience with the concepts discussed in this chapter.

3. Role-play interactions between different age groups.

4. Analyze your own stage of growth and development as described by Erikson.

5. Analyze people you know in terms of Erikson's theory.

6. Observe children at different ages and identify the cognitive stages of growth.

7. Conduct interviews with people in different stages of growth and development using new information learned in this chapter. Record the differences in the responses you get from the interviewees.

CITED REFERENCES

Aldwin CM, Sutton KJ, Chiara G, Spiro A. Age differences in stress: Coping and appraisal. Findings from the normative aging study. *J Gerontol Psychol Sci.* 1996;51B(4): 179–188.

Anderson JR: *Cognitive Psychology and Its Implications.* 3rd ed. New York: WH Freeman, 1990.

Angulo JF: Foodways, ideology, and aging: A developmental dilemma. *Am Behav Sci.* 1988;32(1):41–49.

Bayer LM, Bauers CM, Kapp SR: Psychosocial aspects of nutrition support. *Nurs Clin North Am.* 1983;1(1):119–128.

Biehler RF, Snowman J: *Psychology Applied to Teaching*. 4th ed. Boston: Houghton Mifflin, 1982.

Berger KS: *The Developing Person Through the Life Span*. 3rd ed. New York: Worth, 1994.

Bloom M (ed): *Life Span Development: Bases for Preventive and Interventive Helping*. 2nd ed. New York: MacMillan Publishing Co, 1985.

Bronfenbrenner U: Is early intervention effective? Facts and principles of early intervention: A summary. In Bloom M (ed): *Life Span Development: Bases for Preventive and Interventive Helping*. 2nd ed. New York: MacMillan Publishing Co, 1985.

Brown MH: Innovations in the treatment of bulimia: Transpersonal psychology, relaxation, imagination, hypnosis, myth, and ritual. *J Hum Educ Dev*. 1991;3:50–60.

Campbell SF (ed): *Piaget Sampler: An Introduction to Jean Piaget Through His Own Words*. New York: John Wiley and Sons, 1976.

Chernoff R: President's page: Nutrition and health for older Americans. *J Am Diet Assoc*. 1996;96(10):1053.

Donaldson SI, et al: Resistance-skills training and onset of alcohol use: Evidence for beneficial and potentially harmful effects in public schools and in private catholic schools. *Health Psych*. 1995;14(4):291–300.

Erikson E: *Childhood and Society*. 2nd ed. New York: WW Norton, 1963.

Eckerling L, Kohrs MB: Research on compliance with diabetic regimens: Applications to practice. *J Am Diet Assoc*. 1984;84(7):805–809.

Fieldhouse P: *Food and Nutrition: Customs and Culture*. 2nd ed. New York: Chapman Hall, 1995.

Gutierrez Y, King J: Nutrition during teenage pregnancy. *Pediatr Ann*. 1993;22(2):99–108.

Hamacheck DE: Evaluating self-concept and ego development within Erikson's psychosocial framework: A formulation. *J Couns Dev*. 1988;66:354–360.

Jenkins CD: An integrated behavioral medicine approach to improving care of patients with diabetes mellitus. *Behav Med*. 1995;21:53–65.

Johnson SB: Psychological aspects of childhood diabetes. *J Child Psychol Psych*. 1988;29(6):729–738.

Kart CS: *The Realities of Aging: An Introduction to Gerontology*. 4th ed. Boston: Allyn Bacon, 1994.

Kart CS, Metress SP: *Nutrition, the Aged, and Society*. Englewood Cliffs, NJ: Prentice-Hall, 1984.

Kastenbaum R: *Human Developing: A Lifespan Perspective*. Boston: Allyn & Bacon, 1979.

Kotre J, Hall E: *Seasons of Life: Our Dramatic Journey from Birth to Death*. Boston: Little, Brown, 1990.

Kubler-Ross E: *Death, the Final Stage of Growth*. Englewood Cliffs, NJ: Prentice-Hall, 1975.

Lidz T: *The Person: His and Her Development Throughout the Life Cycle* (revised edition). New York; Basic Books, 1976.

Littlejohn SW (ed): *Theories of Human Communication*. 2nd ed. Belmont, CA: Wadsworth Publishing Co, 1983.

Maslow AH: *Motivation and Personality*. 2nd ed. New York: Harper and Row, 1970.

McKelvey J, et al: Family support for diabetes: A pilot study for measuring disease-specific behaviors. Community Health Care 1989;18(1):37–41.

Peters RG, Rappoport L: Behavioral perspectives on food, nutrition, and aging. *Am Behav Sci*. 1988;32(1):5–16.

Pipes P, Trahms C: *Nutrition in Infancy and Childhood*. 5th ed. St. Louis: Mosby-Year Book, 1993, p. 26.

Rees JM, Worthington-Roberts B: Position Paper: Nutrition care of pregnant adolescents. *J Am Diet Assoc*. 1994;95(4):449–450.

Rogers CR: *On Becoming a Person*. Boston: Houghton Mifflin, 1961.

Satter ES: *How to Get Your Kid to Eat, But Not Too Much*. Palo Alto, CA: Bull Publishing Co, 1987.

Schaie KW: Toward a stage theory of adult cognitive development. *Int J Aging Hum Dev*. 1977–1978;8:129–138.

Sheehy G: *New Passages: Mapping Your Life Across Time*. New York: Random House, 1995.

Sue DU: *Counseling the Culturally Different: Theory and Practice*. New York: John Wiley & Sons, 1990.

Tischler HL: *Introduction to Sociology*. 5th ed. Fort Worth, TX: The Harcourt Press, 1996.

Thomas RM: *Counseling and Life-Span Development*. Newbury Park, CA: Sage, 1990.

Whitney EN, Hamilton EM, Rolfes SR: *Understanding Nutrition*. 5th ed. St. Paul, MN: West Publishing Co, 1990, p. 461.

Williams SR, Worthington-Roberts BS: *Nutrition Throughout the Life Cycle*. 3rd ed. St. Louis: Mosby-Year Book, 1996.

Zemen F: *Clinical Nutrition and Dietetics*. 2nd ed. New York: MacMillan Publishing Co, 1991.

ADDITIONAL REFERENCES

Gordon AM: Nutritional status of Cuban refugees: A field study on the health and nutriture of refugees processed at Opa Locka, Florida. *Am J Clin Nutr.* 1982;35:282–290.

Hayes R, Aubrey R: *New Directions for Counseling and Human Development.* Denver: Love Publishing Co, 1988.

Mussen PH (ed): *Carmichael's Manual of Child Psychology.* 3rd ed. Vol II. New York: John Wiley & Sons, 1970.

Rossi AS: *Gender and the Life Course.* New York: Aldine, 1985.

CHAPTER 7

Cross-Cultural Counseling

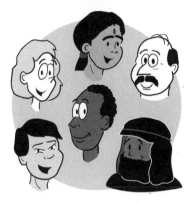

GOALS

Major goals of this chapter are (1) to increase the reader's awareness of his or her own cultural values and beliefs, (2) to provide a basic knowledge on how to study cultures, and (3) to develop skill in counseling individuals from cultures other than their own through:

- Awareness of the influence culture has on lifestyle, including nutrition lifestyle.
- Appreciation of the values of diverse cultures and individuals.
- Flexibility in interventions so that clients' values can be utilized to institute an appropriate nutrition lifestyle.
- Increased perceptiveness in listening to clients and in responses to them.

Learning Objectives

At the end of this chapter the reader will be able to:

1. Define cross-cultural counseling.

2. Describe a competent cross-cultural counselor.

3. Identify personally held values.

4. Identify cultural influences and biases that influence personally held values.

5. List ways to learn about other cultures.

6. Recognize client expressions of cultural influences.

7. Identify values of individuals from other cultures by listening to them.

8. Learn about culture by listening, study, and observation.

9. Begin to apply techniques described.

Key Terms

▶ Cross-Cultural Counseling: counseling a person with significant cultural differences from the counselor—often, but not necessarily, a difference in ethnic background.

▶ Cultural Groups: nonexclusive groups that have a set of values in common—an individual may be a part of several cultural groups at the same time.

▶ Cultural Sensitivity: the recognition that cultural differences and similarities are valued: there is no right or wrong culture; they are just different.

▶ Culture: learned patterns of thinking, feeling, and behaving that are shared by a group of people.

▶ Dominant Culture: the cultural group that has the power to dominate subcultures or other cultures within its domain. For example, in the United States, Americans of European descent currently make up the dominant culture.

▶ Ethnic Group: a group linked by race, nationality, and language with a common cultural heritage.

▶ Multicultural: a description of situations in which two or more distinctive cultures interact.

▶ Values: attitudes and beliefs that are held in high esteem and that guide behavior.

▶ World View: the perception of the world as biased by culture and personal experience.

American society has undergone great changes over the last four or five decades. Major changes in demographics have occurred and communications have developed that make it clear that we live in a multicultural society. These changes will continue into the 21st century. It is expected that the proportion of people of color in the US population will increase significantly over the next 20 years (Lee & Richardson, 1991). The civil rights movement of the 1960s was a major factor in raising awareness of the pluralism of our society. In its wake, people have begun to recognize that those who are culturally different from the dominant culture need not be viewed as inferior (Copeland, 1983). Many cultural groups have been recognized as offering values and customs that can enhance the dominant culture (Pedersen et al, 1996). They have changed and will continue to change the world view of our society.

WORLD VIEW

The world view of groups and individuals is closely correlated to culture. Sue (1981) defines world view as our attitudes, values, opinions, and concepts and how these affect how we think, make decisions, behave, and perceive events. Counselors who hold views different from their clients and are unaware of reasons for this basis may consider the difference in a negative way. For instance, consider the counselor with a world view that holds inner control as an essential characteristic and does not recognize that as a cultural bias. He is likely to consider a world view that life is controlled by outside forces, that is, fate, as a negative characteristic rather than simply a different one. Vontress (1988) refers to the world view as a "person's comprehensive personal philosophy or conception of human life in the universe." For instance, the world view of power is very influential in counseling. People who live in environments in which they have personal power tend to be more optimistic about their ability to change than those who have less power and struggle to survive in difficult environments.

Our shrinking world has the effect of increasing both cultural diversity and multicultural influences on individuals. For instance, people often perceive that keeping ethnic food habits helps to retain their identities, yet the influence of the dominant culture also leads to assimilation into the larger culture. Rice and beans may have been a staple for a recent immigrant from Jamaica, yet mass media advertisement of pizza is very likely to result in less consumption of beans and increased consumption of pizza. Kastenbaum (1988; p. 56) stated that "Navajo foodways are inseparable from their encompassing and coherent view of life. This statement has only limited application to those who have abandoned or become alienated from their heritage. Furthermore, many Navajo have accepted some aspects of the mainstream society . . ." This suggests that assuming that a Navajo client has a traditional Navajo nutrition lifestyle can as easily lead to misunderstanding as assuming that a Navajo client has assimilated a dominant culture nutrition lifestyle.

Population Distribution of Dietetic Practitioners

Dietetic practitioners more heavily represent the dominant culture than the general population. The American Dietetic Association completed a membership database report in 1995. It was found that dietitian members were predominately non-Hispanic whites (90.5%) and women (97.6%). Table 7–1 shows data from the 1995 study of demographic characteristics of ADA members (Saracino & Michael, 1996).

In contrast, it has been predicted that by the year 2000, 70% of the workforce will be composed of people of color, women, and other currently nondominant groups (Johnson & Packer, 1987). Typically, dietetic practitioners work with clients of different ethnic groups in proportion to their representation in the general population (Kittler & Sucher, 1989). The dietetics and nutrition community has long recognized that knowledge about ethnic food habits is necessary. The need re-

TABLE 7 – 1

1995 Demographic Characteristics of Members of the American Dietetics Association		
Characteristics	Registered Dietitians (*n*/%)	Dietetic Technicians, Registered (*n*/%)
Gender		
Men	918/2.4	69/3.9
Women	36,814/97.6	1701/96.1
Total	37,732/100.0	1770/100.0
Race/ethnic origin		
Non-Hispanic White	33,811/90.5	1524/87.4
Asian or Pacific Islander	1838/4.9	72/4.1
Non-Hispanic Black	943/2.5	101/5.8
Hispanic	618/1.7	40/2.3
American Indian, Alaskan Native, or Hawaiian Native	161/0.4	6/0.3
Total	37,371/100.0	1743/100.0

From Saracino J, Michael P: Positive steps toward a multicultural association. Copyright American Dietetic Association. Reprinted by permission from *Journal of the American Dietetic Association*, 1996;96(12):1242–1244.

mains, however, to further develop understanding and appreciation of different cultures in all of their aspects (Terry, 1994).

To this end, the American Dietetic Association included diversity of members as part of its 1996–1999 strategic framework. A truly multicultural association can influence the general public's food choices and nutrition lifestyles. A diverse membership of dietetic practitioners is also required to effect change and shape future food policies and legislation.

DESCRIPTIONS OF CULTURE

Culture itself is not easy to define because of its many meanings and its fluid, always changing nature. Many authors define culture—some very technically, others so vaguely as to be almost meaningless. "Culture" often refers to ethnic groups, political groups, nationality, or socioeconomic groups. However, there are a variety of other groupings that can bind people together as a cultural group, such as age, gender, education, occupation, religion, and geographic location. These groups are not mutually exclusive, and the effects of this overlapping are evident when issues or problems related to a particular grouping come up. For instance, an individual may identify with an ethnic group, but in his or her reactions to health care may find that the culture of age or gender has a stronger influence. For our purposes, we have defined culture as "learned patterns of thinking, feeling, and behaving that are shared by a particular group of people."

Each individual is influenced uniquely by personal experience and feels identity with a different cultural group depending on the situation. For instance, an individual may have a nutrition lifestyle that reflects mainstream culture, but in illness may retreat to a nutrition lifestyle of childhood or ethnicity (or both). People in the helping professions need to be acutely aware of each person individually and simultaneously be aware of some major cultural values that may be influential in that person's world view and coping strategies. The general process of effective communication is to respond to an individual tentatively as a member of a group, then as you continue to listen, respond more specifically to the individual. Poor communicators tend to filter communication so as to support a stereotype (DeVito, 1995).

CROSS-CULTURAL PSYCHOLOGICAL COUNSELING CONCEPTS

The last two decades have seen burgeoning literature in cross-cultural, sometimes called multicultural, counseling. Pedersen and coauthors (1996) describe this as a fourth force in counseling, a force equal with the forces of psychoanalytical counseling, behavior modification, and humanistic counseling. The role that culture plays in how people change and cope with life began to be addressed in the late 1970s. Pedersen, Sue, and others challenged the psychological community to take note of cultural biases of counselors, most of whom are products of the dominant American culture (Pedersen et al, 1996; Sue, 1981).

CASE EXAMPLE ·

A patient seemed psychotic and complained in a listless ramble, "My soul is not with me anymore and I can't do anything." She was deemed seriously disturbed and was taken to a psychiatric hospital. The psychiatrist who interviewed her found out the problem started when she received news of the unexpected death of a close uncle in her native Ecuador. The psychiatrist realized that her clinical picture fit a syndrome known in Latin America as *susto,* or loss of the soul. When facing this tragedy, the soul of the woman departed with the dead person, leaving her "soul-less." In American psychiatric terms, she was depressed. (The Miami Herald, Science section, 12/10/95, p. 1M.)

. . . .

Today, there is general agreement that the culture both of the counselor and of the client has a significant influence on the counseling relationship and the outcome of counseling (Pedersen, et al, 1996). In fact, Burn (1992) discussed these as core ethical issues relating to counselor bias, welfare of the client, and counselor preparedness. Five criteria for a culturally competent provider are as follows (Pedersen et al, 1996):

1. Be aware of and accept cultural differences.
2. Be aware of your own cultural values.
3. Understand that people of different cultures have different ways of communicating, behaving, and solving problems.
4. Have basic knowledge about a client's culture.
5. Be willing to adjust the way you work with people to take into consideration cultural differences.

It is not the intent of this chapter to emphasize this psychological position, but it is relevant for a professional group already quite aware of the strong influences of culture on their clients. It is important for MNTs to gain insight into overall cultural psychological counseling because nutrition counseling concepts are derivative of this approach.

Cultural Influences on Counseling

In the psychological counseling field, awareness has arisen that counseling itself is largely a product of certain Western-oriented (dominant US culture) philosophical assumptions. According to Sue (1981; p. 3), a pioneer in cross-cultural counseling, these include:

(a) concern and respect for the uniqueness of clients, (b) the worth of the individual, (c) a high priority placed on helping others to attain their own self-determined goals, (d) the freedom and opportunity to explore one's characteristics and to develop one's potential, and (e) a future-oriented promise of a better life.

Carl Rogers, the psychologist discussed in the previous chapter who exerted major influence on counseling practices, effectively articulated these ideas in the 1950s when client-centered counseling was developed. Social focus at that time was on the development of the individual. This philosophy, however, did not always prove successful among minority groups (Sue, 1981).

Sue outlined three major characteristics of counseling: language variables, class-bound values, and culture-bound values. Many of these values are inappropriate for groups he categorized as *third world groups*. The generic characteristics of mainstream counseling are shown in Table 7–2.

Sue, Pedersen, and others in the counseling field began comparing Western thinking with that of other cultures and discovered that differences in values between counselor and counselee could result in conflict and misunderstanding (Pedersen et al, 1996). For instance, differences in the perception of whether counseling interventions are even appropriate can lead to conflict. A counselor with a belief in independence and assertiveness may not understand a person with a belief that the family's needs come before the individual's needs, and thus approach the client ineffectively by suggesting assertiveness as a technique for solving problems. Counselors began to view it as important to use the cultural orientation of the client, rather than that of the counselor, as the basis of change (Copeland, 1983). Without suggesting that any counselor's values and beliefs were undesirable, counselor education began to use learning experiences to help counselors recognize that their values and belief systems are culturally bound and create biases in their perceptions of clients (Copeland, 1983).

Development of Cross-Cultural Psychological Counseling

The influence from many cultures has enriched the profession of counseling by bringing forth diverse ideas about how to help people function in a problem-solving way, rather than attempting to force clients into a western set of assumptions. Diversity has also tended to provide "a bewildering variety" of approaches and concerns in cross-cultural counseling (Pedersen, 1996). An increase in social responsibility and recognition that problems are not always attributable to inadequacy among clients, especially those who live in restrictive environments, has led counselors to become less blaming of clients, especially those from strata of society that are less powerful (or see themselves as less powerful). Cross-cultural counseling tends to consist not only of helping clients cope, but also of counselors' making

TABLE 7–2

Generic Characteristics of Counseling		
Language	**Class**	**Culture**
Standard English	Middle	Individual-centered
Verbal communications	Adherence to time schedules (50-minute sessions)	Verbal/emotional/behavioral expressiveness
	Long-range goals	Client-counselor communication
	Atmosphere of ambiguity	Openness and intimacy
		Cause-and-effect orientation
		Clear distinction between physical and mental well-being

Modified from Sue DW: *Counseling the Culturally Different: Theory and Practice.* New York: John Wiley & Sons, 1981. Reprinted by permission of the publisher.

efforts to change conditions that are restrictive (Lee & Richardson, 1991). There is now an emphasis on identifying the experiences and values the client holds important rather than assuming that the counselor's experiences and motivations are the same as the client's.

The Culturally Skilled Psychological Counselor

The culturally skilled psychological counselor is one who "is able to view each client as a unique individual while, at the same time, taking into consideration his or her common experiences as a human being (ie, the developmental challenges that face all people), as well as the specific experiences that come from the client's particular cultural background" (Lee & Richardson, 1991; p. 5). To a certain extent, every counseling situation is cross-cultural because each person, having been uniquely influenced by his or her life experiences, has a unique "culture."

To become culturally skilled, counselors have to examine their own cultural backgrounds, recognize their biases, and become aware of the potential effects those biases have on the counseling relationship. Understanding of and sensitivity to another person's culture is an equal part of the development of a skilled cross-cultural counselor. Cross-cultural empathy, the "only absolutely necessary but not sufficient variable" in a counseling relationship would be impossible without some understanding of other cultures (Pedersen et al, 1996).

Dangers in Cross-Cultural Counseling

The dangers in cross-cultural counseling include the possibility that learning about other cultures may increase stereotyping and may tend to accentuate differences. It is therefore important to become culturally sensitive first before attempting to learn about other cultures. An internal acceptance that there is no right or wrong cultures, just different cultures, is vital if stereotyping is to be avoided. There is also the danger of using political identification of groups as an indication of culture (Copeland, 1983) because so much literature is written and so much research is conducted using political groupings (eg, Hispanics, African Americans). Individuals within a group may not share attitudes, behaviors, values, or other cultural attributes of the culture with which they are identified.

The skilled cross-cultural counselor is the one who takes the responsibility to become aware of his or her own cultural views, to become culturally sensitive, and then to learn about other cultures. This person never forgets that the most important factor in being an effective cross-cultural counselor lies in appreciation of diversity and in listening carefully to the individual client for his or her own expression of cultural values and beliefs.

CROSS-CULTURAL COUNSELING IN THE HEALTH-CARE ARENA

There is no area of life in which there is more cultural upheaval than in health care in the 1990s. Americans are changing their views of health and health care. Technology has had an influence and has also increased costs. Political initiatives to reduce the economic crisis of health-care delivery have created turmoil as to what kind of treatment is best and who should receive care. Prejudice against immigrants is rising at the same time that there is heightened interest among health-care professionals to become more attuned to people's ethnic backgrounds. Values seem in conflict.

Dominant Cultural Values in Health Care

Currently, the dominant culture sees wellness as a positive entity, not just the absence of illness. The idea of self-responsibility for health is on the rise. People seem to be becoming disenchanted with the mainstream medical system (O'Donnell, 1988), perhaps because of irritation with the prescriptive model of health-care delivery. In the health-care community, too, the prescriptive mode of treatment without real regard to the individual has been questioned over the last few years. Models of treatment tend more toward participation by the patients. In addition, support groups for people with various problems or disorders have become popular (Stanford & Perdue, 1988). Such groups also reflect the dominant culture and may not be appropriate in cross-cultural counseling.

Attention to Culture in the Health-Care System

More attention is being paid to cross-cultural skill among the health-care professions. As a first-year medical student, Natow (1994) wrote of the challenge of working in the emergency room where, for the first time, he became an authority figure for people older than himself. He found that health and nutrition beliefs are a significant part of culture, and working effectively with people from different cultures requires suspension of value judgments. He noted that there was a time in America when immigrants strove to become Americanized and this was a motivation toward change. The tendency now is more toward resisting acculturation.

Cultural groups outside the mainstream may or may not share the attitudes of the dominant culture. The lack of power among people belonging to minority groups makes them less apt to use the health-care system and reduces their ability to consider that they can effectively assume direct responsibility for their health (Falvo, 1994).

The nursing profession has been active in developing cross-cultural skills among practicing nurses and students. Falvo has contributed much to understanding cultural issues in health care. She reminds us that cultures differ as to definitions of illness and wellness and what type and from whom health care is acceptable. The health beliefs of each patient/client need to be probed to determine the most effective approach with each patient. For instance, non-Hispanic whites perceived illness as a concrete entity, while some other cultures think of illness as a long-term condition, as a dysfunction of a family, the community, or nature (Marin, 1993).

Models for cross-cultural care have been developed that help to clarify complex interpersonal relationships. Errors in assumptions can create communication problems that diminish the effect of health care (Arnold & Boggs, 1995). Purtilo and Haddad (1996) address both cultural considerations and issues that are important at different stages of the life cycle. Both indicate the concern arising in health care that cultural diversity be addressed.

CROSS-CULTURAL NUTRITION COUNSELING

By the 1970s, the dietetics and nutrition community was also beginning to regard ideas of self-management and self-responsibility in nutrition care with favor. The need to know not only information, but also effective communication skills was evident and became a part of dietetics and nutrition education (Mason et al, 1977; Snetselaar, 1983; Curry Bartley, 1987). Methods were very much in line with dominant culture counseling precepts, and a very valuable step in nutrition counseling was taken in these years toward understanding individuals and focusing on people more than on medical conditions.

Recognition of the cultural meanings of food had long been a tradition in dietetics and nutrition. Much emphasis had already been placed on understanding food habits within a lifestyle. The added factor was the effort to understand human behavior as well, to recognize that focusing on the individual and his or her nutrition lifestyle would have an impact on the process for promoting change rather than simply prescribing diets.

Cultural Influences on Nutrition Lifestyle

It is well known that food choices are neither random nor haphazard. They exhibit patterns and regularities that provide not only biological sustenance, but also a material means for expressing the more abstract significance of social systems and cultural values. People's attachments to certain eating habits reveal social and cultural identities (Lowenberg et al, 1979). Food is an important aspect of identity in at least three ways: (1) in beliefs about how food turns into the self (ie, "you are what you eat"), (2) in how the amount of food consumed and the enjoyment of it expresses character, and (3) in the social aspect of eating, such as rules about what is eaten, when, and with whom (Back, 1977). Numerous other concepts of the meaning of food are discussed in Chapter 2.

It is the cultural milieu in which we grow up that determines our values and behavior and subsequently our lifestyles and nutrition lifestyles. Food, originally chosen because of availability, soon comes to represent our cultural heritage. For instance, it could be speculated that a religious belief in the sacredness of cows may have been established from a logical thought process that using the milk of scarce cattle would provide longer-lasting nutrition than killing the cows for meat. Over generations, such original reasoning may have become a cultural dictate and an expression of deep religious belief. The modern expression "sacred cows" refers to strongly held beliefs that should not be tampered with in attempts at social change. In any multicultural communication, care taken to avoid trampling on a "sacred cow" helps to establish good rapport.

Cultural heritage offers not only a sense of collective identity, but also a sense of pride and dignity. It provides purpose and stability to everyday life. No person lightly relinquishes habits and customs that help structure life and give it meaning.

Cultural Groupings that Have Meaning in Medical Nutrition Therapy

Sociologically and politically described cultural groups are generally ethnic, as in Hispanic, African American, or American Indian. These divisions do not suffice for identifying cultural influences on food habits. Hispanics, for instance, are stereo-typically thought of as Mexicans in some parts of the country, as Cubans in other parts of the country, and as Puerto Rican in other parts of the country. In fact, there are many more groups who are "Hispanic," such as Brazilians who have a European heritage from Portugal. This group was often influenced by intermar-riage with Native Americans and immigrants from the Far East. All of these groups have distinct food habits as well as cultural traditions. A much closer inves-tigation of an individual beyond an ethnic category is necessary before a real un-derstanding can be gained about a "Hispanic's" food culture. Native American cul-ture is also very diverse. For instance, a professional working with Native Americans needs to learn about the specific cultural factors among people in their precise geographic location. Asians may share some common cultural values, yet even among Chinese people there are significant differences in food culture, de-pending on the geographic location.

Cultures of gender, age, economics, urban or rural habitat, and geographic lo-cation also cross ethnic lines. For instance, a person who is in the middle class eco-nomically may find that she has more in common with a middle-class person of an-other ethnic culture than with a very poor or a very rich person of the same ethnic background. On the other hand, a person from a very rich or a very poor segment of society may have difficulty understanding some middle-class values, despite a shared ethnic background. Literature on cross-cultural counseling suggests that white counselors of the dominant middle class tend to assume that clients from ethnic minorities are of the lower class. Although this may sometimes be true, this perception is more often the result of the client's use of a language that is different from the counselor's (Sue, 1989; Farkas, 1986). Religious and philosophical cul-ture are also not always apparent by ethnic identification. Educational level tends to be an important factor in world view and cultural orientation.

In nutrition counseling, cultural groupings such as age or gender may be very im-portant. Different nutrition lifestyles may be expected during different stages of life or according to gender. Certain foods may be stereotyped as "for children" (milk), "for men" (steak), "for women" (yogurt), or "for the aged" (cooked cereal for sup-per) in spite of knowledge to the contrary. Each generation has its own food fa-vorites. For instance, a campaign by McDonald's centered around a sandwich for "adults," the concern being that food from McDonald's was perceived by the public as for children only. There has been increasing attention given to women's issues and cultural perspectives (Douglas, 1984). In a world of plenty almost everything we eat can be culture-bound if we choose, and every intervention into a person's nu-trition lifestyle is an intervention into cultural values, beliefs, and behaviors.

There are even those who perceive cultures of cuisine. In *The Sociology of Food* (1992), Mennell describes the gradual emergence of recognizable national cuisines as being "broadly parallel to the formation of nation-states." In a discus-sion of the parallel cultures of "two tastes," Belasco (1989) describes the food cul-tures of "Healthy Gourmet" and "American Standard"—which are really descrip-tions of two aspects of the dominant culture—and the supposed conflicts between taste and good health. The idea expressed is that there are two distinct cultures: that which is obsessed with (not just talking about) eating "right," and that which clings with bravado to older more traditional food habits. One group espouses pleasure; the other seems to be suffering from nutritional "nihilism," the complete destruction of pleasure. People influenced by the latter culture seem afraid to eat almost anything because every food has been in some way identified as being "bad." Pleasure from food is viewed with suspicion and relationships between food and disease are exaggerated. Foods are seen as causes as well as magical cures for medical conditions. Belasco calls this the "medication of nutrition."

At the same time, cultural differences in food habits and nutrition lifestyles in our society seem to be diminishing. In an international study, pizza was found to be popular among several cultures (Curry Bartley, 1985). Lieberman and Bobroff (1991) found that in Florida there is hardly any ethnic cuisine that has not been influenced by other cultures in the same geographic locations. "Ethnic" foods also have cross-cultural influence as Americans develop interest in "eating Chinese, French, Italian, Vietnamese," and so on. An excellent example of cross-cultural dining is a popular Cuban-Chinese restaurant in Miami, Florida, that employs only transvestites as food servers.

The population of the United States has often been described as a melting pot, but there is now recognition that our population has not melted or melded into one homogeneous culture. More reference is being made to America as a salad bowl, with each ingredient clearly definable yet held together loosely by a dressing. Perhaps it is becoming more like a soup, in which the different ingredients have softened somewhat, and flavors have been exchanged through the broth.

Developing Cross-Cultural Counseling Competence

Cross-cultural counseling competence has three elements: (1) awareness of your cultural background, biases, and world view; (2) knowledge about, and sensitivity to others' cultural background, biases, and world view; (3) and skill in cross-cultural communication. The need for skill in cross-cultural communication has been recognized among dietitians and nutritionists. Increasing numbers of articles and books are appearing that address the issues in (nutrition) counseling (Kittler & Sucher, 1989; Burn, 1992; Terry, 1994; Bronner, 1994. They reveal both perspectives of the dominant culture and the issues that confront individuals who are engaged in cross-cultural counseling. Terry (1994; p. 501) states that "all individuals live in households, communities, and regions, and in times and circumstances that determine nutritional health or disease with greater certainty than access to all the nutrition education and services that dietitians can envision. In short, we are what we eat culturally as well as physiologically."

Awareness of One's Own Cultural Background

Perhaps you have already recognized that there are different world views. Perhaps you have always assumed that everyone sees the world as you do, that your culture is *the* culture. Most of us see our own culture as generally "right." Observing one's own culture objectively can be an exercise of immense learning. For example, what were your thoughts after reading about the transvestite restaurant in the preceding section? Recognizing that your own culture creates bias does not require that it be seen as negative. Objectivity will enable you to evaluate your cultural beliefs as neither right nor wrong, simply as phenomena. You are likely to appreciate your own culture as well as acknowledge the positive value of other cultures.

Each person reading this book has a unique combination of cultural influences. As you study this chapter, it will be helpful to analyze your own values, beliefs, and behaviors and determine the cultural influences that have impinged on your development.

Cultural Orientation of the Dietetics and Nutrition Profession. The cultural background shared by most readers of this book is that of health-care professional. Health-care professionals represent, most often, middle- to upper-class culture (Purtilo & Haddad, 1996). Even among those who represent other cultural entities, the educational processes for health-care professionals create a shared culture as part of the system of higher education, a product of the dominant culture. Each reader shares some of these cultural values. You may recognize some as a part of the culture and disagree with them. Some you may not see as a part of the culture, even though others do. For instance, some dietitians and nutritionists value a vegetarian lifestyle, others believe that all foods can be included in a healthy lifestyle.

Dietetic practitioners do not represent a cross section of American culture (Kittler & Sucher, 1989). For instance, there are more women, the educational level is higher than average, and representatives of minority groups are in smaller proportion than in the general population. In addition, the educational experience is influenced by the health-care culture.

Currently, most dietetics and nutrition professionals grew up in the dominant American culture of European descent. Because educational institutions of higher learning are primarily influenced by this same culture (Sue, 1981), students from all cultural backgrounds become influenced by the dominant culture as schooling progresses. The following list of values common to middle-class Americans of European descent was produced by students studying cultural aspects of nutrition over the years.

Those most commonly mentioned are:

▍ Work is good. Those who work are more valuable. Material wealth is good and is a consequence of work.
▍ Independence is a sign of maturity, and a goal to be achieved.
▍ The use of Standard English is expected among professionals.
▍ Logic and cause-and-effect thinking are fostered.
▍ Health is a personal responsibility.
▍ A connection is made between a "good nutrition lifestyle" and "good health and longevity."

Among these values, the connection between nutrition and a good life is a common value that is a major identifier of the profession. It is the one that has induced professionals and students alike to undertake efforts to influence others to our value system.

Adapting Psychological Counseling Skills to Medical Nutrition Therapy and Nutrition Counseling

Because nutrition counseling concepts have been adapted from psychological counseling culture, many of the same cultural biases abound. Sue identified four general characteristics of counseling: "(a) monolingual orientation, (b) emphasis on long-range goals, (c) distinction between physical and mental well-being, and (d) emphasis on cause-and-effect relationships" (Sue, 1989). Awareness of the potential for these factors to influence nutrition counseling is important. They are all characteristics that could diminish the effect of nutrition counseling with clients of different cultures.

Even the event of nutrition counseling is subject to cultural influences. The dominant culture expects intervention (Richardson & Molinaro, 1996). Native American culture, for instance, often supports ideas of nonintervention and the value of protecting autonomy. This difference in and of itself can lead to problems of communication (Farkas, 1986).

The curricula of dietetics and nutrition programs provide insight into the values of the profession. Curriculum mandates from universities, governments, and professional organizations generally express the world view of the dominant culture. Terry (1994; p. 501) states that "the scientific, prescriptive, and technical aspects are given high prestige, respect, and recognition, while those aspects related to the art of delivery have generally been undervalued." Dietetic practitioners have begun to value the "art of delivery" more in recent years, yet the need remains to focus additional resources on developing skill in counseling.

Becoming Aware of Other Cultures

Another process in becoming a skilled cross-cultural nutrition counselor is to learn about other cultures. Communication between individuals of different cultures varies from those who have few cultural difference to those who have extreme cultural differences. Samovar and Porter (1991) provide examples from maximum differences to minimum differences. The wider the difference between cultures, the more difficult the task of effective communication.

The influence on one's culture creates *culture bias*, a tendency to perceive both language and nonverbal behavior in the light of its meaning in one's own culture, In addition, each person develops *personal bias*, a tendency to perceive language and nonverbal behavior in terms of the personal significance attached to it (Purtilo & Haddad, 1996). Becoming aware of these biases will assist in preventing misinterpretation of the communication of people from other cultures.

Components in Learning About Cultures. There are three components in learning about cultures—listening to clients, studying the literature describing various cultures, and observing the milieu in which your own clients live.

The nutrition lifestyle of all cultures is probably influenced most by ethnicity and the economic availability of food. Nutrition lifestyle is the product of all the cultural influences throughout an individual's life. Given an opportunity, each client will express his or her cultural habits and values. The task is to listen carefully to hear what may often be subtle hints rather than straightforward revelations of values. Techniques of listening were discussed in Chapter 4.

Research literature can provide many insights into cultural influences on nutrition and nutrition lifestyles. Many good studies are cited at the end of this chapter that address the specifics of some cultures. It is also important to study about culture from the perspectives of the fields of sociology, anthropology, and economics (Douglas, 1984.) The field of literature also has much to offer in revealing the meanings of food. The popular media, radio, print, and television provide insight into popular ideas about food and culture. The caveat is to beware of the tendency to stereotype. No individual exactly embodies the description of the culture with which he or she identifies.

A few comments about major cultural groups in the United States are included in this chapter, but it is not our intent to provide comprehensive information. We believe this should be done within the local environment.

African American clients have lines of heritage tracing back to slavery and deprivation. Many remain in poverty today and feel some lack of trust in the dominant culture (Sue, 1981). They feel the prejudices of the dominant culture against them because of race and their socioeconomic level.

Hispanic Americans suffer under negative perceptions because of current political attitudes regarding government support of aliens. Hispanic Americans perceive their identity as national rather than ethnic much more strongly than do people from the dominant culture (Arnold & Boggs, 1995).

Asian American describes as many as 32 different cultures of people from Asian countries living in the United States. Typically, Asian Americans are emotionally restrained and family oriented, and perceive illness from the yin-and-yang perspective. The family is crucial, usually being considered much more significant than the individual (Arnold & Boggs, 1995).

Native Americans are often more comfortable with long silences than are people from other cultures. In addition, they may respond better to a slow approach to the main subject of an interview. For many, healing practices have important religious aspects (Arnold & Boggs, 1995). Some Native Americans are alienated from their cultural heritage and may resent approaches based on their supposed cultural background (Sue, 1981; Pedersen et al, 1996).

Going about in the community observing the cultural milieu provides invaluable understanding of cultural expectations as well as of the availability of food. Foods available in grocery stores and restaurants in close proximity to a client are the foods most likely to be consumed. Awareness of the environment can help you interpret what you hear from the client. It can help fill the client's memory gaps of what was eaten and alleviate hesitancy on the part of the client to reveal food intake that he or she may think will meet with disapproval.

Terry (1994) devised a format for determining the food behaviors and food environment that need to be understood to effectively provide services that have application in cross-cultural settings. Table 7–3 displays these factors.

Overcoming Barriers to Effective Cross-Cultural Counseling

Values. The assumption that one's own culture has the right values and solutions to problems of people from all cultures can result in attempts to impose one's own values on others. For instance, assertiveness is often valued in the dominant American culture and is seen as an excellent problem-solving technique. Assertiveness is not a value in all cultures. Attempting to develop assertiveness in a client whose culture does not place high value on assertiveness may increase anxiety in the client because of cultural conflict. Work with the client to discover which of the cultural values he or she embraces can foster a way to reach desired goals. There may be indirect ways of assertion that are acceptable in a nonassertive culture.

TABLE 7 – 3

Aspects of the Food Behavior and Food Environment that Must be Understood for Delivering Nutrition Services that Meet the Needs, Desires, and Lifestyles of Clients

Aspects of the Food Behavior and Food Environment	What the Dietitian Needs to Know	Example
Food Environment of the Household and Community		
Availability	What types of food are available both in the environment and economically	Note foods available from local food sources and their relative price
Acceptability	What items are accepted as food and under what conditions	Differentiate those foods preferred from those available but not preferred
Safety	What is the short-term and long-term safety of the foods eaten	Note short-term and long-term health problems related to the safety of the food supply
Nutritive quality	What is the nutrient profile of the total diet and the nutrient composition of major foods in the diet	Calculate the adequacy of the diet for providing the kilocalories and nutrients needed for optimum health and for reducing the risk of disease; note specific foods that make substantial contributions to nutrient intake
Food Behavior of the Household and Community		
Selection	Which foods are most commonly chosen for consumption, and who makes food selection decisions	Differentiate those foods chosen consistently that make up a substantial proportion of the food supply from those eaten inconsistently or seasonally
Procurement	How and where are foods obtained by the household and community	Note foods obtained from grocery stores, home gardens, vending machines, restaurants, and other sources and determine how often these sources are used
Distribution	How are foods divided among household and community members	Determine who decides what and how much will be eaten
Manipulation	How is food prepared before eating	Find out common cooking and preparation methods for major foods
Consumption	Which foods are eaten, how much, when, with whom, and where	Ascertain typical daily eating patterns and special event patterns
Storage	How is food put away for future use	Determine which foods are commonly stored or preserved, for how long, and using what facilities and methods; determine whether food storage practices are adequate and safe
Disposal	Which food is disposed of, how, when, where, and why	Note those foods commonly rejected for consumption and how they are disposed of

CASE EXAMPLE ·

A client has been to the nutrition counselor twice and a satisfactory rapport has been established. The client has expressed feelings of powerlessness in getting his mother to prepare meals consistent with the nutrition therapy goals.

C L I E N T: "She just won't buy the foods I want. She likes to cook the way she did in the old country. Lots of frying and no fruits and vegetables."

M N T: "Have you made it plain to her that you need to change your food intake?"

C L I E N T: "I could never do that, it would hurt her feelings."

M N T: "Oh, I see. There are many ways to let people know what you want. Let's brainstorm and come up with a few of them."

They did "brainstorm" and the client decided that the first action he would take would be to bring home some very pretty fruit (his mother liked esthetic arrangements) and make an arrangement on the table. Actually, the whole family liked it and began eating the fruit. Mother apparently "got the message" and began making the fruit arrangements herself. No direct assertiveness ever occurred.

· ·

Interpersonal Barriers. There are some problems in competence that tend to become more pronounced the greater the cultural differences between client and counselor. These include:

1. Discounting the sincerity of what is said. Sometimes this happens because of nonverbal communication patterns that are different. For instance, if you expect people to look you straight in the eye when talking, you may distrust someone who looks away. Unless you recognize that in the client's culture it is not polite to look into another's eyes, you may determine that the client is lying. Mirroring and matching verbal and nonverbal client behaviors, as described in depth in Chapter 4, are profoundly effective in dealing with people from other cultures.
2. Misinterpreting clients' words and gestures because they mean different things in respective cultures. For instance, words such as "staple foods" are not easily understood or translated. The word *boniato* means one food to a Cuban person and a different food to a Jamaican person.
3. Misjudging when to tell a client what to do and when to use a counseling style in which the client takes major responsibility. For instance, a well-educated, middle-class homemaker with a good knowledge of nutrition would likely not respond to a prescriptive style, whereas a person who sees the health-care professional as an authority who will tell them what to do would become frustrated by a participative style (Samovar & Porter, 1991).

Language Barriers. Language barriers can exist between speakers of the same language as well as between speakers of different languages. Clients from different cultures do not speak the standard language of the health-care professional (Falvo, 1994). There may be a native language difference. In trying to be cooperative with the health-care professional, a client may use simple language because he or she is unfamiliar with English or the technical language, or both. That simple language may then be interpreted by the counselor as a sign of limited intelligence (Falvo, 1994). Cases in which counselor and client do not know each other's language occur occasionally, often in institutional settings. An interpreter is then essential. Use of language may also differ among subcultures of the same larger culture. "Although foreign sounding to the health professional, the language of the subculture may be highly developed and structured and quite adequate for conveying ideas" (Falvo, 1994; p. 142).

Contextual Barriers. Flexibility is the key to effective cross-cultural communications: being able to adjust your style to the other person's style. Two concepts are of particular concern in adaptation of style. One regards issues of locus of control; another, differences between high- and low-context cultures.

Locus of control refers to beliefs about internal or external control of human destiny. People with an internal locus of control believe their own actions are primary in shaping their fates. People with an external locus of control believe that their fates are contingent on chance or luck. In some cultures, internal control is valued; in others, there is a belief that fate is determined through external control such as the will of God. Planning for change should be handled differently for clients who believe differently. Following are two examples:

CASE EXAMPLE ·

Client with Internal Locus of Control

Client and counselor have been working together for some time and have a good rapport.

CLIENT: "I know the reasons for my high blood sugar are related to my food habits. I probably even know what to do about it."

MNT: "What do you think you could do about it?"

Client with External Locus of Control

CLIENT: "My high blood sugar just won't seem to go away. I guess it is just my fate."

MNT: "Yes, I see. I have worked with some people with high blood sugar and it has been possible to control blood sugar fairly well. There is a nutrition plan that could have some effect on your blood sugar. Would you like to try it?"

· ·

A survey in the July/August 1994 issue of the *Diabetes Educator* described the influence of spiritual and religious factors on Hispanic adults with diabetes. Of 104 Hispanic adults surveyed, 68% believed it was God's will that they had diabetes and 28% believed that their diabetes was a punishment from God. Seventeen percent of those surveyed used herbs to treat their diabetes (ADA, 1994). Generally speaking, the dominant American culture values an internal locus of control, but minority cultures are more likely to value an external locus of control (Sue, 1989).

Communication with people in high- or low-context societies also requires flexibility. Low-context cultures rely heavily on the verbal aspects of communication. There is a tendency to formalize communication with contracts, protocols, and so on. High-context cultures rely more on nonverbal aspects of communication. There may be a distrust of formal contracts because the culture would expect an oral commitment to be sufficient (Sue, 1981). Forcing rigid procedures on an individual from a high-context culture, for example, would probably not be effective. Completing a contract for change verbally instead of filling out a written one would be more acceptable. MNTs who may be low-context–oriented will find it beneficial to practice observing nonverbal communication and restricting their own verbalizations when dealing with a high-context–oriented client.

Simply exposing clients to new ways does not automatically result in adoption of the new ways. Clients must believe that the new way will be an improvement. With all clients, and particularly with clients from cultures different from your own, the new ways must be compatible with their values (Kittler & Sucher, 1989). Often the difference between client acceptance and rejection is the communicative effectiveness of the counselors in perceiving nonverbal messages. This is especially true in cross-cultural counseling because clients rarely feel secure enough to make their real attitudes known directly.

Body Movements. Cultures vary in their standards of physical activity in communication. For instance, in the British upper class, hand and body are expected to remain fairly rigid, whereas Italians expect a great deal of body movement. Cross-cultural communication skill includes becoming comfortable with a range of bodily movements. Mirroring and matching can be an excellent technique to use (see Chap. 4).

Eye Contact. Rules about eye contact vary from culture to culture. Many European Americans have learned that they should look others "straight in the eye" when communicating. In some cultures, including some Native American and Asian cultures, this is considered impolite (Wilson, 1979; Dillard, 1983).

Facial Expression. The face is the most expressive part of the body, but all cultures do not support free expression of emotion. All people have emotions. Do not assume that when they are not expressed the way you would express them, a client does not have emotions. Some cultures require stoicism in the face of difficulties while others allow much expression (Harwood, 1981).

Time. Cultural differences in the perception of time can be a real hazard in cross-cultural communication. Time can refer to speed of talk, meeting time restraints, or the time frame for making change. In the dominant culture we live by the clock. Being late is a serious social error. Other cultures do not perceive time in this way. For instance, some Hispanic cultures view arriving at the stated time for a meeting as rather strange behavior. There is also great variation regarding time orientation toward the past, the present, and the future. In this respect there are often great differences within the same culture even as much as there are between cultures.

Teaching Aids. Teaching aids that are prepared for mass distribution are by necessity based on generalizations about cultural appropriateness. The skilled cross-cultural counselor limits the use of mass-produced materials in individual cases. Not until the widespread availability of the computer was individualization of teaching materials truly feasible. Language or pictorial representation needs to be suited to the culture and educational level of clients. Often knowledge of the appropriateness of materials is a combination of careful observation of the immediate cultural milieu and trial and error. One tool for evaluating the educational level of written materials is described in *Teaching Patients with Low Literacy Skills* by Doak, Doak, and Root. Detailed methods for evaluating materials is provided.

Issues Facing the MNTs Whose Backgrounds Are Not That of the Dominant American Culture

No one culture has more need than another to become aware of itself in preparing for cross-cultural counseling. However, little has been written about individuals who share relatively few of the values of the dominant culture. For instance, some cultures value being on time while others do not. How is a counselor whose culture does not value being on time adjust to deal adequately with being on time for counseling appointments when it is expected? Such an individual needs to deal with prejudices he or she may have toward the dominant culture and its pressures. How will a counselor who is not accustomed to functioning in the context of long-term goals be effective with a client whose thinking orientation is toward the future? Questions such as these have yet to be answered and represent a prime area for discussion and research.

There is also the issue of the power differences between the dominant culture and subcultures within our society. Even though much has been accomplished toward sharing of power over the last few decades, there is still a perception regarding glass ceilings that limit women and minorities in the power structures of society. Issues remain regarding the shifting of power from one group to another as our society shifts from the historically dominant European American culture to a more pluralistic power structure. Because of such ideas a client from the dominant culture may not perceive the MNT as powerful and may have a tendency to discount the intervention.

A dietetic practitioner can take steps to develop a strong positive self-concept and high self-esteem as a way to overcome these problems. Indeed, the entire profession will have increased success in cross-cultural counseling through efforts to establish confidence and competence among professionals.

Characteristics and Behaviors of Skilled Cross-Cultural Medical Nutrition Therapists

Positive Regard for All Cultures. Appreciation of different cultural values underlies the development of skill and the willingness to focus counseling on the cultural background of the client. If the MNT remains alert to the expressions of the values the client holds and uses them to motivate the client to establish a healthy nutrition lifestyle or modify his or her food habits in response to disease, the potential for change on the part of the client is increased. Appreciation is an elusive goal, one that is recognized more by inference than by direct observations. In addition, being alert to barriers to effective communication and ways to overcome them is an essential skill. The client will likely perceive appreciation as a sense that the nutrition therapist is empathic to him or her.

Flexibility. Techniques of counseling should be adjusted to meet the expectations of clients. For instance, the flexible counselor is able to work with the client's value system, present material in a variety of formats, and use a participative or an authoritative style depending on the situation.

Awareness. Without necessarily discarding his or her own value system, the MNT should be able to recognize both cultural and personal biases, since they exist in the value systems of all cultures. She or he uses the resources available to learn about clients and their cultures.

Samovar and Porter (1991) describe the following skills of the aware MNT:

1. Nonjudgmental attitude: This can be shown verbally and nonverbally. Do not interrupt your client.
2. Tolerance for ambiguity: This is the ability to react with little discomfort to new or poorly understood situations.
3. Respect: Displaying respect is important in all aspects of counseling and particularly imperative in a cross-cultural situation. It can give clients status and contribute to their self-esteem as well as foster a positive regard for your counseling relationship.
4. Personalized knowledge and perceptions: People who recognize values, beliefs, and attributes as their own, and as not necessarily shared by others, are more successful than those who know "the truth." You can begin phrases with "I think," "I feel," or "In my experience."
5. Empathy: Put yourself in your client's shoes to understand another's point of view.
6. Turn-taking: Make sure conversations are two-way. Do not monopolize interactions.

Cultural competence enhances the credibility of the MNT. When it is clear to a client that he is going to be able to "do things my way," he will be more willing to listen and plan for changes in his nutrition lifestyle. If a client believes that the MNT will accept her beliefs and values, the client is released from spending energy defending the culture and can then spend that energy solving problems (Falvo, 1994).

Summary

Concepts of nutrition counseling and understanding of cross-cultural counseling are derived from concepts of psychological counseling. A strong influence has been exerted by the dominant American culture, which is based on European ancestry. Every counseling situation is to some extent cross-cultural, because each individual's world view is uniquely influenced by that person's exposure to his or her cultural environment. The skilled cross-cultural MNT is the one who has become aware of his or her own cultural background and the biases in perception that are the result. She or he appreciates and learns about others' cultures and utilizes the clients' values to help motivate the development of a nutrition lifestyle in both wellness and in response to disease states.

Suggestions for Further Learning

1. Make a list of your own values.

2. In a group, make a list of perceived values among cultural groups in your community.

3. As a group, list and discuss difficulties that may arise in cross-cultural communication and how to combat them.

4. As a group, list and discuss ways in which you can learn about cultures in your community.

5. Practice interviewing individuals from several cultural groups, identify the values you perceive them to have, and then check with the individual to confirm (or correct) your perceptions.

6. Discuss the following dialogue wherein an inaccurate assumption is made by the counselor. What was effective and why? What would you have done differently? Think of other dialogues and role-play them with a partner.

MNT: "Please tell me what you ate on Friday."

Client: "I didn't eat anything. I only had water."

MNT: "That's not very healthy. Do you understand the physiological implications when you do that?"

Client: (says nothing; looks down; face turns red)

MNT: "Is this a regular practice for you?"

Client: "No. I only do it on Friday during Lent. It is the practice of my religion."

MNT: "I'm very sorry! I didn't consider that. I assumed you were doing it to help with your weight loss. Let's pick another day, a typical one—this time you choose one."

Client: " OK, let's do Thursday. For lunch I had *ropa vieja* and *congri*."

MNT: "I'm not familiar with *ropa vieja*. Can you tell me how that is made?"

CITED REFERENCES

Anonymous. Role of religion and folk medicine in Hispanics' view of diabetes. *J Am Diet Assoc.* 1994; 94(12):1397.

Arnold E, Boggs KU: *Interpersonal Relationships: Professional Communication Skills for Nurses.* 2nd ed. Philadelphia: WB Saunders, 1995.

Back TK: Food, sex and theory. *In* Fitzgerald (ed): *Nutrition and Anthropology in Action.* Amsterdam: van Gorcum, 1977; pp 24–34.

Belasco WJ: The two taste cultures. *Psych Today.* December 1989; p. 29–36.

Bronner Y: Cultural sensitivity and nutrition counseling. *Top Clin Nutr.* 1994:9(2):13–19.

Burn D: Ethical implications in cross cultural counseling and training. *J Counsel Devel.* 1992;70:578–583.

Copeland EF: Cross cultural counseling and psychotherapy: A historical perspective, implications for research and training. *Pers Guid J.* 1983;Sept:10–15.

Curry Bartley K: *Dietetic Practitioner Skills: Education, Counseling and Business Management.* New York: Macmillan Publishing Co, 1987.

Curry Bartley KR: Ethnic influences on food habits of teenagers in England, New Zealand and the United States. *Sch Food Service J.* 1985;10:6–9.

DeVito JA: *The Interpersonal Communication Book.* 7th ed. New York: Harper Collins Custom Books, 1995.

Dillard JM: *Multicutural Counseling.* Chicago: Nelson-Hall, 1983.

Doak CC, Doak LG, Roof JH: *Teaching Patients with Low Literacy Skills.* Philadelphia: JB Lippincott, 1985.

Douglas M: Fundamental issues in food problems. *Curr Anthro.* 1984;25(4):498–500.

Falvo DR: *Effective Patient Education: A Guide To Increased Compliance.* 2nd ed. Gaithersburg, MD: Aspen Publishers, 1994.

Farkas CS: Ethnic-specific domination patterns: Implications for nutrition education. *J Nutr Educ.* 1986;18(3):99–103.

Goleman D: Psychiatry makes room on the couch for culture. *Miami Herald.* 12/10/95; p. 6M.

Harwood A: Ethnicity and Medical Care. Cambridge, MA: Harvard University Press, 1981.

Holli BB, Calabrese RJ: *Communication and Education Skills.* Malvern, PA: Lea & Febiger, 1986.

Johnson WS, Packer AM: *Workforce 2000: Work and Workers for the Twenty First Century.* New York, Hudson Institute, 1987.

Kastenbaum R: Old food for fast people. *Am Behav Sci.* 1988;32(1):50–60.

Kittler PG, Sucher K: *Food and Culture in America: A Nutrition Handbook.* New York: Van Nostrand Reinhold, 1989.

Lee CC, Richardson BL: *Cross Cultural Issues in Counseling: New Approaches to Diversity.* Alexandria, VA: American Association for Counseling and Development, 1991.

Lieberman LS, Bobroff LB: *Cultural Food Patterns of Florida: A Handbook.* Gainesville, FL: Florida Cooperative Extension Service, 1991.

Lowenberg ME, Todhunter N, Wilson ED et al: *Food and People.* 3rd ed. New York: John Wiley & Sons, 1979.

Marin G: Defining culturally appropriate community interventions: Hispanics as a case study. *J Commun Psych.* 1993;21:149–161.

Mason M, Wenberg B, Welsh P: *The Dynamics of Clinical Dietetics.* New York: JW Wiley & Sons, 1977.

Mennell S: *The Sociology of Food: Eating, Diet and Culture.* London; Sage Publishing; 1992.

Natow SJ: Cross cultural counseling. *J Nutr Elderly.* 1994;14:(1):23–31.

O'Donnell JM: The holistic health movement: Implications for counseling theory and practice. *In* Hayes R, Aubrey R (eds): *New Directions for Counseling and Human Development.* Denver: Love Publishing Co, 1988; pp 365–382.

Pedersen PB, Dragunz N, Lonner WJ, Trimble JE (eds): *Counseling Across Cultures.* 4th ed. Thousand Oaks, CA: Sage Publications, 1996.

Purtilo R, Haddad A: *Health Professional and Patient Interaction.* 5th ed. Philadelphia: WB Saunders, 1996.

Richardson TQ, Molinaro KL: White counselor self-awareness: A prerequisite for developing mulicultural competence. *J Couns Dev.* 1996;74:238–242.

Samovar LA, Porter RE: *Intercultural Communication: A Reader.* 6th ed. Belmont, CA: Wadsworth Publishing Company, 1991.

Saracino J, Michael P: Positive steps toward a multicultural association. *J Am Diet Assoc.* 1996;96(12):1242–1244.

Snetselaar L: *Nutrition Counseling Skills.* Rockville, MD: Aspen Publishers, 1983.

Stanford G, Perdue J: *In* Hayes R, Aubrey R (eds): *New Directions for Counseling and Human Development.* Denver: Love Publishing Co, 1988; pp 397–417.

Sue DW: *Barriers to Effective Multicultural Counseling* (videotape). Hayward, CA: California State University, 1989.

Sue DW: *Counseling the Culturally Different: Theory and Practice.* New York: John Wiley & Sons, 1981.

Terry RD: Needed: A new appreciation of culture and food behavior. *J Am Diet Assoc.* 1994;94(5):501–504.

Vontress CE: Social class influence on counseling. *In* Hayes R, Aubrey R (eds): *New Directions for Counseling and Human Development.* Denver: Love Publishing Co, 1988; pp 346–364.

Wilson C: Food customs and nurture: An annotated bibliography on socio-cultural and bio-cultural aspects of nutrition. *J Nutr Educ.* 1979;11(suppl):27–28.

ADDITIONAL REFERENCES

Anderson R, Ross V: *Questions of Communication: A Practical Introduction to Theory.* New York: St. Martin's Press, 1994.

Bronner Y, Burke C, Joubert BJ: African-American/soul foodways and nutrition counseling. *Top Clin Nutr.* 1994;9(2):20–27.

Brooks GE: The art of integrating diversity: Addressing treatment issues of minority women in the 90's. *Renfrew Perspec.* 1994;Winter:1.

Brown LK, Mussle K (eds): *Ethnic and Regional Foodways in the United States: The Performance of Group Identity.* Knoxville, TN: The University of Tennessee Press, 1984.

Chernoff R: *Communicating as Professionals.* Chicago: The American Dietetic Association, 1986.

Claudio VS: *Ethnic and Regional Food Practices.* Chicago: The American Dietetic Association, 1994.

Davis WN: Gender, race, culture and eating disorders. *Renfrew Perspec.* 1994;Winter:2.

DeBruyne LK, Sizer FS, Wolfes SR: Ethnic diets and health. *Nutr Clin.* 1991;6(6):1–16.

DeVito JA, Hecht ML: *The Nonverbal Communication Reader.* Prospect Heights, IL: Waveland Press, 1990.

International Food Information Council: Celebrating with food. *Food Insight Curr Top Food Safety Nutr.* 1990;Nov/Dec:1.

Lseong FTL, Helen HWK: Going beyond cultural sensitivity on the road to cross culturalism: Using the intercultural sensitizer as a counselor training tool. *J Couns Dev.* 1991;70:112–118.

O'Brien MJ: *Communications and Relationships in Nursing.* St. Louis: The CV Mosby Co, 1974.

Rodriquez JC: Diet, nutrition, and the Hispanic client. *Top Clin Nutr.* 1994;9(2):28–39.

Ray EB, Donohew L: *Communication and Health: Systems and Applications.* Hillsdale, NJ: Lawrence Erlbaum Associates, 1990.

Samolsky S, Dunker K, Hynak-Hankinso MT: Feeding the Hispanic hospital patient: Cultural considerations. *J Am Diet Assoc.* 1990;90(12):1708–1710.

Scheller MD: *Building Partnerships in Hospital Care.* Palo Alto, CA: Bull Publishing Co, 1990.

CHAPTER 8

Emotional Factors

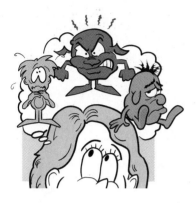

The goals of this chapter are (1) to present a discussion of common and normal emotions that may be barriers to changes in nutrition lifestyle, and (2) to review the process of grieving and dying that may be faced by individuals who are counseled by medical nutrition therapists.

Learning Objectives

At the end of this chapter the reader will be able to:

1. Describe symptoms of anxiety, depression, and anger.

2. Describe interventions that can help reduce the intensity of emotions.

3. Identify common emotions expressed in role-playing.

4. In role-playing (or in practice settings), conduct counseling sessions, identify the emotions expressed, and make note of interventions and their effects on clients.

5. Compare the descriptions of grieving and dying presented in the chapter.

6. From case studies or practice, identify the stages of grieving and dying being expressed by patients/ clients.

7. Begin to address clients' emotions, and dying patients and their families, comfortably.

Key Terms

▶ Anxiety: a state of heightened awareness of danger resulting from unrealistic fears.

▶ Depression: feelings of helplessness, hopelessness, sadness, and other signs of a low mood.

▶ Process of dying: psychological stages that accompany the physiological dying of the body.

Most emotions that clients exhibit are normal and can be effectively addressed when they are pertinent to medical nutrition therapy. When emotional tension reaches a level that interferes with problem solving, the emotion itself becomes a problem that needs to be faced if progress is to be made in finding solutions and establishing a desirable nutrition lifestyle. In some cases, the MNT can address emotional issues with the client; at other times, a referral is needed. For instance, a normal reaction to the diagnosis of a life-threatening disease includes some anxiety, depression, and grieving over loss of health. An MNT has the skills to help a client reduce moderate anxiety and depression. However, when either the intensity or the duration of strong feelings is more than normal, psychotherapy professionals need to participate. If the MNT is to guide clients effectively, it is important that he or she recognize the expression of feelings and recognize certain traits and symptoms of emotional disorders. This chapter does not intend to suggest that the MNT attempt to diagnose emotional disorders. She or he simply needs to be aware of factors that suggest the need for intervention either by the MNT consulting with a psychotherapist or by direct referral to the client's physician or other appropriate professional.

Negative feelings are a normal part of changing a nutrition lifestyle. A person who has been told that she or he needs to modify food choices will exhibit some anxiety from anticipation of the unknown. If the person believes that the future will make demands for which she or he is unprepared, higher levels of anxiety occur. Real losses that accompany ill health will be smaller barriers to problem-solving if emotional factors are effectively addressed. Anxiety and depression will probably be present as part of the processes. People grieve over losses, not just in death, but also with losses of health, desired lifestyle, favorite foods, inability to exercise, and so on. The concept of loss of any kind can summon grieving. Every client functions better by acknowledging the emotional aspect of changing a nutrition lifestyle, and by being given reassurance that he or she will be able to cope with the future.

The grieving processes described in this chapter were the result of work with patients who were dying from long-term illnesses, but they can also be fruitfully applied to patients with nonterminal illnesses. In addition, families of the terminally ill grieve for the person they are about to lose. In situations such as long-term-care facilities, part of the MNT's tasks may be to counsel families of dying patients.

This chapter discusses three emotional factors that may warrant psychological counseling prior to or along with medical nutrition therapy. They are *anxiety, depression,* and *grieving.* Each client will exhibit one or more of these reactions, or perhaps all of them. Emotions play a significant role in adjustments in nutrition lifestyle, particularly in life-threatening diseases such as diabetes, cancers, cardiovascular disease, and renal disease.

The literature emphasizes that symptoms of pathological levels of emotion overlap or confound one another. Individuals have more than one emotion at a time, or express a socially acceptable emotion rather than the one they really feel. For instance, an individual who is learning to be assertive may need to be a little angry to overcome feelings of anxiety before assertive behavior can take place.

ANXIETY

Social scientists of the 1950s "discovered" anxiety, and it is now so popular that "everyone" can have "free floating anxiety." Anxiety is generally distinguished from fear, which is logically based, by a lack of evidence that the anxiety is logically based. Rather, anxiety seems to be based on anticipation of disaster in situations in which logic does not suggest disaster. Anxiety is also characterized by a general sense of impending disaster. Some anxiety is thought to be motivating, but when the level of anxiety becomes intense, it becomes a hindrance to problem-solving. When this occurs, the level of anxiety must be reduced before a client can address rational problem-solving.

Incidence

Probably about 25% of the US population (about 50 million people) suffer from anxiety and about 15% have a clinical anxiety disorder (Leon et al, 1995). The result of widespread anxiety is societal anxiety. An example of societal anxiety that is significant to nutritionists and dietitians is *nosophobia* (excessive fear of disease), which is evidenced by the widespread use of fad diets as "preventive" or "cure-all" measures. People may attribute magical properties to food as a cure for this or that disease regardless of whether there is scientific evidence to link that food to disease. On the other hand, people may fear a particular food as a killer, such as red meat. On one level nosophobia, such as fear of heart attacks, may be useful in making societal changes; however, it is not useful on the personal level. Real concern about maintaining good health and establishing a healthy nutrition lifestyle is based in reality. Nutrition lifestyle includes food choices both logical and pleasurable and comfortably exists as a part of overall lifestyle. Obsession with food intake suggests anxiety or phobia, and the resulting physiological stress may be as bad or worse on health than poor food habits.

Description

Anxiety, a feeling of heightened awareness and anticipation in its mildest form, is an unavoidable condition of life. Though uncomfortable, it is considered to be functional in avoiding danger and as a motivator in problem-solving activities. As feeling intensifies, anxiety becomes a vague threat to one's safety and self-concept, progressing to the intense feelings associated with a state of panic. When anxiety reaches the level of intensity that prohibits effective functioning its difference from fear becomes clear (Arnold & Boggs, 1995). Fear is heightened alertness in the face of a clear and present danger, whereas anxiety is a sense of impending doom that does not seem justified by circumstances or a vague notion of a threat to one's self-concept that cannot be identified. In *Women and Anxiety* the nature of anxiety is described:

> Anxiety is a feeling of dread, a nameless fear that distracts the minds and hearts of people of all ages. It is a constellation of physical symptoms, of uncomfortable, troubled feelings and thoughts, that may be relatively mild or reach the point of utter panic. It is a reaction to frustration and to unresolved anger that seems to burn a hole into your very being. It is a response to unbearable stress. It represents an inability to maintain the neurobiochemical balance essential to a sense of well-being. It is a beacon light signaling the existence of unconscious emotional conflict.
>
> *de Rosis, 1979, p. 10*

Even reading the paragraph relays a sense of stress created by the feeling of anxiety.

Symptoms of Anxiety

Life patterns indicate the ways in which people cope with the stress of everyday living, or the more intense stress that is caused by unresolved inner conflicts. An excessive need to be liked by everyone or excessive needs to be alone may be ploys to control anxiety. Hostility, over-competitiveness, excessive needs to control, physical illness, sexual impotence, overwork, eating disorders, alcoholism, drug addiction, and other symptoms may signal anxiety levels that are a hindrance to good health, including healthy eating habits.

In a study of approximately 500 undergraduate students at the University of Calgary, the behaviors most frequently described by anxious students were to worry, talk, fidget, pace, tremble, perspire, and run. When medical clinicians surveyed the evidence of anxiety, they noted in diagnoses such things as "tense muscles, palpitations, pallor, faintness, increased blood pressure, nausea, vomiting, diarrhea, frequent urge to urinate, headaches" (Costello, 1976). These two viewpoints provide guidelines for observing ourselves and our clients to detect anxiety. In ourselves we also can recognize anxiety by such things as a feelings of tightness in the chest, a lump in the throat, butterflies in the stomach, a feeling of dread, shortness of breath, and nervousness. Each of us has a unique way of feeling and expressing anxiety.

Signs of motor tension, autonomic hyperactivity, vigilance, and scanning are present in the anxious person. The level of anxiety can be determined by the intensity of behaviors. When a very high level of anxiety is reached, panic results. Even a generally mentally healthy person can occasionally reach the panic state. When this happens, problem-solving stops until the anxiety is quieted.

Signs of Anxiety

Motor Tension: trembling, twitching, feeling shaky; muscle tension and aches or soreness; restlessness.

Autonomic Hyperactivity: shortness of breath or smothering sensations; palpitations or accelerated heart rate; sweating or cold clammy hands; dry mouth, dizziness, or lightheadedness; nausea, diarrhea, or other abdominal distress; flushes or chills, frequent urination; difficulty swallowing.

Vigilance and Scanning: feeling keyed up or on edge, exaggerated startle response, difficulty concentrating or the mind going blank because of anxiety, trouble falling asleep, and irritability.

Perceptual ability decreases as anxiety increases. Table 8–1 (Arnold & Boggs, 1996) shows how perceptual ability, coping ability, and behaviors change as anxiety increases. When anxiety is high, problem-solving is not possible.

An Anxiety Model

A model of anxiety that can be usefully applied in medical nutrition therapy is presented in *Women and Anxiety* (de Rosis, 1979). It is shown in Figure 8–1. The author considers anxiety to result from the evolution of a set of standards, or "shoulds," during the developmental years, which serves to unconsciously influence and control our lives. These "shoulds" are unrealistic expectations of perfec-

TABLE 8 – 1	Levels of Anxiety with Degree of Sensory Perceptions, Cognitive and Coping Abilities, and Manifest Behaviors		
Level of Anxiety	**Sensory Perceptions**	**Cognitive/Coping Ability**	**Behaviors**
Mild	Heightened state of alertness: increased acuity of hearing, vision, smell, touch	Enhanced learning, problem-solving; increased ability to respond and adapt to changing stimuli; enhanced functioning	Walking, singing, eating, drinking, mild restlessness, active listening, attending, questioning
Moderate	Decreased sensory perceptions: with guidance, able to expand sensory fields	Loss of concentration; decreased cognitive ability Cannot identify factors contributing to the anxiety-producing situation. With directions can cope, reduce anxiety, and solve problems Inhibited functioning°	Increased muscle tone, pulse, respirations Changes in voice tone and pitch; rapid speech Incomplete verbal responses Engrossed with detail
Severe	Greatly diminished perceptions: decreased sensitivity to pain	Limited thought processes: unable to solve problems even with guidance Cannot cope with stress without help. Confused mental state; limited functioning	Purposeless, aimless behaviors Rapid pulse, respirations: high blood pressure; hyperventilation Inappropriate or incongruent verbal responses Immobilization
Panic	No response to sensory perceptions	No cognitive or coping abilities; without intervention death is imminent	

°Functioning refers to the ability to perform activities of daily living for survival purposes.
From Arnold A, Boggs KU: *Interpersonal Relationships: Professional Communication Skills for Nurses.* Philadelphia, WB Saunders, 1995.

tion that cannot be met, which results in tension (anxiety) and self-hatred, disgust, and persistent anger. For instance, if you "should" be a nice woman who is never angry, this expectation will conflict with angry feelings that will inevitably arise from time to time. The psychologist Paula Levine, in a 1996 presentation to dietitians, stated that the phenomenon of little girls being pressured to be "nice" frequently occurs around the age of 8 years. This also appears to be about the time that girls begin to feel a sense of general anxiety. This anxiety, left unresolved, is quite likely to become a barrier to effective problem-solving later in life.

Further complicating the picture is the fact that not only do we have a list of "shoulds" about what to feel and think and how to behave, but sometimes the "shoulds" conflict with reality as well as with themselves. For instance, if you should be both submissive and stand up for yourself, you have a perfect set-up for failure.

Angry you→   conflicts with   ←Nice you
↓
and leads to
↓
ANXIETY

FIGURE 8–1. Anxiety. (From DeRosis HA: *Women and Anxiety: A Step-by-Step Program for Managing Anxiety and Depression.* New York: Delacort Press, 1979.)

CASE EXAMPLE ·

The client is in charge of a clerical pool in a law firm. She is overweight and has identified conflict between being submissive with her bosses and assertive with those she supervises. She believes that this accounts for part of her eating problems.

CLIENT: "I really have a problem with confrontation. I know I shouldn't argue with my bosses, but I should be strong with my staff. I never seem to do it right. Yesterday, I had to fire someone and I worried all day. I was okay in the interview, but I was so anxious. I could hardly breathe. I eat a lot, too." (client is breathing shallowly, muscles are tense, speech is rapid.)

MNT: "OK, now, take three deep breaths . . ."

CLIENT: (takes three deep breaths)

MNT: "Now do you feel a little calmer?"

CLIENT: "Yes, in another minute I'll be able to think again."

The MNT waits a moment before continuing, meanwhile monitoring the client's breathing to be sure that shallow breathing does not return.

· ·

The long-term goal in this situation probably will be to find some way besides eating for the patient to reduce anxiety.

Anxiety Disorders

Certain levels of anxiety indicate an emotional disorder. Generalized anxiety disorder is characterized by the presence of chronic, persistent anxiety, with no specific cause (APA: DSM-IV, 1994). The person with generalized anxiety disorder seems to have a sense of impending doom even when everything is going well. Diagnosing generalized anxiety disorder is not within the skills of the MNT because of its complexity. Signs that a referral is needed include client expressions of fear with nonspecificity of source, and a combination of several of the following chronic physical symptoms:

Shakiness
Shortness of breath

Dizziness
Chronic diarrhea
Difficulty with concentration
Irritability
Sleeplessness
Rapid heartbeat

It is apparent that a person exhibiting these symptoms needs a referral to a physician. Not only are the symptoms serious, but they also could be the result of many medical problems other than anxiety.

Implications for Medical Nutrition Therapy

Much of the anxiety that an MNT encounters in the self and in clients is a normal part of life, and the MNT can take everyday tactics to cope with it and use it to advantage. Often, the mere recognition that anxiety is present is helpful in focusing the anxiety into motivation and success. Clients may express a feeling of nervousness or insecurity about their ability to follow a food intake pattern that is different from their previous one. People who must feed others may also have some anxiety about being able to take care of themselves and also keep feeding patterns for the family normal.

Techniques to address anxiety include education, thought-stopping, breathing exercises, talking about anxiety, and developing coping mechanisms. A few words of encouragement and education to teach clients skills they need will go a long way to reduce anxiety. The role of negative cognition can be addressed, and thought-changing techniques can be effective (Beck et al, 1985). Simply having the client breathe more deeply can help. In the example cited, this technique was used, followed by a discussion of the thoughts and feelings and completion of a contract regarding the action to take instead of eating when the level of anxiety begins to interfere. If an intervention does not result in anxiety reduction, consideration must be given to referring the client to a physician or a psychotherapist.

Pursuing nutrition instruction that focuses on too many changes at one time is one way in which an MNT can harm a person who is prone to anxiety. Anxiety will develop as the client becomes overwhelmed by the prospect of making many changes. The MNT may need to address her or his own anxiety about what she or he "should" do as an MNT (eg, accomplish counseling all in one session).

DEPRESSION

A simple definition of depression is sadness, gloom, and emotional dejection. Emotional dejection greater than what is warranted by any objective reason suggests a disease entity. Since some depression in any illness is normal, coping with depression is a significant aspect of medical nutrition therapy. Surprisingly enough, the MNT may be among the first to become aware of both normal and abnormal depression among people who seek treatment for weight control, because the nutrition problem is an easy way to avoid addressing the emotional problem (Ryan & Shea, 1996).

Incidence

Depression is about as prevalent as anxiety, and depressingly popular. Many medications are on the market to treat depression, for both clinical conditions and for normal responses to life events. It is estimated that anywhere from 5 to 25% of all Americans suffer from severe depression at some time in their lives (Wolberg, 1988). Less that half of these are ever treated for it. Depression is considered the most common problem in older people (Ryan & Shea, 1996).

Symptoms of Depression

Anxiety and depression have many characteristics in common, and some authors describe anxiety as a symptom of depression or depression as a symptom of anxiety (Last, 1993). It is often true that they go together and there is evidence that both have genetic factors in their etiology. Drugs frequently seem to be an effective treatment for both (Kendall & Watson, 1989). However, depression seems to be more of an immobilizing emotion than anxiety and is linked with decreased interest in life and disincentive to activity. People who are depressed often also look depressed, exhibiting sagging shoulders, a fallen face, and a slow step. Descriptive phrases used by depressed people include being "weighted down," "heavy with burdens," or feeling "helpless" and "tired." Crying, sulking, and withdrawing are behaviors associated with depression. Almost without exception, people who are depressed express low self-esteem (Costello, 1976).

Additional signs that help identify a depressed mood include loss of interest or pleasure in activities and expressions of being sad, discouraged, or "down in the dumps." Associated symptoms include appetite disturbance, changes in weight,

TABLE 8–2

Psychological Symptoms of Depression Found in General Medical Patients	
Symptom	Percentage of Patients
Irritability	78
Anxiety	75
Depressed mood	50
Crying	36
Loneliness	36
Guilt	31
Feelings of dissatisfaction	29
Pessimism	25
Indecisiveness	22
Helplessness	22
Self-hate	18
Feelings of failure	15
Suicidal thoughts	14
Feelings of being punished	10
Hopelessness	7

From Schwab JJ, Bialow MR, Clemmons RS, Holzeer CE: The affective symptomalogy of depression in medical inpatients. *Psychosomatics.* 1966; 7:214–217.

sleep disturbance, psychomotor agitation or retardation, expressions of guilt, difficulty concentrating, and suicidal thoughts or statements.

Both the "blues," which are considered to be a normal and necessary response to unpleasant events, and an extended period of depressed mood that would lead to a diagnosis of clinical depression are fairly common among individuals seeking medical nutrition therapy. For one thing, a person often seeks, or is referred to, counseling in the wake of diagnosis of a serious and often life-threatening illness, following which it is normal to be depressed. In addition, chronic illness tends to result in depression. Since both life-threatening and chronic illness more frequently afflict the elderly, symptoms of depression are more likely to occur among the elderly. Both psychological and physical symptoms of depression have been reported among general medical patients and they are described in Tables 8–2 and 8–3.

Regardless of circumstances, it is common practice among health-care providers to address symptoms. For those cases in which there seems to be a lack of evidence of a known cause for a prolonged depressed mood, actual diagnosis of clinical depression does not have to occur before action is taken. The symptoms are much the same regardless of cause or duration. The intensity of symptoms is significant. Severe symptoms need to be addressed, especially because depression is one of the most treatable of emotional problems.

Clinical Depression

A synopsis of the symptoms of depression that are described in DSM IV (APA, 1994) include the following:

Adults can usually identify a depressed mood. In children, an irritable mood or loss of interest in all, or almost all, activities may indicate depression. Vocabulary that suggests a depressed mood includes *sad, hopeless, discouraged, helpless, who cares, what's the use, down in the dumps,* and similar words and phrases. Clients

TABLE 8–3

Occurrence of Physical Symptoms of Depression Among General Medical Patients	
Symptom	Percentage of Patients
Fatigue, lethargy	70
Insomnia	68
Upper gastrointestinal disturbances (indigestion, etc.)	52
Headache	42
Anorexia	40
Lower gastrointestinal disturbances (constipation)	39
Recent weight loss	32
Chest tightness or pain	29
Tachycardia	29
Generalized pain	22
Recent loss of libido	21
Urinary disturbances (frequency, dysuria)	21

From Schwab JJ, Clemmons RI, Bialow M, Duggan V, Davis B: A study of somatic symptomatology of depression in medical inpatients. *Psychosomatics.* 1963; 6:273–277.

who are depressed may describe feeling that even the most simple task is difficult or impossible, or express indecisiveness, brooding, and preoccupation with death (but not fear of death). Actual reference to wanting to die or kill oneself should be taken quite seriously as a symptom to be immediately addressed by a qualified professional.

Nonverbal symptoms of clinical depression include sad or depressed affect, withdrawal, poor hygiene, slow walking, and refusal to engage in activities that are fun. Additional symptoms include changes in eating habits—either eating more or less than usual—usually resulting in loss or gain of weight, sleep disturbances, psychomotor agitation or retardation, decreased energy, feelings of worthlessness or excessive or inappropriate guilt, difficulty thinking or concentrating, recurrent thoughts of death, and suicidal ideation or attempts. Specific psychomotor signs of agitation include the inability to sit still, pacing, hand-wringing, and pulling or rubbing of hair, skin, clothing, or other objects. Psychomotor retardation includes slowed speech, increased pauses before answering, soft or monotonous speech, slowed body movements, a markedly decreased amount of speech, muteness, and fatigue in the absence of physical exertion. Other behaviors associated with depression may be chronic tearfulness, anxiety, irritability, brooding, excessive concern with physical health, panic attacks, and phobias. Although anxiety has been discussed in its own entity, it is also classified as a most important symptom of depression (APA: DSM-IV, 1994).

Food intake can be both a symptom and a factor in depression. Extremes of weight often result in depression. When clinical depression is diagnosed, food intake can certainly be a factor in a client's recovery. Taking steps to eat regularly and in moderate amounts can help a client recover from both psychological and physical symptoms.

CASE EXAMPLE ·

Anna, an 80-year-old immigrant from Norway, attended a nutrition program for the elderly. She had recently lost her husband. She was frail and depressed and was losing weight. The consultant registered dietitian noticed that she rarely ate her meal at the center, and learned through questioning her that she ate little at home also. The first counseling strategy of the dietitian was to sit next to Anna at meal time, to eat something along with her, and to encourage Anna to eat. When the dietitian felt she had gained enough rapport, she asked Anna to agree to eat something at home in the evening, which Anna did, every day for a week. Anna reported that she felt better and a bit stronger. At this point, the dietitian suggested to the social worker that it might be timely to address the depression issue directly.

· ·

People who are depressed almost universally express low self-esteem and report having been unmotivated for several months. Grievers are more likely to have a low or angry mood and may see the world as impoverished, but they do not see themselves as impoverished. Many authors described this attitude as *grieving* rather than depression. The distinction is important because people with low self-esteem are especially in need of counseling strategies to raise their feelings of self-worth before they will be motivated to change. A person grieving over loss of health or impending death needs empathy and patience as he or she works through adjustments.

Implications for Medical Nutrition Therapy

Simply listening to the client express her or his emotions is the first line of treatment for depression. After that, efforts to point out evidence that the client is not helpless, hopeless, or powerless may help mobilize clients to do something. Doing something subsequently helps to bring about recognition of power and control. In some very debilitating diseases, such as terminal cancer, doing something about food intake may be the only avenue of control and power the individual has left, and changes in food intake can have ramifications on the entire emotional outlook of such patients.

The MNT needs to be alert to events to which the normal response is depression and be prepared to respond appropriately to clients. Bereavement and threatened bereavement, physical illness, and in general all losses of sources of self-esteem lead to depression. In addition, events that change significant routines and interpersonal relations, such as marriage, births, and changing jobs or domicile sometimes result in symptoms of depression. Losses are more likely to occur in middle-aged or older individuals and may be a more important factor in depression among the elderly than among younger people. Post-traumatic stress, the response to a stressor that would be markedly distressing to almost anyone, is usually experienced with intense fear, terror, and helplessness that may settle into depression. Heart attacks, strokes, emergency surgery, and acts of violence are examples of events after which the intensity of feelings has major implications for the way in which a client is approached. Post-trauma is a very likely time for MNTs to become included in a case team. Dietitians in acute-care institutions need to be acutely aware of the likelihood that their patients are experiencing post-traumatic stress. The stages of change model discussed in Chapter 5 is an excellent reference to use in guiding the approach to patients.

For instance, a diagnosis of diabetes, a life-threatening disease, is very likely to result in some symptoms of depression. Weight-control regimens are also likely to result in depression because of the necessity to control, some degree of loss of routine food habits and foods, and the slowness of change in weight. Responding appropriately and recognizing the situations in which referral is needed is an important factor in a satisfactory outcome of medical nutrition therapy.

Since significant levels of emotional intensity result in diminished capacity, it often falls to the dietetic practitioner to address symptoms presented during a therapy session and to have a sense of situations in which a referral is needed (Ryan & Shea, 1996). Encouraging the client to talk about feelings can help reduce the level of intensity in an immediate situation, and in many cases no intervention is needed other than listening. Instructing a client to take some deep breaths may also be useful in reducing intense feelings.

It is not the function of the MNT to help the person understand why she or he is depressed. However, since disturbed eating behavior is frequently a symptom of depression, the MNT might need to help a client choose alternative behaviors to replace eating as a response mechanism to feelings of depression.

LOSS AND GRIEF

Life events have expected emotional results, since each event entails both a gain and a loss. Many psychologists consider grief to be a part of the adjustment to any loss in life. Others consider that even desirable events such as marriage, getting a new job, or achieving a goal can lead to depression because the loss of an old routine is involved. Still others recognize that change of any sort brings about a loss of structure as a person moves from one set of habits to another, and postulate that grief and depression are the adjustment to loss of structure.

Each person you see as an MNT has likely experienced a significant event related to nutrition and also in some other aspects of life. The nutrition lifestyle is only one aspect of the entire lifestyle. The MNT needs to keep in mind that there are times when changes in nutrition lifestyle are not a priority. Other concerns and issues need to be resolved before nutrition is addressed. Times of significant losses rank among situations in which deferring medical nutrition therapy may be appropriate.

Even in situations in which it is important to address nutrition, the MNT needs to regard the client and the situation holistically. A healthy person deciding to change a nutrition lifestyle will feel the loss of old eating habits, which were part of the structure of their lives. For people who have suffered a loss of good health and have received a diagnosis of a life-threatening disease, the treatment of which entails modification of lifestyle, the pattern of reconciliation will be much the same as the process of grieving for the loss of life, and it may lead to depression. Furthermore, elderly patients face other losses, such as loss of self-esteem because they are no longer working or have diminished incomes, or the loss of family and friends.

Two models of loss and grief are described in this chapter, the Kübler-Ross model of death and dying and Leming and Dickinson's description of stress reaction to loss.

Death and Dying

Working on nutrition support teams was probably the first situation in which dietetic practitioners began to recognize their role in helping patients deal with death and dying. This recognition has spread to all of those who provide nutritional care or medical nutrition therapy to dying patients and their families. Indeed, awareness is developing that the processes by which the dying cope with the loss of everything, even their lives, are also used by people who have suffered a loss of health. Understanding these processes will increase sensitivity, communication skills, and the wisdom with which you face the dying patient (Kübler-Ross, 1975).

Perceptions of Death and Dying

There is often a conspiracy of silence among personnel who work with the dying. It is probably an attempt at denial that fails to hide the prognosis of death, and, at the same time, tends to isolate the patient and prevent the supportive environment that the patient needs. Interactions are stilted and uncomfortable, which makes facing death more difficult for the patient.

Changing this situation requires both an intellectual examination of death and dying and a personal examination of one's own beliefs, attitudes, and feelings about death. Death and dying is not pleasant for anyone, yet to become an effective MNT, you must come to grips with the place of death in life. Becoming more aware of general human responses to the prospect of death, your own response to the contemplation of your own death, and your response to the dying client is part of counseling competency.

Death, the last scene in the drama of life, comes in many ways. Each person's story is her or his own, just as is the rest of life. Death can be sudden or slowly drawn out, painful or peaceful, from a clearly defined disease, or from old age. Most people fantasize about their deaths, and want a "good" death, whatever that may be (Nuland, 1994). The scenario of death in which the MNT is likely to play a role is that of a patient with a terminal illness, or that of a patient who dies slowly from general disintegration of the life forces. When people who have a terminal illness are cognizant of what is happening, they have the opportunity to experience the stages of dying that are described by Kübler-Ross. If they are not cognizant, such as in Alzheimer's disease, or if they die suddenly or unexpectedly, it is the family and caregivers who may experience the stages of dying as stages of grief. When people are diagnosed with a life-threatening illness, they may experience some or all of the stages of grief, even though death is not imminent.

Elisabeth Kübler-Ross on Death and Dying

Elisabeth Kübler-Ross, MD, is unquestionably the most prominent pioneer in the psychology of death and dying and in helping health-care professionals understand the phenomenon of loss with which we all so often work. Dietetic practitioners recently have begun to recognize their responsibility in coping with death and dying and helping dying patients and their families meet the challenges they face in this facet of human growth and development. Ethical issues may arise in terms of feeding dying patients, but more frequently MNTs face the issue of psychological support in addition to provision of food. The next few pages address the Kübler-Ross theoretical concepts of the processes involved when people die from long-term illness, and offer some perspectives on the role of MNTs in providing care.

In setting the stage for the processes through which people journey toward death from long-term disease, Kübler-Ross described the attitudes toward death that are prominent in this country. Technology has tended to make death remote, because dying people are most frequently removed from the family setting. There is a pervasive attitude of denial and attempts to master death, as if we could eventually overcome it altogether (Kübler-Ross, 1975). For instance, we talk of preventing heart disease and cutting down on deaths from heart disease, as if those who would be rescued from dying of heart disease would not die at all, or even become sick. Furthermore, we tend to blame people for their illness. Such attitudes result in a health-care system that is poorly equipped to help dying people and their families face this stage of life (Nuland, 1994). These attitudes make it difficult for the elderly, whose habits have been classed as "bad" retrospectively, and especially devastating for young people, such as those with AIDS.

Humans have always feared death and thought of it as an outside force, a frightening happening. The unconscious mind has difficulty accepting non-existence, and therefore, death is the most fearsome and ultimately undesirable of all possible horrifying events. A basic denial of one's mortality is a necessary defense in living.

Death is a taboo subject for discussion, and references to death are generally oblique. "If something happens to me . . ." is said rather than "If I should die. . . ." Avoiding talk of death has become pronounced in American society, in which death from acute disease has become rare, and most of us expect to live long and healthily. Tolerance for grief is also low. We expect the grieving to get back to work within a few days. Indeed, when a socially unacceptable death occurs, some people regard grieving at all with disdain (Nuland, 1994).

The stages of dying, as described by Kübler-Ross, include denial, anger, bargaining, depression, and acceptance. Kübler-Ross does not see these stages as progressions in a straight line, but more as a dynamic model in which a person moves among the various stages. Other theorists have described the process as a range of emotions felt by the individual as opposed to sequential stages (Purtilo & Haddad, 1996). Kübler-Ross (1969) also recognized that not all people enter all stages and that a person may move very quickly or slowly through stages. Some people may experience all stages in one day; others get stuck in one stage and stay there. Variables that play a part in this dynamic move through the stages include personality (how one deals with the problems of life is usually similar to how one deals with the problems of death), the quality of the support system, and the duration of the illness. So, in some ways, the model is a description of a desirable process of growth and development in this the last important life process.

Denial and Isolation

For the individual who has been diagnosed with a terminal illness, there is a need to establish a buffer against the shocking news that will allow the person time to collect himself or herself, and as time passes develop other less radical defenses with which to face his or her own personal death. The first reaction to the news that one is suffering from a fatal illness is usually "No, not me." There are a number of ways of acting this out. One is to go from doctor to doctor to faith healers to religion or to any other "authority," such as a nutrition quack, who might help with the denial. Another way that people use denial is to refuse to talk about dying and to refuse treatment. Instead, people will make plans for the future, perhaps pretend they are cured, and take on a false gaiety. The use of food and diet may also be a method of denying impending death. People may be vulnerable to nutrition treatments that promise cure, they may refuse appropriate nutritional treatment, or they may insist that a dietary regimen they are following is curing them in spite of evidence to the contrary. An example that Kübler-Ross used was that of a young woman with terminal liver disease who refused the appropriate dietary treatment even though her food intake frequently resulted in pain and suffering and at times led to a comatose state. Dr. Kübler-Ross described her approach as one of never contradicting the patient when she insisted that she was getting better, yet refusing to help her deny her illness by insisting that she follow her diet. "There were days when she stuffed herself with forbidden foods, only to suffer twice as much the next days. This was intolerable and we told her so. This was a part of reality that we could not deny with her." (Kübler-Ross, 1969, p. 123). This was the method used by Kübler-Ross and her staff to tell the patient implicitly that she was dying because they did not think she would tolerate being told explicitly. Kübler-Ross went further, describing the overeating of forbidden foods as suicide attempts, indicating a fluctuation between denial and a wish to get death accomplished. This example highlights the multifaceted meanings of food and the sensitivity needed by a MNT involved with dying patients.

Implications for Medical Nutrition Therapy. Some of the following indicate that a patient is in the denial stage.

> Seeking "healers" and miracle cures
> Believing that a diagnosis is in error
> Refusing nutrition treatment or counseling
> Talking about the illness as if it is insignificant

Caretakers and friends who are also in the denial stage frequently avoid the dying person, making things worse. During this stage, the role of the MNT is to develop rapport. The Stages of Change Model (Chap. 5) would suggest that the client is in the precontemplation stage, a time to refrain from putting pressure on the client to change.

Anger

When the "not me" denial can no longer be maintained, "why me?" becomes the question, and anger, rage, envy, and resentment envelop the patient and the environs. This is a difficult stage for caretakers, because the anger is directed toward them, often without justification. Food and diet are often a target of the dissatisfaction being felt, and the dietetic practitioner becomes involved either in an inpatient setting or in counseling the individual and family. The patient becomes intolerant, and it is often only real understanding of anger as a natural aspect of dying that will provide caretakers with enough motivation to continue visiting the patient and to continue efforts to provide the attention and respect so badly needed by the patient.

Implications for Medical Nutrition Therapy. Anger is very hard for caretakers of dying people because they tend to take the anger personally. The patient may ask for special food and then not like it, complain about the service, even if the food is fine, or in other ways find fault with even the most intensive effort to be pleasing. Food and nutrition may be a weapon in dealing with anger toward death in a productive way. Control of one's food consumption may be a way of keeping control in a world where one is losing control of everything. The dying person, especially one in the hospital, may focus on controlling his or her diet as a last grasp on self-control. Tactics that include pressuring the patient to eat "properly" are likely to result in anger and rebellion. Patience and allowing the patient time to reconcile his or her feelings are more likely to result in a practical decision to accept a nutritional change, and also serve to assist a patient to move forward in the process of dying.

As in the denial stage, the MNT's role is generally to maintain rapport with the client. The task of maintaining rapport is not easy and may depend upon the ability of the MNT to keep her or his own emotions calm and cool. If the MNT recognizes that his or her own feelings are intense and uncomfortable, she or he needs to obtain help. The following case example provides one way in which this stage can be resolved.

CASE EXAMPLE ·

A 75-year-old woman with diabetes, recovering from open heart surgery in a rehabilitation facility, seemed to be moving through the process of dying as described by Kübler-Ross. She was angry, would not eat hospital foods, and was getting candy brought in by friends. Her blood glucose level ranged between 200 and 300 and could not be controlled by oral medication. The patient berated both the physician and the dietitian; she wanted to die. The only time of the day that she became calm was when her granddaughter, who had just come to live with her, visited. In consultation, the physician and MNT made the following plan for encouraging the woman, who was not physiologically dying, to enjoy life again. They discussed the presence of the granddaughter as motivation for living, deciding that in spite of patient protest, insulin would be prescribed to control blood glucose during the hospitalization; the granddaughter would be asked to become involved in medical nutrition therapy, and follow-up medical nutrition therapy would be arranged when the patient went home. The patient did indeed realize that her granddaughter's presence was a reason for living. Reports from the MNT indicated that the social support in the home was having a positive effect on the woman's knowledge about nutrition care in diabetes, as well as on her general lifestyle.

· ·

Bargaining

The bargaining stage is described as recognition that anger and rage have been ineffective against death, and there is hope that maybe the inevitable can be postponed if postponement were asked for nicely. This attitude is not unlike that of a child who has thrown a tantrum to no avail and has begun to manipulate a parent by wheedling, simpering, and begging, "If only you'll let me, I promise to be good and do as I am told." In this case, the promise is to "die as I must." Bargaining includes promises to accept what is coming later for "just one more" and is an empty promise, with a new bargain ready as soon as a wish is granted.

Implications for Medical Nutrition Therapy. This is not a stage often observed by dietetic practitioners among dying people because it is often an internal process. However, in chronic disease states, it is common. There are situations in which bargaining occurs for just "one more chance" to enjoy some beloved food. More often than not the wished-for food is not enjoyed after all. In inpatient settings, it can result in resentment among the staff for "trying so hard to please the patient" and then not being appreciated or being concerned that a "forbidden" food might cause harm.

CASE EXAMPLE ·

A young woman of 16, on dialysis and ineligible for a kidney transplant, was close to death. She may have made her bargain to die gracefully in a food-related method. One day during medical nutrition therapy, as she was undergoing dialysis, this conversation took place.

C L I E N T: "You know, I've been eating almost nothing. Do you think a nice slice of apple pie with cheese would hurt me?" (she knows the answer to this question already).

M N T: "What do you think?"

C L I E N T: "If you'd just tell me I could have it I wouldn't ask again. Maybe you'd even bring me some from the cafeteria. I promise I'll be good if you'll just do that for me."

M N T: "It means a great deal to you, doesn't it?"

C L I E N T: "Yes, oh, please, it would be so good."

In this case, the MNT brought the requested pie. The patient ate two bites of the pie and reported that it tasted good, gave the MNT a hug, and finished the dialysis. The next day she died.

· ·

In this example, it cannot be known for sure that the client was bargaining, but it is clear that what she was asking of the MNT was to grant a dying wish. It may be that this patient died in the bargaining stage, or perhaps as the result of the interchange came to an acceptance stage.

Depression

When energy for denial, anger, and bargaining can no longer be mustered, the dying patient will have a rising sense of loss that is felt keenly. Loss may be felt in every facet of life as the patient recognizes all of the many things he or she must surrender, until finally everything, including life, will be lost. Physical attributes will be lost through surgery or through the ravages of disease, and in almost all cases financial losses will be significant if not disastrous. Patients who are breadwinners may have great stress from their inability to provide for their families, while older people may lose their homes and possessions and, in fact, feel guilty that they have nothing to leave their children.

In addition, the patient must grieve in preparation for his or her loss of life. Too much "cheering up" by friends, family, and professionals can prevent the dying person from reconciling the loss of all loved ones, all lost opportunities to have lived differently, and loss of all potential for the future.

During this phase it is important to allow expression of depression and sorrow with responses that let the patient know that it is acceptable to be sad. Often no response at all is needed except presence, a touch of the hand, or minimal verbal acknowledgment that you are receiving the message. It is necessary for patients to work through this stage successfully if they are to die in the stage of acceptance.

Those attending the patient, including the MNT, usually find this stage and the last stage of acceptance very difficult because the urge to "do something" for the patient is strong. Our own guilt feelings may arise from a sense of being helpless over our own loss of control in the face of death. We are in anguish over missed opportunities to do something for the patient before it is too late (Nuland, 1994).

Implications for Medical Nutrition Therapy. During this stage, a patient often is not hungry and not satisfied by food. Rather than proceeding with medical nutrition therapy or pressuring patients to eat, energy should be focused on helping families cope with losing their loved one and helping them to stop "trying." The MNT may need to let go of the patient also. Caretakers have difficulty discontinuing efforts to maintain life for the patient; yet in many situations, if the dying person is to finish the process of dying with dignity, discontinuation of efforts is the greatest gift that caretakers can give (Nuland, 1994). Nutrition counseling per se is probably rarely conducted. However, counseling techniques are needed in helping a family realize that the patient is probably not in pain from lack of food, even though she or he is drinking and eating little or nothing. This can have a significant effect in letting people know that they have done all that they could and give them "permission" to stop. One of the points of concern with friends, family, and medical professionals is that they have "done everything possible" for the patient. Dietitians who work in facilities where people die frequently have the opportunity for this kind of counseling as members of teams in which care decisions of a life-and-death nature are made.

Patients who are depressed will respond to nutrition care with little enthusiasm much of the time. The following case example describes one dietitian's sensitivity to the patient's needs in a holistic manner.

CASE EXAMPLE ·

The dietitian visited the bedside of a 30-year-old man in the last stages of AIDS. His tray had been returning to the kitchen largely untouched. Upon arriving at his bedside, she detected that he was depressed and unenergized.

C L I E N T: "I just can't eat the food. Nothing agrees with me except chocolate pudding."

M N T: "Would you eat some chocolate pudding if I sent some to you?"

C L I E N T: "Yes, I'd eat some chocolate pudding every hour if you would send me a supply. I get so full that I can only eat a little at a time. I'd really feel good about that."

The patient did eat chocolate pudding every hour for the next 4 days, ignoring his regular meals. The fifth day he began to eat a little of the food on his tray. He ate chocolate pudding the rest of his life, diminishing in quantity only during the last 3 days before he died.

• •

The dietitian recognized the responsibility to respond to the patient's needs in a broader sense than strictly nutritional needs. The decision had already been made not to prolong life with enteral or parenteral feedings, and there was no need to become concerned over the nutritional value of his diet. She could sense that his soul was better fed with chocolate pudding.

Acceptance

Acceptance of death results from the passage of time as the patient slowly comes to contemplate death as an expected, and even desirable, event. It does not seem to be a resigned and hopeless stage, but rather a peaceful time of letting go of the world. Not eating is often an important part of this stage. It is often not recognized that giving up food, that is, the loss of the pleasure of food, as well as the sustenance that food brings, may be a significant part of the process of dying. Those who do not understand the acceptance phase of dying may continue to press patients to eat. There are also ethical issues that often involve the participation of dietetic practitioners in questions of feeding and hydrating patients. There is a great need for professionals to pay attention to what patients have to say about their wishes during this stage. It is often the family that needs support more than the patient, so that they can let go of the patient and help him or her to die in peace rather than with a sense of failing the family by not living any longer. It is important to help family members recognize that they need to look beyond their own needs to those of the patient as death approaches.

There seems to be a real difference in the way that the very old accept death as compared with the young, who may feel as if they are being cheated of a part of their lives. Not all people progress through all of the stages, but more could if those around them became aware of the process and the responses that can help patients work through the stages, enabling them to die in peace and dignity.

Implications for Medical Nutrition Therapy. At the end of a long-term illness, friends and family often gather to share the time for dying. It may not be a time when the medical nutrition therapist is likely to be part of the scene. However, it is a time to say good-bye to the patient if your relationship with the person calls for it. Often, very close relationships are formed during the course of a long illness. Sharing good-byes with the patient and the family is respectful of the acceptance of death and can help bring about closure or completion for you and for those involved.

Stages of Dying as Compared to a Stress Response

Others have set forth concepts regarding the process of coping with dying which also are of value in working with dying people. Leming and Dickinson (1985) used the basic physiological stress-response processes of anticipation, onset of a stressful event, disorganization, organization, and resolution to help understand dying. Following is a summary of their concepts.

Anticipation

Very early in childhood, each of us, in a remote way, has learned of death and recognized that each of us will die sometime. The way in which each of us anticipates personal death, this most difficult of all things to imagine, is culture-bound, usually limited to intellectual activity, and often based primarily in fear of the unknown. When we develop symptoms of illness that are commonly known to be related to fatal illness, or when we have symptoms that we do not understand, we usually develop a heightened state of anticipation that the diagnosis of our problems will be "a death sentence."

The patient may anticipate the possibility of a foreseeable death with a mixture of emotions; anxiety, curiosity, even excitement that another stage of life is about to begin. There is probably little focus on nutrition in this process. It is probably not appropriate to conduct medical nutrition therapy at this time.

Onset of a Stressful Event

When the moment arrives that the most feared diagnosis is confirmed, the result is shock. The individual perceives a threat, and defenses must be raised to prevent the person from being overwhelmed by the unthinkable. Denial is almost always the initial response.

Physical symptoms of stress or shock include the following (Mason, 1985):

- The heartbeat increases to pump blood throughout the necessary tissues with greater speed, carrying oxygen and nutrients to cells and clearing away waste products more quickly.
- As the heart rate increases, the blood pressure rises.
- Breathing becomes rapid and shallow.
- Adrenaline and other hormones are released into the blood.
- The liver releases stored sugar into the blood to meet the increased energy needs of survival.
- The pupils dilate to let in more light; all the senses are heightened.
- Muscles tense for movement, either for flight or protective actions, particularly the skeletal muscles of the thighs, hips, back, shoulders, arms, jaw, and face.
- Blood flow is greatly constricted to the digestive organs.
- Blood flow increases to the brain and major muscles.
- Blood flow is constricted to the extremities, and the hands and feet become cold. This protects you from bleeding to death quickly if the hands or feet are injured in fight or flight, and allows blood to be diverted to more important areas of the body.
- The body perspires to cool itself, since increased metabolism generates more heat.

This physiological stress-reaction may happen when bad news (a threat to life) is received, even though it is not needed as it is when a physical threat occurs. This is not the time for medical nutrition therapy, yet it is not uncommon for the MNT to be called upon to conduct a nutrition consultation; for instance, after a patient has been told he is at high risk for a heart attack. A patient may initially respond with a demeanor of compliance. This attitude is rarely long-lasting because the patient probably was not able to listen, so remembers little. In addition, when the immediate threat of death is over, motivations other than fear of death are needed to make changes in nutrition lifestyle.

Disorganization

As denial begins to fail and awareness increases, a set of physiological processes occurs that produces signs of physical distress, a breakdown of logical thought, distorted feelings, and changes in interactive behavior. Those who suffer overtly are more likely to receive comfort than silent sufferers because it is almost impossible for others to ignore an obviously distraught individual.

Implications for Medical Nutrition Therapy. When a person is in a stage of disorganization, which many are as they face the confusing task of dying or adjusting to a life-threatening disease, she or he will probably respond to direct interventions better than to more ambivalent strategies that help a person become aware of long-term solutions. The patient/client will be relieved by being told some things to do for the short run; the long run can be dealt with at a later time.

Organization

As this stage occurs, individuals begin to take stock of their resources, begin to realize that they have work to do before they die, and realize that they are still living. They can no longer tolerate their own disorganization. During this stage, energy is turned to completing the task of dying as well as possible. Often communication with others with more experience in dying, or with professionals, is sought as the individual searches for adequate resolution.

Implications for Medical Nutrition Therapy. This stage is most productive for gaining client commitment to reasonable changes. The rigidity of nutrition lifestyle is disease-specific, and related to the expected longevity. For instance, people with end-stage renal disease are faced with the need for very limited food choices.

Resolution

A person who has reached resolution can be thought of as feeling a sense of accomplishment, perhaps even a sense of exhilaration and invulnerability, no longer fearing death. Often, the adequacy of the support system is a major factor in the ability of people to reach this stage.

Implications for Medical Nutrition Therapy. Counseling parallels those ideas discussed following the Kübler-Ross model.

Dying

Summary of Implications for Medical Nutrition Therapy. Both models of the process of dying have implications for dietetic practitioners. The stage in which patients are working toward completing the tasks of their lives has a significant impact on the success of medical nutrition therapy. Patients who are in shock/denial are likely to reject nutrition information. When a patient is in the stage of disorganization, the logical processes necessary to assimilate nutrition information and put it to practice are likely to be lacking. Patients who are in the organization stage may well be receptive and eager to listen to nutrition education and to consider nutrition lifestyle changes as an effective way of continuing to live fully during the time they have left. As part of the needed support system for patients in the resolution stages, dietetic practitioners function to reassure patients, allowing the patient's desires regarding eating to be the determining factor in how nutrition care is handled, either through counseling or feeding. In all stages, awareness and strategies to support the patient through times when she or he is receptive, as well as when she or he is not receptive to nutrition education and counseling, need to be in the repertoire of the MNT. This requires self-discipline. The desire to help can lead to anxiety resulting in poor timing in the presentation of either ideas or food.

Another factor in which the relationship between the MNT and patient may be affected is the cause-and-effect relationship that may be perceived when a person is dying from a disease that may have a diet-related cause. Many "if only" thoughts may plague patients and families, and result in complex judgmental guilt and anxiety (Leming & Dickerson, 1985). For instance, a woman with terminal breast cancer may be dealing with guilt from a lifetime of consuming high-fat foods, or resentment at getting breast cancer even though she ate a low-fat diet most of her life. Rebellion about specific nutrition prescriptions, experimentation with extreme diets, or productive attempts to sensibly control the diet may all result from efforts to cope with dying. A very positive way that people can deal with the inevitable loss of health and control over one's life is to eat nutritiously—it is a wonderful way to care for oneself during this time. Food is sometimes one of the very last things that is finally given up by patients. At some point, eating favorite foods seems to be an expression of still living, still wanting pleasure, still able to control what is accepted into the body. Among the elderly who seem to be dying because the body has worn out rather than from any well-defined disease, refusing to eat is often a signal that the work of giving up worldly things has been completed and they have accepted death.

Coping with Living Among Dying People

In a discussion of coping with the dying patient, it is appropriate to remember that every person is still living until they have died, and treating the living as if they are living is important. Rainey and coauthors identified adaptive and maladaptive behaviors that may be expected among persons with a diagnosis of terminal cancer. These are described in Table 8–4. This chart is best used as a guide for likely responses rather than as a tool to use for specific patient behavior expectations.

TABLE 8–4

Adaptive and Maladaptive Behavioral Responses by Phase of Illness (Terminal Cancer)

Normal: Adaptive Behavior	Abnormal: Maladaptive Behavior
Prediagnostic Phase	
Constant or overconcern with the possibility of having cancer	Development of cancer's symptoms without having the disease
Denial of the disease's presence and delay in seeking treatment	
Diagnostic Phase	
Shock	Complete denial with refusal of treatment
Disbelief	Fatalistic refusal of treatment on the basis
Initial, partial denial	that death is inevitable
Anxiety	Search for other opinions or unproved
Anger, hostility, persecutory feelings	("quack") cures
Depression	
Initial Treatment Phase	
Surgery	
Grief reaction to changes in body image	Postoperative reaction depression
Postponement of surgery	Severe, prolonged grief reaction to changes
Search for nonsurgical alternatives	in body image
Radiotherapy	
Fear of x-ray machine and side effects	
Fear of being abandoned	Psychotic-like delusions or hallucinations
Chemotherapy	
Fear of side effects	Residual drug-induced psychoses
Changes in body image	Severe isolation-induced psychotic distur-
Anxiety, isolation	bances
Altruistic feelings and desire to donate body or organs to science	Severe paranoia
Follow-up Phase	
Return to normal coping patterns	Mild depression and anxiety
Fear of recurrence	
Recurrence and Retreatment Phase	
Shock	
Disbelief	Reactive depression with insomnia,
Partial denial	anorexia, restlessness, anxiety, and irri-
Anxiety	tability
Anger	
Depression	
At Point of Progressing Disease	
Frenzied search for new information, other consultants, and quack cures begins	Depression
Terminal-Palliation Phase	
Fear of abandonment at death by others, pain, shortness of breath, and facing the unknown	Depression
Personal mourning with anticipation of death and a degree of acceptance	Acute delirium

From Rainey LC, Wellisch DK, Fawzy I, et al: Training health professionals in psychosocial aspects of cancer: A continuing education model. *J Psychosoc Oncol.* 1983; 1:41–60.

Abandonment is a realistic fear that people with prolonged terminal illnesses have, as related by Purtilo and Haddad (1996, p. 366–367).

> . . the first weeks following a person's [hospitalization] are attended by flowers, cards, numerous visitors, and constant encouragement. But the able-bodied grow weary. Their responsibilities are many and varied. They are disillusioned by the afflicted person's inability to return to the real world of involvement, independence, and responsibility. Sometimes they are even angry that the afflicted person "refuses" to come back home where she or he "belongs," or return to the job in order to lighten the work load. Then, just about the time the [terminally ill] person comes to full grips with the stunning reality . . . the room is bare, the phone silent and the flowers have long since wilted."

Supportive relationships often taper off, leaving the dying to die alone. As a result, health-care professionals may need to see a patient even when it is not warranted on a professional service basis. A brief "hello, how are you feeling today?" or a caring touch serves as a much needed human contact. Sometimes a phone call after discharge is a good source of comfort and encouragement.

The family is not a group merely to be tolerated by professionals. They are an integral part of the team (Purtilo & Haddad, 1996). If a patient has several family members who come into the picture as death gets closer, the MNT will discover that these newcomers to the scene are not in the same stage of grieving as those who have been there longer. It will be important to allow each person his or her own process. This means that sometimes things that have been decided will have to be decided again. The MNT and the entire team need patience in working with all the different individuals as each works through the process in his or her own manner.

CASE EXAMPLE ·

The patient was a 91-year-old woman who was deteriorating bit by bit. Her children had worked together with each other and the medical professionals over the years making decisions to let their mother die as naturally and peacefully as possible. Yet, during the last days of her life, when the extended family came together, several of the newcomers expressed strong feelings and concerns that everything possible was not being done for her. One was particularly concerned that the patient was not receiving nourishment. Fortunately, the family and the health-care team, including an MNT, were able to retrace the decision-making course and treatment strategies used thus far. This helped the entire family spend their last moments with the patient satisfactorily.

· ·

Interactions to Avoid

When a patient is expressing concern about his or her situation it is best *not* to say things such as "Oh, everything will be OK" or, "I'm sure you have nothing serious."

Other platitudes often heard that are nonsupportive are such statements as "Now, now, don't cry" and "I'm sure things are not all that bad."

It is nonsupportive to ignore a patient's discussion of what may be troubling him or her. A patient will feel ignored if the MNT insists on talking about the diet when the patient is expressing emotion and concern.

It is important not to tell the patient something you know that he or she may not already have been told. Often silence and a listening stance are all the patient needs as a sign of support.

After a Patient/Client Dies

Little has been written for the MNT for guidance after a patient or client dies. Especially during the care of a patient who has suffered a long-term illness, a very caring relationship can develop between the MNT and the patient. When the death of that patient occurs, the effect on the MNT can be intense. The MNT needs to be aware that she or he also needs to go through the process of grieving. Emotional support is often needed at this time. To whom should one turn for support? How is closure accomplished? How are respect and condolence expressed to the family? There are no definite answers to these questions. They depend on the MNT's own personality, views on death, and relationship with the patient and the family.

One of the authors worked with pediatric oncology patients for many years. In the beginning, she did not allow herself to become too close to any of the patients, knowing that they would probably die. As time passed, she became more accepting of this process of care and came to love many children who eventually died. Each time, the grieving process was present but different, depending on the particular relationship that had developed. One adolescent boy, who died of complications of a bone marrow transplant for leukemia, came to her house often over the course of years of hospitalizations, and the patient gave her son his Nintendo game set to play with while he was away getting his transplant. This was years before Nintendo was wildly popular and was a unique treasure at that time. He never returned for it and she has since given it (with permission from his mother) to another patient she treated. Whatever the level of involvement is with the person, some degree of loss will be felt by all who participated in care. The pediatric oncology nurses (a rare breed!) were a great source of emotional support and guidance throughout the courses of patients' illnesses and deaths. Social workers and fellow dietetic practitioners can also be part of good support systems.

Closure is also important. What is appropriate and satisfying depends on the MNT and his or her relationship with the person who died. Condolence cards, flowers, and prayers can be given to the family, and funerals can be attended. The authors have gone to a number of funerals of clients throughout the years. As well as serving as a vehicle for completion with the person who died, funerals are also rich in cultural nuances. Much can be learned about how differently death is processed from culture to culture.

Summary

Emotional responses are a normal element in the decision to change a nutrition lifestyle, whether by choice or in the treatment of illness. Anxiety and depression are among the most troubling responses. Although they are not mutually exclusive, anxiety is generally expressed by symptoms of agitation and increased activity. Depression is generally expressed by slowed reaction and an appearance of melancholy. The overt expression is the one that the MNT should address initially. If the intensity of emotion is not easily reduced, the MNT needs to consult with a psychotherapist or refer the client to the attending physician.

For those who die from a long illness, there is time for an orderly process for this last stage of life. Kübler-Ross described the stages of denial, anger, bargaining, depression, and acceptance. Leming and Dickinson described stages of anticipation, onset of a stressful event, disorganization, organization, and resolution.

The dying person, caretakers, and friends go through these processes. During the final stages, the dietetic practitioner may need to provide support for those still living more than for the dying person. When working with people who are dying or who have recently lost a loved one, it is important to be aware of where they are in the process of dealing with loss and to appropriately time nutrition interventions.

Suggestions for Further Learning

1. In small groups, discuss the feelings of anxiety and depression. Write words that best fit these feelings. Compare them among yourselves and to the material in the book.

2. In groups of three, act out feelings of anxiety and depression that might be expressed in a medical nutrition therapy session. Role-play client and counselor. The third group member observes. After the role-play, the "counselor" should first disclose her perceptions, then the "client," then the observer.

3. In a mock session or practice setting, use intervention techniques that may help reduce anxiety, depression, or feeling levels in a dying patient. Take note of the effect of the interventions. Compare them to situations in which you or someone else may have used less effective interventions.

4. As a group, discuss experience, beliefs, and attitudes about death and dying.

CITED REFERENCES

American Psychiatric Association: *Diagnostic and Statistical Manual of Mental Disorders.* 4th ed. Washington, DC: American Psychiatric Association, 1994.

Arnold A, Boggs KU: *Interpersonal Relationships: Professional Communication Skills for Nurses.* Philadelphia: WB Saunders, 1995.

Beck AT, Emery G, Greenberg A: *Anxiety Disorders and Phobias: A Cognitive Perspective.* New York: Basic Books, 1985.

Costello CG: *Anxiety and Depression: The Adaptive Emotions.* Montreal, Canada: McGill-Queen's University Press, 1976.

de Rosis HA: *Women and Anxiety: A Step-by-step Program to Manage Your Anxieties and Depressions.* New York: Delacorte Press, 1979.

Kendall PS, Watson D (eds): *Anxiety and Depression: Distinctive Overlapping Features.* San Diego: Academic Press, 1989.

Kubler-Ross E: *Death, the Final Stage of Growth.* Englewood Cliffs, NJ: Prentice-Hall, 1975.

Kubler-Ross E: *On Death and Dying.* New York: MacMillan, 1969.

Last CG (ed): *Anxiety Across the Lifespan: A Developmental Perspective.* New York: Springer Publishing Co, 1993.

Leming MR, Dickinson GE: *Understanding Dying, Death, and Bereavement.* Fort Worth, TX: Holt, Rinehart and Winston, 1985.

Leon AC, Portera L, Weissman MM: The social costs of anxiety disorders. *Br J Psych.* 1995;166(suppl 27):19–22.

Levine: *Eating Disorders.* Continuing Education, Baptist Hospital, Miami, FL; April 1996.

Mason LJ: *Guide to Stress Reduction.* Berkeley, CA: Celestial Arts, 1985.

Nuland SB: *How We Die: Reflections on Life's Final Chapter.* New York: Alfred A. Knopf, 1994.

Purtilo R, Haddad A: *Health Professional and Patient Interaction.* 5th ed. Philadelphia: WB Saunders, 1996.

Purtilo RB: Similarities in patient response to chronic and terminal illness. *Phys Ther.* 1976;56:282.

Rainey LC, Wellisch DK, Fawzy I, et al: Training health professionals in psychological aspects of cancer: A continuing education model. *J Psychosoc Oncol.* 1983;1:41–60.

Ryan C, Shea ME: Recognizing depression in older adults: The role of the dietitian. *J Am Diet Assoc.* 1996;96(10):1042–1043.

Wolberg LR: *The Techniques of Psychotherapy.* 4th ed. Part 2. Philadelphia: Grune & Stratton, 1988.

ADDITIONAL REFERENCES

Ayd FJ (ed): *Mood Disorder: The world's major public health problem.* Baltimore: Ayd Medical Communications, 1978.

Barlow DH: *Anxiety and Its Disorders: The Nature and Treatment of Anxiety and Panic.* New York: The Guilford Press, 1988.

Beck AT: *Cognitive Therapy and the Emotional Disorders.* New York: International Universities Press, 1976.

Chaisson S, Maureen G (eds): *Depression in the Elderly: An Interdisciplinary Approach.* New York: John Wiley & Sons, 1985.

Dean A: *Depression in a Multidisciplinary Perspective.* New York: Brunner/Maxel, 1985.

Despelder LA, Strickland AL: *The Last Dance: Encountering Death and Dying.* 4th ed. Mountain View, CA: Mayfield Publishing Co, 1996.

Gallant DM, Simpson GM (eds): *Depression: Behavioral, Biochemical, Diagnostic and Treatment Concepts.* New York: Spectrum Publications, Inc, 1976.

Hulce M: *Women and Mental Health: New Directions for Change.* New York: Harrington Park Press, 1985.

Jack DC: *Silencing the Self: Women and Depression.* Cambridge, MA: Harvard University Press, 1991.

Kastenbaum R: *The Psychology of Death.* 2nd ed. New York: Springer Publishing Co, 1992.

Keitner GI (ed): *Depression and Families: Impact and Treatment.* Washington, DC: American Psychiatric Press, 1990.

Kendall PC, Watson D: *Anxiety and Depression: Distinctive and Overlapping Features.* San Diego, CA: Academic Press, 1989.

Kline NS (ed): *Factors in Depression.* New York: Raven Press, 1974.

Scharf M: *Unfinished Business: Pressure Point in the Lives of Women.* Garden City, NY: Doubleday & Co, 1980.

Taylor DB, Arnow B: *The Nature and Treatment of Anxiety Disorders.* New York: The Free Press, 1988.

Weissman MM, Paykel ES: *The Depressed Woman: A Study of Social Relationships.* Chicago: University of Chicago Press, 1974.

Wells KB: *Depression as a Tracer Condition for the National Study of Medical Care Outcomes: Background Review.* Santa Monica, CA: Rand, 1985.

CHAPTER 9

Eating Disorders

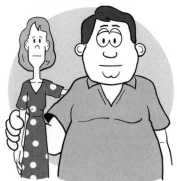

"...Jack Sprat's wife could eat no fat, and he could eat no lean, yet what they really needed was something in between..."

GOALS

The major goals of this chapter are (1) to review the historical background and current information on eating disorders, (2) to develop an understanding of the issues involved in counseling a person with an eating disorder, and (3) to discuss the implications for the MNT.

Learning Objectives

At the end of this chapter the reader will be able to:

1. Summarize current theories and facts about eating disorders.

2. Recognize warning signals of eating disorders.

3. Explain the diagnostic features of anorexia nervosa, bulimia nervosa, and binge eating disorders.

4. Describe nutrition counseling strategies and treatments used.

Key Terms

▶ Anorexia Nervosa: characterized by a refusal to maintain a minimally normal body weight as defined in the Diagnostic and Statistical Manual of Mental Disorders, 4th edition (DSM-IV).

▶ Binge: to eat an amount of food in a discrete period that is definitely larger than most people would eat in a similar period of time under similar circumstances as defined in DSM-IV.

▶ Binge Eating Disorder: characterized by recurrent episodes of uncontrolled eating, without purging or other compensatory behavior as defined in DSM-IV.

▶ Bulimia Nervosa: characterized by repeated episodes of binge eating followed by inappropriate compensatory behaviors as defined in DSM-IV.

▶ Eating Disorders: severe disturbances in eating behavior as defined in DSM-IV.

In recent years, the incidence of eating patterns that are contrary to good health has increased dramatically among Americans. Nutrition lifestyles that result in overweight or underweight are a significant problem. Increased weight among Americans conflicts with an enormous emphasis on being physically attractive in general and on being thin in particular. Siever (1994; p. 252) reports that "many observers have suggested that the enormous pressure placed on women to be physically attractive puts them at increased risk for developing eating disorders."

The current expectation of thinness in American society has led to questioning the distinction between "normal" eating and eating disorders. Ellyn Satter, a pioneer in nutrition counseling, described normal eating as follows in her 1987 book, *How to Get Your Kid to Eat . . . But Not Too Much* (pp. 69–70):

> Normal eating is being able to eat when you are hungry and continue eating until you are satisfied. It is being able to choose food you like and eat it and truly get enough of it—not just stop eating because you think you should. Normal eating is being able to use some moderate constraint in your food selection to get the right food, but not being so restrictive that you miss out on pleasurable foods. Normal eating is giving yourself permission to eat sometimes because you are happy, sad or bored, or just because it feels good. Normal eating is three meals a day, most of the time, but it can also be choosing to munch along. It is leaving some cookies on the plate because you can have some again tomorrow, or it is eating more now because they taste so wonderful when they are fresh. Normal eating is overeating at times; feeling stuffed and uncomfortable. It is also undereating at times and wishing you had more. Normal eating is trusting your body to make up for your mistakes in eating. Normal eating takes up some of your time and attention, but keeps its place as only one important area of your life.

In short, normal eating is flexible. It varies in response to your emotions, your schedule, your hunger, and your proximity to food. But this is not the way normal eating was described by Polivy and Herman (1987; p. 635). They pointed out in an article in the Journal of Consulting and Clinical Psychology that "a normal lifestyle now requires periodic exercise; normal eating now requires periodic dieting." It seems that society demands that a person eat enough to maintain an acceptable body size and no more. These expectations have so distorted attitudes toward weight, body image, and food that more people than not have developed disruptive eating patterns. Admiration for a thin physique and criticism for a rounded physique are pervasive enough that even people whose weight is within the recommended range are sometimes perceived and perceive themselves as overweight (Polivy & Herman, 1987).

A recent study indicated that registered dietitians do not differ from the public in their ability to perceive body weight accurately. Two thirds of the study participants of normal weight perceived themselves to be overweight (McArthur & Rose, 1997). An ideal body image that often is not possible, even for a very disciplined individual, has tended to distort both scientific and common-sense awareness of healthy food intake. The result has been the increase of disordered eating patterns to the point that eating disorder diseases have been identified and diagnostic criteria and treatment plans have been established.

Anorexia nervosa and bulimia nervosa are primarily psychological disorders and are discussed in detail in this chapter. Binge eating disorder is also discussed. Although it was not included as a full criteria set in the 1994 fourth edition of the Diagnostic and Statistical Manual of Mental Disorders (DSM-IV), binge eating disorder was included in the appendix as a disorder worthy of further study. Simple obesity is not explored in this chapter. It does not appear in the DSM-IV because "it is not clear that it is consistently associated with a psychological or behavioral syndrome" (APA, 1994).

Although considered to be mental disorders, eating disorders are notable for their nutrition-related aspects. For a person with disordered eating to fully recover, issues concerning food intake and related behaviors, body image, and weight regulation need to be resolved. This amounts to resolving the entire nutrition lifestyle. A medical nutrition therapy approach to a lifestyle change is appropriate. The MNT is the logical member of the treatment team to address nutrition lifestyle issues with people recovering from eating disorders. The American Dietetic Association (ADA, 1994; p. 902) stated in the position paper on nutrition intervention in the treatment of anorexia nervosa, bulimia nervosa, and binge eating disorder that "those who treat persons with eating disorders should be cognizant of the psychological and nutritional aspects of eating disorders throughout the recovery process."

Throughout this text, emphasis has been placed on understanding the multidimensional aspects of food consumption, client behavior, and change. It is especially important in this context of counseling people with eating disorders that the skills of counseling and the confidence to deal with emotional issues be employed. The problem-solving method is an appropriate approach. A dietetic practitioner who is skilled in counseling will be effective in counseling clients with psychologically based diseases. In fact, a new dietetic practice subgroup, nutrition therapists, under the dietetic practice group, Dietetic Entrepreneurs, originated from, among others, a group of dietitians dealing with clients with eating disorders. These dietetic practitioners realized that eating disorders were a specialty, and that, indeed, they were therapists for their clients. Reiff and Lampson-Reiff (1992) suggest that people with eating disorders want a nutrition therapist who:

- Is flexible.
- Understands their fears about food and weight.
- Has spent time learning to understand what eating disorders are.
- Will work at a pace they can handle.
- Does not have unrealistic expectations.
- Will make sensitive comments.
- Is patient.
- Is caring and nonjudgmental.
- Has experience in working with people with eating disorders.
- Does not demand perfection or compliance.
- Is optimistic and hopeful about recovery.
- Works with them in a collaborative rather than in a controlling manner.

Also of interest regarding MNTs are studies of the incidence of eating disorders among dietitians. Drake (1989) found that 24% of a group of college students majoring in dietetics possessed characteristics of anorexia nervosa. The author indicated that students may choose dietetics as a major because of their personal issues and obsessions with food. Crockett and Littrel (1985) also found that a group of dietetic majors practiced some degree of purging after eating. Two later studies by Johnston and Christopher (1991) and Howat and coauthors (1993) did not cor-roborate these findings. A 1997 study indicated that dietitians who counseled over-weight individuals were more critical of themselves regarding weight than they were of their clients (McArthur & Ross, 1997).

To enhance practical application, discussion of each eating disorder in this chapter begins with the specific diagnostic criteria published by the American Psy-chiatric Association and concludes with a sample chart note describing an actual client with each eating disorder.

HISTORICAL BACKGROUND

Anorexia Nervosa

Many medical historians have credited the English philosopher Sir Thomas Hobbes with the "discovery" of anorexia nervosa. This is because Hobbes wrote of a woman who had fasted for 6 months, and whose "belly touch(ed) her backbone." Although this woman's neighbors considered her to be a saint, Hobbes, a rational-ist, felt there was an underlying disorder, and pronounced her "manifestly sick." Other historians think it was Dr. Richard Morton, who in 1694 published a "Treatise on Consumptions," who first discovered anorexia nervosa. He described two skeletal adolescent young women who closely match the symptoms we associ-ate with the disease today (Maxmen, 1986).

> Although Hobbes and Morton are certainly among the first two men to view anorexic behavior as a sickness, the behavior itself is actually centuries old. Reference is made, for example, to a serf in 895 A.D. named Friderada, who starved herself, while denying that she was starving and refusing help. However, there was not much evidence help was fully offered. It was believed that women such as Friderada who starved were inspired by God. In fact the original term "anorexia" is based on the Latin anorexia mirabilis, or miraculous loss of appetite.
>
> *Rauch, 1993; p. 5.*

By the 19th century, however, the idea that fasting was of divine origin was be-ginning to be questioned. For those women whose motives were not necessarily spiritual, the term "fasting girl" had entered into both the European and American language (Jablow, 1992). As is true for many other diseases, anorexia nervosa was first classified as a disease in the 19th century. At first it was associated with any number of other illnesses (eg, cancer, tuberculosis), but in the 1870s, anorexia ner-vosa was regarded as a discrete disease. In England and France, two medical scholars (Sir William Gull and Charles Lasegue, respectively) independently iden-tified anorexia nervosa as including such symptoms as the refusal to eat, severe weight loss, constipation, amenorrhea, low body temperature, low pulse rate, and obsessive exercising. The two scholars differed, however, in their focus. Gull con-centrated on the physiological aspects, and Lasegue on the psychological (Brum-berg, 1988).

Lasegue stressed that the "emotional cause" of starvation may be hidden, but that any description of a person with anorexia would be incomplete without refer-ence to family interactions (Brumberg, 1988). Lasegue had the earliest record of linking a patient's symptoms with her family dynamics. Subsequently, in the late

19th and early 20th centuries, the adherents to the Lasegue school of thought believed that the cure for women with anorexia nervosa was removal of the girl from her home environment until such a time as she had gained the desired amount of weight. In other words, remove the patient from the environment that is causing her psychological discomfort, and she will once again resume a healthy appetite (Rauch, 1993).

With time, however, the illness was seen as more complex, as it was often resistant to this treatment. In the 1940s, post-Freudian scholars began explaining anorexia nervosa in terms of unconscious fantasies and aversion to sexuality. By the 1980s not only were family interactions examined, but many feminists began to look at links between eating disorders and women's roles in society. In recent years, biobehaviorists have returned to Gull's physiological rooting of the disease, searching for neuroendocrine changes and genetic and physiological aspects that may determine the etiology of eating disorders (Eades, 1990).

Social attitudes toward weight in Western society have taken a turn in recent years. Although gluttony has been criticized historically, there was also wide social support for a rounded figure because it was seen as a sign of prosperity and considered attractive through the eyes of artists and writers who described beautiful women as robust. Today, severe underweight may be criticized, yet the saying persists, "It is impossible to be too rich or too thin." The media now depict very thin women as beautiful.

Bulimia Nervosa

Bulimia nervosa does not have as detailed a history as anorexia nervosa, but it also dates back early in human history, the earliest record being the 2nd century AD. We have records of Galen writing of the disease "bulimis," which translates from the Greek to "great hunger" (Jablow, 1992). The Romans had "vomit halls" where group vomiting occurred as an acceptable answer to the gluttony manifested in the upper society. Medical literature throughout the years speaks of bulimia nervosa only sporadically. In France in the 19th century, it was linked to diabetes. It was not until the mid 1970s that bulimia nervosa was recognized as a distinct eating disorder.

Binge Eating Disorder

Binge eating has no written record as such, except perhaps in descriptions of gluttony. Through the years it might have been thought to be merely symptomatic of someone with a "hearty appetite." It is expected that binge eating disorder will be entered into the DSM-V because the sheer numbers of patients dictate that the medical profession examine the disorder. Recent studies have shown that, currently, those who compulsively overeat outnumber both those with anorexia nervosa and those with bulimia nervosa (Spitzer, 1993).

The social standards and attitudes that have developed over time seem to influence the approach of health-care providers in the treatment of eating disorders. Generally speaking, there is more empathy evident in treatment plans for the underweight than for the overweight, and more evidence that the physiological effect of change in caloric intake is taken into consideration for the underweight than for the overweight. No one would suggest a drastic overload of the system of the underweight, yet drastic approaches to reduction of caloric intake are common. Even though small changes work more satisfactorily, only weight increase regimens seem to follow this dictum. Weight loss regimens tend to be based on severe changes in diet. Patients themselves and health-care providers often seem willing to "punish" the overweight with deprivation regimens.

THE ETIOLOGY OF EATING DISORDERS

Biopsychosocial Model

The biopsychosocial model originated by the noted psychiatrist George Engels has evolved as a comprehensive attempt to understand the "whole person." It is "a scientific model constructed to take into account the missing dimension of the biomedical model" (Engel, 1980; p. 535). The model is based on a systems approach and takes into account all systems relevant to humans. Figure 9–1 illustrates Engel's biopsychosocial model.

In its application to eating disorders, this model strives to uncover and integrate biological, psychodynamic, and sociocultural components of the mental illness of eating disorders. For example, people are "in" nature and a part of it, hence *human nature* (psychological). We connect with each other and change each other (social), and the environment then changes us. Neuronal tissue grows in response to its environment to create a genetic mechanism (biological) (Pies, 1994). Successful treatment of the person with eating disorders often integrates all of these aspects.

Psychodynamics

The psychodynamic element focuses on the idea that an abnormality in childhood or in the families of individuals who later develop anorexia nervosa or bulimia leads them subconsciously to develop bizarre eating behaviors to control an otherwise internalized chaotic situation. For example, clinicians often uncover significant abuse patterns in the victim's family—drug, alcohol, and sometimes sexual (Shuie, 1990). A history of sexual abuse is as high as 80% in bulimia nervosa patients. In one of the few publications that looked at psychodynamics between father and daughters, Dr. Margo Maine, director of the Eating Disorders Program at the Institute of Living in Hartford, Connecticut, expressed the concept of anorexia nervosa as a result of the emptiness young girls have experienced because their fathers were emotionally absent (Maine, 1991).

Sociocultural

The sociocultural factors that contribute to the development of eating disorders are pressures of our culture on young people, especially young women. Currently, society has expectations of thinness that are widely unrealistic. In fact, extremes in weight tend to hide a woman's physical femaleness. In recent years, some have viewed eating disorders as a femininity issue and treatment plans have been devised with this in mind. Accordingly, in some residential treatment programs, the known psychology of women is being used. An emphasis on relationship develop-

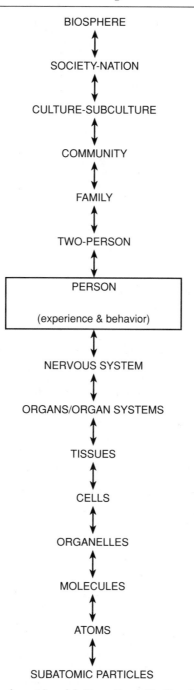

FIGURE 9–1. Engel's biopsychosocial model. (From Engel GL: The clinical application of the biopsychosocial model. *Am J Psych.* 1980; 137(5):535–543. Copyright 1980, the American Psychiatric Association. Reprinted by permission.)

ment, fostering a sense of belonging to a community, and mutually interactive treatments are being employed with success. Other aspects of female psychology used at one facility, the Renfrew Center, include (Davis, 1992):

■ An intensely collaborative, egalitarian treatment structure
■ A focus on personal and nurturing psychotherapeutic experience
■ A woman's ability to find her own inner voice

Biological

Research into biological causes for eating disorders has focused primarily on malfunction of neurotransmitters or genetics. Malfunction of neurotransmitters or their receptors within the hypothalamus of the brain may form a biological basis for major eating disorders.

Nash (1996) reported that Dr. Walter Kaye, professor of psychiatry at The University of Pittsburgh, has been evaluating serotonin disturbances to see whether they contribute to the pathogenesis of eating disorders. He has found increased levels of a major serotonin metabolite in patients a year after they had recovered from anorexia nervosa or bulimia, which might indicate a suboptimal level during the course of the disease. He also discovered that their first-degree relatives had core eating-disorder symptoms themselves. More research in this interesting area is ongoing.

Diagnostic Criteria for Eating Disorders

The DSM-IV, published by the American Psychiatric Association, has been developed to assist in the diagnosis of mental disorders by individuals with appropriate training and experience. The criteria are guidelines in helping health-care workers to make clinical diagnoses. MNTs can use the manual to better understand clients and in some cases to recognize the need for psychological consultation. In addition, it can help MNTs recognize clients who exhibit preclinical symptoms and take action that may prevent the development of the serious conditions that constitute a diagnostic eating disorder. A summary of diagnostic criteria for each eating disorder in DSM-IV is included in the text.

ANOREXIA NERVOSA

The diagnostic criteria for anorexia nervosa are listed in Box 9–1 (APA, 1994; p. 544).

Profile of Women with Anorexia Nervosa

Before they become afflicted by anorexia nervosa, most victims are described as "the best little girls in the world." They are often viewed as bright, helpful, conscientious, and eager to please. However, despite this appearance to the outside world, even to those who know them best, the young women are filled with feelings of inadequacy and self-doubt. Perfectionists, even superachievers, they may suffer terribly from low self-esteem. In addition, they seem unwilling to grow up. Compliments are rejected by them as flattery, and self-criticism is constant. They

Box 9–1	**Diagnostic Criteria for Anorexia Nervosa**

DSM-IV 307.1 Anorexia Nervosa

A. Refusal to maintain body weight at or above a minimally normal weight for age and height (eg, weight loss leading to maintenance of body weight less than 85% of that expected or failure to make expected weight gain during period of growth, leading to body weight less than 85% of that expected).
B. Intense fear of gaining weight or becoming fat, even though underweight.
C. Disturbance in the way in which one's body weight or shape is experienced, undue influence of body weight or shape on self-evaluation, or denial of the seriousness of the current low body weight.
D. Amenorrhea in postmenarchal women, that is, the absence of at least three consecutive menstrual cycles. (A woman is considered to have amenorrhea if her menstrual periods occur only after administration of hormones such as estrogen.)

Specify type:

Restricting type: During the episode of anorexia nervosa, the person does not regularly engage in binge eating or purging behavior (ie, self-induced vomiting or the misuse of laxatives, diuretics, or enemas).
Binge eating/purging type: During the episode of anorexia nervosa, the person regularly engaged in binge eating or purging behavior (ie, self-induced vomiting or the misuse of laxatives, diuretics, or enemas).

Reprinted with permission from the *Diagnostic and Statistical Model of Mental Disorders*. 4th ed. Copyright 1994 American Psychiatric Association.

seemingly strive to please others, relinquishing control except in their food intake (Reiff & Lampson-Reiff, 1992; Maine, 1991; Jablow, 1992).

No matter the age, the woman with anorexia nervosa is striving to bolster her self-esteem. Believing that a thin body will miraculously establish a high self-esteem and make her popular, she begins to diet. Society encourages her. As she becomes thinner, she is often told how good she looks and she feels more popular. Perhaps for the first time in her life she begins to acknowledge her success. It is present in the mirror and on the scale. She feels more secure and begins to perceive that weight control is the answer to low self-esteem. She denies her hunger, even to herself, and often becomes excessively preoccupied with thoughts of food, calories, and grocery shopping. Malnutrition will eventually weaken her body and dull her mind. High self-esteem becomes hard to maintain, but she is loath to give up the idea that being thin is the panacea for all that troubles her. Her sense of body image becomes distorted, and she will insist and believe that she is much too fat, even when close to death. Being thin is "something to die for" (Lawrence, 1993).

Treatment Strategies

Modalities for working with people with anorexia nervosa include the addiction model and the recovery model. Both are modifications of approaches to substance abuse. They have been applied more widely in treating eating disorders that require weight gain than in those requiring weight loss. However, there are organizations, such as Overeaters Anonymous and Eating Disorders Anonymous, whose support structure is based on the addictive model.

Addictive Model

The addictive model utilizes the Twelve Steps of Alcoholics Anonymous modified for eating disorders. It assumes that there are certain foods that are toxic to the body and cause depression, which must be eliminated from the diet permanently. Refined sugar and flour are the primary targets for elimination from the diet. The treatment features the idea that the person is always "sick" but recovering, a life-long task, and always susceptible to relapse (Reiff & Lampson-Reiff, 1992).

Recovery Model

The recovery model assumes that eating disorders result from unresolved issues within the individual or between the individual and the environment. A greater emphasis is placed on the family and its role in the development of the eating disorder. The goal of the recovery model is personal growth and the development of life management skills. Success focuses on feelings of personal worth and acceptance of one's self rather than on weight. This treatment's foundation is that recovery *is* possible, the individual is not always susceptible to relapse.

Cognitive Behavioral Therapy

Cognitive behavioral therapy is generally used as part of the treatment plan for clinicians who advocate the recovery model. Much of the irrational behavior observed in anorexia nervosa is a direct result of the person's set of beliefs, attitudes, and assumptions about food, weight, and body image. Most clinicians accept that, at some point, causal factors converge at the patient's belief that "it is absolutely essential that I be thin." People with anorexia nervosa tend to develop a set of responses to comments made regarding obvious irrational behavior, particularly their restrictive eating. They include the following (Reiff, Lampson-Reiff, 1992):

"I don't like desserts."
"I'm a vegetarian."
"I don't like Italian food."
"Fatty foods just don't agree with me."
"I'm allergic to sugar."
"If I eat at night, I have trouble sleeping."
"I have food allergies."

When beginning the use of these responses, the individual knows they are not true, but as time goes on, she starts believing her own lies. Reiff and Lampson-Reiff developed a Belief Challenge Form for people to use during recovery (Fig. 9–2). It enables the person to challenge distorted beliefs about food, food behavior, and weight.

Unfortunately, the MNT's telling a client that something is true does not change the beliefs. As we have explained in previous chapters, knowledge alone rarely changes behavior. Cognitive therapy is discussed in more detail later in this chapter.

Outcome studies show that for patients with anorexia nervosa, 44% have an overall good outcome, about 30% have an intermediate outcome, and about 25%

have a poor outcome, rarely reaching a normal weight. From 5 to 20% of patients die as a result of complications of anorexia nervosa (Levine, 1995).

Transference and Countertransference Issues

The nutritionist needs to be aware of the potential for transference and counter-transference. Even though the MNT is not doing psychotherapy, she or he is not immune to these issues. Transference and countertransference issues are more likely to arise during treatment of eating disorders because of the psychological nature of the disease.

Transference

Transference occurs when the client's feelings are directed toward the MNT as though the MNT were the original source of the feelings (Gilliland, 1989). The client has "transferred" feeling from some previous significant individual to the MNT, and is usually dealing with the present situation with reactions from the past. This usually happens unconsciously in the client, so it needs to be identified and confronted by the MNT. Discrepancies in verbal and nonverbal behavior, a client's response that is irrational, and intense feelings that do not seem to correspond with the issue at hand are all signs of possible transference issues.

Some transference is a natural part of a therapeutic relationship. The client may seek your approval as he or she seeks his or her parents' approval. Regular consultations with team members or a psychology specialist, or both, can help in the recognition and resolution of transference issues.

Countertransference

Countertransference is the transfer to the patient of feelings from the original source by the professional. The professional's own repressed feelings may be aroused through identification with the patient's experiences and problems, or through responding in kind to the patient's expressions of love or hostility toward him or her. This tendency will distort the objective attitude of the therapist, but it may also serve as a source of insight into the patient (Reiff & Lampson-Reiff, 1992; p. 110). If the MNT has unresolved issues, such as anger with parents or a need to be in control, they affect the relationship with the client. Some common issues are those regarding the progress of therapy and unresolved issues about men or women or authority figures.

CASE EXAMPLE ·

The MNT had unresolved issues with authority figures. At one point in the treatment of a client with an eating disorder, she disagreed with the team leader's suggestions. Unconsciously, she formed an alliance with the client in treatment issues. If she had resolved her own issues with authority, she would have resolved her issues with the team leader.

· ·

NAME _____   DATE _____

BELIEFS ABOUT FOOD, HUNGER, & WEIGHT

INSTRUCTIONS: Please fill in the boxes beside each statement according to the following directions:
Column A: Write T for true if current scientific thought holds the statement to be true.
 Write F for false if current scientific thought holds the statement to be false.
Column B: Write T for true if **you** believe the statement is true.
 Write F for false if **you** believe the statement is false.
Column C: Write T for true if you **behave** as if the statement is true, regardless of whether you believe it or not.
 Write F for false if you **behave** as if the statement is false, regardless of whether you believe it or not.
Please fill in every box.

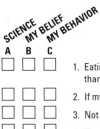

SCIENCE MY BELIEF MY BEHAVIOR
A   B   C

☐ ☐ ☐ 1. Eating certain combinations of food at the same time will cause me to gain weight faster than if the same foods are eaten individually at different times.

☐ ☐ ☐ 2. If my body feels bloated, it means I have gained weight.

☐ ☐ ☐ 3. Not feeling hungry means I have eaten too much and am going to gain weight.

☐ ☐ ☐ 4. The longer I go without eating each day, the less total food I will eat that day.

☐ ☐ ☐ 5. The lower my percent body fat, the healthier I will be.

☐ ☐ ☐ 6. If I use laxatives after binging, I will not gain weight.

☐ ☐ ☐ 7. Excessive exercise prevents weight gain.

☐ ☐ ☐ 8. If I eat food containing sugar, I will gain weight.

☐ ☐ ☐ 9. Vitamin and mineral supplements are not safe to take because the caloric content of the tablets is unknown.

☐ ☐ ☐ 10. Not eating foods containing high quality protein is a good way to maintain a low weight or to lose weight.

FIGURE 9–2. Sample form to record beliefs about food, hunger, and weight. (Copyright 1990, Dan W. Reiff, MPH, RD.)

To become aware of countertransference issues, take note of feeling intense or irrational feelings toward the client. Consult with other team members to help to identify these issues and resolve them.

Additional examples of beliefs about treatment that can affect the MNT's reactions include the following (Reiff & Lampson-Reiff, 1992):

1. The person with the eating disorder should accept me as an authority regarding all aspects of food and nutrition, and I should not be questioned.
2. The person with the eating disorder should not demonstrate that she has more knowledge than I do of certain aspects of nutrition, such as the caloric content of foods.

☐ ☐ ☐   11. Exercise decreases appetite.

☐ ☐ ☐   12. The combination of foods I eat, not the total calories I consume, is responsible for the amount that I weigh.

☐ ☐ ☐   13. I will gain weight if I eat right before I go to sleep because my body is inactive all night.

☐ ☐ ☐   14. Not having menstrual periods has nothing to do with percent body fat.

☐ ☐ ☐   15. If I feel bloated, I need to restrict liquids.

☐ ☐ ☐   16. I tell people I am a vegetarian so I can avoid eating foods I feel will cause me to gain weight.

☐ ☐ ☐   17. The lower my percent body fat, the healthier I will appear to others.

☐ ☐ ☐   18. If I stop using laxatives, the weight I gain will be fat, not water.

☐ ☐ ☐   19. If I use laxatives after I eat, the food will move more quickly through my body, fewer calories will be absorbed, and I will not gain weight.

☐ ☐ ☐   20. If I have any sugar at all, I will lose control of the ability to eat limited amounts of food containing sugar and will not be able to stop.

☐ ☐ ☐   21. The lower my weight is, the better my athletic performance.

☐ ☐ ☐   22. I can have a healthy vegetarian diet that excludes complex carbohydrates and high quality protein.

☐ ☐ ☐   23. The only reason that I have my food and weight related behaviors is to control my weight.

☐ ☐ ☐   24. Other people can eat more food than I can and maintain their weight.

☐ ☐ ☐   25. Eating at the salad bar rather than ordering the main meal results in consuming fewer calories.

☐ ☐ ☐   26. The reason that I binge is because I am addicted to sugar.

☐ ☐ ☐   27. The longer I restrict my food intake, the more likely I am to binge eat.

FIGURE 9–2. *Continued.*

3. The person with the eating disorder feels more powerful than I do because she weighs less than I do.
4. I feel intimidated by the person with the eating disorder because I am overweight and she is thin.
5. If she takes my advice, she respects me. If she questions me, she obviously does not respect me.
6. The changes in behavior I suggested she make are really simple. If she is not making progress, it means she is not trying.

It is important to be aware of the area of countertransference. It can be used positively in therapy to help discuss issues and to strengthen the relationship between the MNT and the client.

Form 9–1 is a sample of an MNT's chart note for an actual client with anorexia nervosa (courtesy of Tammy Beasley, RD, LD, CEDS).

BULIMIA NERVOSA

A summary of the diagnostic criteria for bulimia nervosa in DSM-IV is given in Box 9–2 (APA, 1994; p. 549).

Form 9–1

Chart Note for a Client with Anorexia Nervosa

CLIENT PROFILE REPORT

Initial Nutrition Assessment

PATIENT:
DIAGNOSIS: Anorexia Nervosa
THERAPIST:
PHYSICIAN:
DIETITIAN:

Subjective. Patient reports that "extreme eating behaviors" began @ age 19 after death in the family. Steadily progressed w/increase in abnormal behavior: 1981 (115#); 1985–87 (approx. 100#); 1988 (88#)—began seeing therapist; 1990 hospitalized (86# post-admission—lowest adult wt). Saw nutritionist 6–7 mon afterwards w/minimal results. Does note occasional episodes of vomiting over past 1.5 y. Exercises intensely avg of 2 h, 4–5 d/wk (up to as much as 3 h, 6 d/wk on occasion). Drinks 4 L diet soda daily, w/additional 40+ packets of artificial sweeteners used in other beverages. Diet hx: 1 meal/d, in late evenings after exercise; no dairy b/o newly developed lactose intolerance; no fruits/minimal carb/no caffeine. Pt reports 100% preoccupation w/issues of food/wt/exercise.

Objective. yo female seen for medical nutrition therapy re: anorexia nervosa, w/ purging by excessive exercise per pt hx. MED CONDITIONS include irregular periods w/amenorrhea since last June (6 mo trial of birth control pills, but pt had d/c'd over past 8–9 mo); nl labs except elevated cholesterol (b/o lack of estrogen per OB/GYN). MEDS: none except Metamucil; Ca^{2+} (1000 mg/d); megadoses multivitamin; B complex.
HT: 5'5"; WT: 94# today (steady × 3 mo per pt). HIGHEST ADULT WT: 122# (21 yo); LOWEST ADULT WT: 88# (30 yo). IBW based on small frame size = 112.5–115#. CURRENT INTAKE = 375–400 nutrient calories/d, 37 g protein (39%) + 500 non-nutrient calories/d. Based on intake, adjusted Basal Energy Expenditure (BEE) = 840 calories. SOMATIC SXS include: hypothermia, excessive hair loss/thinness of hair; insomnia; inability to maintain concentration; changes in teeth enamel and sensitivity; receding gums.

Assessment. Pt has little knowledge of sxs of starvation/malnutrition, long-term effects on body/organs/metabolism, dangers of exercise purging in combination w/minimal caloric intake except for what she has read on her own; however, she states "I'm ready

Profiles of Women with Bulimia Nervosa

Although there is growing awareness of bulimia nervosa as a significant problem (there are at least 500,000 to one million people with bulimia nervosa in the United States), a clear profile of personality has not been discovered. Many are college or career women in their 20s or 30s, although many start exhibiting problematic behaviors before the age of 20. There is some indication of the presence of depression and low self-esteem, and a greater need for approval than individuals not suffering from bulimia. A family history of depression is very common in these individuals. They may use food to maintain a "nurturing" bond with an unavailable mother. Some describe feelings of chronic emptiness and neediness. Purging has been described as a punishment for expressing anger over neediness and wishes for more closeness with those they love. Several factors may trigger a binge, in-

Form 9–1

Chart Note for a Client with Anorexia Nervosa *(Continued)*

to do something about this . . . I need to be scared." Reviewed somatic sxs w/pt in relationship to malnutrition—noting that "nl" labs are expected as adaptive response of body; however, decrease in muscle mass, increase in somatic changes, amenorrhea are indication that the body compromises itself to maintain life processes. Discussed metabolism and BEE needs in addition to exercise calories expenditures in comparison w/current intake. Concerned that pt's intake (only 48% adjusted BEE) is after all of her daily activities and consists of minimal usable calories, which forces body to use protein she does eat as energy vs. tissue rebuilding/replacement. Also concerned about excessive use of non-nutritive calories and megadoses of supplements. Discussed w/pt. Pt agreed to the following modifications: decrease diet sodas by ½ L/day (replace w/water); drink ½ modified protein shake (per pt's recipe) bid, the other ½ prior to exercise; add carbohydrate snack midafternoon; increase protein calories in PM "protein shake." Changes will be slow but consistent to manage pt's fear while improving nutritional status. Also suggested pt reduce supplementation to 1 multivit/min per day, w/daily Ca^{2+}. Need to watch sxs of withdrawal from sweeteners, blood sugar responses, somatic changes.

Plan. 1) Dietary modifications and increases as above.
      2) Completion of safe food list and expectation handouts per pt.
      3) Discussion w/treatment team prior to next appointment.
      4) Decrease in exercise intensity/duration by 30 min/session.
      5) F/U in 1 week.

Box 9–2

Diagnostic Criteria for Bulimia Nervosa

DSM-IV 307.51 Bulimia Nervosa
A. Recurrent episodes of binge eating. An episode of binge eating is characterized by both of the following:
    1. Eating, in a discrete period of time (eg, within any 2-hour period), an amount of food that is definitely larger than most people would eat during a similar period of time and under similar circumstances, and
    2. A sense of lack of control over eating during the episode (eg, a feeling that one cannot stop eating or control what or how much one is eating)
B. Recurrent inappropriate compensatory behavior in order to prevent weight gain, such as self-induced vomiting, misuse of laxatives, diuretics, enemas, or other medications, fasting or excessive exercise.
C. The binge eating and inappropriate compensatory behaviors both occur, on average, at least twice a week for 3 months.
D. Self-evaluation is unduly influenced by body shape and weight.
E. The disturbance does not occur exclusively during episodes of anorexia nervosa.
Specify type:

Purging type: the person regularly engages in self-induced vomiting or the misuse of laxatives, diuretics, or enemas.
Non-purging type: the person uses other inappropriate compensatory behaviors, such as fasting or excessive exercise, but does not regularly engage in self-induced vomiting or the misuse of laxatives, diuretics, or enemas.

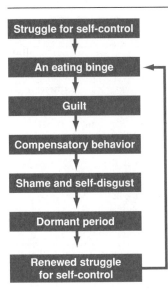

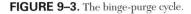

FIGURE 9–3. The binge-purge cycle.

cluding hunger, social disappointment, unstructured activities, anxiety, boredom, anger, and depression (Snetselaar, 1989). Patterns of restrictive eating are also commonly present during the slack period so that feelings of deprivation occur, which justify another binge.

One model of the binge-purge cycle is shown in Figure 9–3. Binging is not universal among those with bulimia nervosa, however.

The term *bulimia* means "ox-hunger" and reflects the way in which individuals are seized by uncontrolled urges to binge. It is possible for one person to consume 10,000 to 20,000 calories in a binge. Binges generally consist of foods high in sugar and fat such as ice cream, cakes, pastries, donuts, pancakes, cookies, candies, chocolates, bread, fast foods, pizza, potato chips, and peanut butter (Snetselaar, 1989). These foods are generally considered "unsafe" or "forbidden" by the person who is binging. Quantities of food can also be enormous. One binge might consist of two large pizzas, one cake, two dozen cookies, one dozen donuts, one box of cereal, and one gallon of milk, although not all binges are this extensive. Vomiting, laxatives, diuretics, exercise, fasting, or a combination of these are used to maintain weight. Some people who overeat in a non-binge fashion also appear to use purging to maintain a desirable weight.

Physical symptoms that can be noted include dehydration, cheilosis, knuckle calluses, mouth and pharynx abrasions, esophagitis and heartburn, and decaying teeth due to vomiting excessively. The frequent induction of diarrhea from the use of laxatives can cause metabolic acidosis. Use of up to 60 laxatives per day has been reported by some clients with bulimia nervosa.

Treatment Strategies

Many approaches to the treatment of bulimia nervosa have been suggested. Some practitioners suggest treating it as an affective disorder and prescribe antidepressants. Others employ family therapy, psychoeducational approaches, feminist therapy approach, and the cognitive-behavioral approach of response prevention. Regardless of treatment approach, the MNT should be aware of the types of beliefs that bulimics commonly share.

Bauer and Anderson (1989) included the following as some of the shared beliefs of bulimia clients:

1. Being or becoming overweight is the worst thing that can happen. Fat is considered disgusting and repulsive and to be fat is to be a failure. Thought-stopping as a technique is useful in breaking this belief.

2. Certain foods are good foods, other foods are bad foods. Good foods are considered diet foods. Bad foods are fattening. Eating good or bad foods makes you a good or bad person. Nutrition education helps in dealing with this belief.

3. You must have control over all of your actions to feel safe. Self-control is considered a sign of discipline and strength. Teaching the client problem-solving skills, assertiveness training, and thought-stopping is effective in this domain of control.

4. You must do everything perfectly or what you do is worthless. Bulimics tend to be perfectionists and negate accomplishments and dwell on failures. If a goal has been accomplished, compliment the client in a way that she will give it to herself. For example, "You must be pleased with the way you did that."

5. Everyone must love you and approve of what you do. Other people must be kept happy regardless of the cost to yourself. A bulimic tends to perceive rejection and think she is basically a bad person. It is very important that a sound, trusting relationship be developed before attempting any interventions that can be interpreted as criticism by the client.

Cognitive Behavioral Therapy

Cognitive behavioral therapy has been reported as an effective treatment strategy for persons with bulimia nervosa (Polivy & Herman, 1985; Wilson, 1986; Hsu, 1990). Cognitive therapy emphasizes some degree of control over eating, which is largely behavioral, and over the identification and modification of dysfunctional thoughts, beliefs, and values, which is the cognitive component.

Treatment techniques may be broadly divided into five categories (Hsu, 1990):

- Cognitive restructuring
- Self-monitoring
- Identification of antecedents to binges
- Nutrition education and meal planning
- Miscellaneous techniques such as
    - Exposure and response prevention
    - Behavioral contracting
    - Social skills training
    - Problem-solving techniques
    - Stimulus control

Except for the following short description of exposure and response prevention, these techniques are described adequately in a host of references (see Additional References) and are therefore not detailed again here.

Exposure and Response Prevention

Exposure and response prevention is a cognitive behavioral technique whereby individuals with bulimia nervosa are exposed to eating "unsafe" or frightening foods in the presence of a therapist. The therapist is present for support during this time of anxiety and also to prevent subsequent vomiting (Leitenberg et al, 1988). The client learns that his or her anxiety can be reduced without recourse to vomiting. Clients also experience that eating normal food without vomiting does not lead to the extreme weight gain predicted. This is a performance-based therapy that involves active and repeated practice in approaching feared situations.

Outcome studies show that for bulimic clients, approximately 70% who complete treatment programs report substantial reduction of bulimic symptoms. However, relapse rates range from 30 to 70% up to 3 years after treatment (Levine, 1995).

Medications: Anorexia and Bulimia

There is no "magic pill" to cure eating disorders. However, medications are often used in conjunction with other therapies. It is likely that treatment will continue to be integrated using nutritional, psychological, and pharmacological modalities. Tricyclic antidepressants (desipramine) are often used if a person has generalized anxiety or panic disorder. The antidepressant Prozac (a serotonin-receptor inhibitor) has proven effective with chronic anorexia nervosa and bulimia nervosa. It reduces the frequency of binging and purging in both depressed and nondepressed bulimic patients. In anorexic patients, it alleviates depressive symptoms and leads to weight gain.

Monoamine oxidase inhibitors are sometimes tried when the tricyclic antidepressants or the antidepressants do not work. However, these carry the risk of side effects because of the associated dietary restrictions. Ondansetron (Zofran) has recently been tested to reduce the frequency of binging and purging among patients with bulimia nervosa (Kim, 1996). Ondansetron has traditionally been used to ease nausea and vomiting due to chemotherapy.

Other groups of drugs have been tried, including antipsychotics (neuroleptics), lithium, appetite stimulants, anticonvulsants, zinc, and naloxone (Narcan), depending on the comorbidities (Agras et al, 1995). The length of time needed on a drug is unknown, although the best data suggest at least 6 months on a trial-and-error basis. If one drug does not produce results, another should be tried.

Forms 9–2 through 9–6 are provided for guidance in the application of treatment techniques in anorexia nervosa, binge eating disorder, and bulimia nervosa.

Text continued on page 258

Form 9–2

Worksheet on Normal Eating

1. What does normal healthy eating mean to you?

_____

_____

2. Basal metabolic rate, or the rate of energy (calories) you use while resting, is not usually below 1200 calories. Where do these calories go?

HEART	12% (144 calories)
KIDNEY	12% (144 calories)
LIVER	23% (276 calories)
BRAIN	23% (176 calories)
MUSCLES	30% (360 calories)

3. Make a list of BENEFITS vs. COSTS/LOSSES from changing or stopping your unhealthy eating habits:

BENEFITS: _____

_____

_____

COSTS/LOSSES: _____

_____

_____

4. Based on your feelings of foods as "Bad" vs. "Good," rate the following groups of foods on a scale of 1 - 5, with (1) = BAD and (5) GOOD:

a. FATS	1 BAD	2	3	4	5 GOOD
b. CARBOHYDRATES	1 BAD	2	3	4	5 GOOD
c. PROTEINS	1 BAD	2	3	4	5 GOOD
d. SUGARS	1 BAD	2	3	4	5 GOOD
e. BREAKFAST	1 BAD	2	3	4	5 GOOD
f. LUNCH	1 BAD	2	3	4	5 GOOD
g. DINNER	1 BAD	2	3	4	5 GOOD
h. SNACKS	1 BAD	2	3	4	5 GOOD

Nutrition Assessment Form for Eating Disorders

NAME: _____   DATE: _____

ADDRESS: _____

_____

PHONE #: _____

MEDICAL RECORD #: _____   DATE OF BIRTH: _____

THERAPIST/PSYCHOLOGIST: _____

PSYCHIATRIST: _____

PHYSICIAN: _____

AGE: _____   HEIGHT: _____   CURRENT WEIGHT: _____

EATING DISORDER BEHAVIOR HISTORY: "TELL ME YOUR STORY":

1. When did your eating disorder begin? _____
   Can you describe what particular event(s) led to your first experience with disordered eating?

   _____
   _____
   _____
   _____
   _____
   _____

2. Which of the following behaviors describe your current pattern of eating?
   a) Restriction of daily calories? _____
   b) Restriction of calories *and* purging? _____
      If yes, how do you purge? _____
      How often? _____
   c) Binge eating without purging? _____
   d) Binge eating followed by purging? _____
      If yes, how do you purge? _____
      How often? _____

WEIGHT HISTORY:

1. Lowest weight: _____   Age: _____
   How long did you maintain this weight? _____

2. Highest weight: _____   Age: _____
   How long did you maintain this weight? _____

3. What is the greatest weight fluctuation you have experienced in:
   1–3 day period of time? _____   1 week? _____   1 month? _____

4. Have you ever participated in an organized diet program? Yes _____ No _____
   If yes, which one(s)? _____
   What was the greatest amount of weight lost? _____ Regained? _____

EXERCISE HISTORY:

1. Do you exercise regularly? No _____ Yes _____

2. What type of exercise do you do?
   Type: _____   Frequency/Duration: _____

3. Did you exercise in the past? No _____ Yes _____ If yes, answer the following:
   Type: _____   Frequency/Duration: _____

4. Have you ever participated in an organized sport? No _____ Yes _____
   If yes, what sport? _____   When? _____

Nutrition Assessment Form for Eating Disorders *(Continued)*

MEDICAL ASSESSMENT:

1. Medical history: _____

_____

2. Are you taking any regular medications?

_____

3. Are you currently taking any vitamin/mineral supplements?

_____

4. **Menstrual Cycle:**
   Age of first menstrual period: _____
   Date of last menstrual period: _____ Age: _____ Weight: _____
   Have you ever been on birth control pills? No _____ Yes _____ If yes,
   when? _____

5. **Overall Somatic Symptoms:**
   Have you ever noticed blood in your vomit? Yes _____ No _____
   Have you ever noticed blood in your stools? Yes _____ No _____
   Do you have problems with constipation? Yes _____ No _____
   diarrhea? Yes _____ No _____
   Do you ever feel bloated? Yes _____ No _____ Frequency? _____
   Do you often feel cold? Yes _____ No _____
   Have you noticed any changes in your hair (thinness, loss of hair, etc)?
   Yes _____ No _____
   Have you noticed any changes in your fingernails? Yes _____ No _____
   Have you noticed any changes in your skin? Yes _____ No _____
   Have you noticed any changes in your sleep? Yes _____ No _____
   Have you noticed any changes in your teeth or gums (sensitivity, loss of, etc)?
   Yes _____ No _____
   Have you noticed any changes in your energy level? Yes _____ No _____
   If yes, how much did you weigh when you noticed the energy changes? _____

FAMILY HISTORY

Have you or any family member had any of the following (please check all that apply)?

1. Anorexia Nervosa?   Self _____   Relative(s) _____
2. Bulimia Nervosa?   Self _____   Relative(s) _____
3. Cancer?   Self _____   Relative(s) _____
4. Compulsive Overeating?   Self _____   Relative(s) _____
5. Depression?   Self _____   Relative(s) _____
6. Heart Disease?   Self _____   Relative(s) _____
7. High Blood Pressure?   Self _____   Relative(s) _____
8. Hypoglycemia?   Self _____   Relative(s) _____
9. Other?   Self _____   Relative(s) _____

How many brothers do you have? _____ Age(s): _____

How many sisters do you have? _____ Age(s): _____

FOOD RELATED BEHAVIORS:

1. Do you use any beverages or foods to decrease or avoid hunger feelings, such as diet sodas or gum?
   Yes _____ No _____ If yes, please list: _____

2. Do you restrict fluids to prevent water weight gain? Yes _____ No _____

3. On a scale of 1–10, in which 1 equals "never" and 10 equals "always," what number describes the amount of time you spend thinking about food, your body weight, hunger, and/or exercise? _____

Safe Food List

FOOD CATEGORY	LIKE	DISLIKE	SAFE	UNSAFE
Animal Protein Foods				
Fish—salmon, tuna				
Fish—cod, snapper, sole				
Shellfish				
Poultry–light meat				
Poultry–dark meat				
Veal				
Beef				
Pork				
Lamb				
Cold cuts				
Liver				
Egg				
Egg white, substitute				
Protein Substitutes				
Tofu				
Peanut Butter				
Sunflower seeds				
Nuts				
Legumes (beans/peas)				
Dairy Foods				
Whole milk				
Lowfat milk (2%)				
Skim or 1% milk				
Yogurt, nonfat plain				
Yogurt, nonfat/sugar-free				
Yogurt, fruit-flavor				

Form 9–4

Safe Food List *(Continued)*

FOOD CATEGORY	LIKE	DISLIKE	SAFE	UNSAFE
Frozen yogurt, nonfat				
Ice milk				
Sherbet				
Ice Cream				
Cottage cheese, nonfat				
Cottage cheese, lowfat				
Cheese, nonfat				
Cheese, lowfat				
Hard cheese, regular				
Fat Condiments				
Butter				
Bacon				
Cream cheese				
Margarine				
Margarine, diet				
Mayonnaise				
Mayonnaise, diet				
Olive or canola oil				
Corn oil				
Salad dressing, oil				
Salad dressing, creamy				
Salad dressing, nonfat				
Avocado				
Olives				
Gravy				
Sour Cream				

Continued

Form 9–4

Safe Food List *(Continued)*

FOOD CATEGORY	LIKE	DISLIKE	SAFE	UNSAFE
Carbohydrate Foods				
White breads				
Whole grain breads				
Bagel				
English muffin				
Fruit/bran muffin				
Pancake/waffle				
Whole grain cereal				
Sugar cereal				
Wheat germ				
Crackers, saltine				
Whole grain crackers				
Snack crackers				
Pastry, croissant				
White rice				
Brown rice				
Oatmeal				
Grits, cream of wheat				
Pasta				
Potato, white				
Potato, sweet				
French fries				
Corn				
Black beans/red beans				
Vegetable Foods				
Asparagus				
Beets				

Form 9–4

Safe Food List *(Continued)*

FOOD CATEGORY	LIKE	DISLIKE	SAFE	UNSAFE
Broccoli				
Brussel sprouts				
Cabbage				
Carrots				
Cauliflower				
Celery				
Cucumber				
Eggplant				
Lettuce, all types				
Mushroom				
Onion				
Spinach				
String (green) beans				
Squash, yellow				
Tomato				
Tomato juice				
V8 juice				
Zucchini				
Fruit Foods				
Apple				
Applesauce				
Apple juice				
Apricots, fresh/dried				
Banana				
Berries, blue/black				
Berries: strawberry				
Cantaloupe				

Continued

Safe Food List *(Continued)*

FOOD CATEGORY	LIKE	DISLIKE	SAFE	UNSAFE
Cherries				
Grapefruit				
Grapefruit juice				
Grapes				
Grape juice				
Honeydew melon				
Mango				
Nectarine				
Orange				
Orange juice				
Papaya				
Pear				
Pineapple				
Pineapple juice				
Plums				
Prune juice				
Raisins				
Tangerine				
Watermelon				
Mixed fruit juices				
Combination Foods				
Pizza				
Macaroni/cheese				
Frozen dinner-regular				
Frozen dinner-diet				
Casseroles				
Hamburger/fast foods				

Form 9–4

Safe Food List *(Continued)*

FOOD CATEGORY	LIKE	DISLIKE	SAFE	UNSAFE
Desserts/Sweet Foods				
Hard candy				
Chocolate candy/bar				
Cookies, regular				
Cookies, nonfat				
Cake, regular				
Cake, nonfat				
Pies, fruit/cream				
Pudding/custard				
Jello				
Beverages				
Soft drink, regular				
Soft drink, diet				
Alcohol (beer/wine)				
Hard liquor				
Coffee/tea, regular				
Coffee/tea, decaf				
Snack Foods				
Gum, with sugar				
Chips, potato or corn				
Microwave popcorn				
Air-popped popcorn				
Pretzels				
Rice cakes, plain				
Rice cakes, flavored				
Sugar-free candy/gum				
Other: _____				

Continued

Form 9-4

Safe Food List *(Continued)*

Are you a vegetarian?   Yes _____   No _____
If yes, how long have you been a vegetarian?

Indicate the type of vegetarian pattern you follow by checking one of the following options:
    No animal foods or products are consumed _____
    Milk products are consumed _____
    Milk and egg products are consumed _____
    Milk, egg, and fish or chicken are consumed _____
    Fish only is consumed _____
    Other _____

Form 9-5

How to Reduce Binge Eating

As you begin to recover from your eating disorder, efforts will be made to reduce or avoid binge eating. Reducing the number of episodes of binge eating can shorten the length of time required for treatment and make it easier for your body to stabilize at your normal body weight.

    Whenever you feel the need to binge, the following suggestions may help you reduce the urge:

1. **WRITE DOWN WHAT YOU ARE PLANNING TO EAT FOR YOUR BINGE.**
   A. This will "buy time" and allow you to THINK ABOUT HOW YOU WILL FEEL after you have eaten your binge foods.
   B. This will help you to PLAN and MAKE A CHOICE to offer yourself an alternative to binge eating, such as calling a close friend to talk about what you are feeling that is triggering the desire to binge.
   C. This will help ELIMINATE or at least REDUCE some of the COMPULSIVENESS that coincides with binge eating.
   D. This will help INCREASE YOUR AWARENESS about WHY you are desiring to binge eat in the first place.

2. **ALWAYS REMEMBER THAT "PART" OF A BINGE IS BETTER THAN "ALL" OF A BINGE!**
   A. Remember that recovery is a PROCESS and every step taken on the road to recovery, whether positive or negative, is an opportunity to LEARN more about yourself.
   B. Try to think about all the POSITIVE CHOICES that you have made recently, especially the choice you made to recover by seeking help from others.
   C. Avoid the self-talk that says "I am a failure because I binged" by changing the message to say "I can learn from this, and I am one step closer to recovery from the knowledge I have gained."

Chart Note for a Client with Bulimia Nervosa, Purging Type

CLIENT PROFILE REPORT

Initial Nutrition Consultation

DATE:
PATIENT:
DIAGNOSIS: Bulimia nervosa, purging type
PHYSICIAN:

Subjective. Pt presents w/6–7 y h/o bulimia nervosa. Notes constant concern about weight throughout childhood and reports that older sister also has compulsive overeating problem (although w/o purging). "I was inspired by a movie on bulimia" @ age 15 and started purging by vomiting. Worsened through high school until 12 episodes/dy. Saw therapist during this time w/little improvement in sxs. Had "close to death" experience @ 17 (weighed 91#); had starved self for days, then purged; hospitalized for hypokalemia. Improved sxs during 1st year of college; however, became "very sick" during sophomore year when involved in serious relationship. Hospitalized several times. Sxs leveled to 2x/d; worsened w/senior year b/o increased stress and bulimia was "only way to get through it." Doing better when arrived home until sister left for Italy. Notes increase in alcohol consumption b/o compensation to avoid food binges. DIET INTAKE: "GOOD" day includes light bkft, grazing on small snack of protein, banana during afternoon, dinner of "big salad" w/proteins or restaurant meat or fish; "BAD" day is binge on leftovers, especially at breakfast, which leads to b/p cycles "rest of day." Avoids fats. TRIGGER foods include breads, bagels, pastas, as well as sweets. EXERCISE SCHEDULE: used to be 2 h/d; now 3–4x/wk, 40 minutes each.

    OBJECTIVE: yo female seen for medical nutrition therapy re: bulimia nervosa, purging type. No other medical problems. MEDS: Prozac x 2 mo. HT: 5′5″; WT today: 115#. IBW based on small/med frame = 115#. Pt's DBW = 100–115#. HIGHEST WT: 128# (2 mo ago) w/recent loss of 13# b/o exercise, dieting. LOWEST WT: 91# (19 yo). BEE = 1350 kcal; ADJUSTED BEE = 945 kcal based on avg cal intake of 630–800 kcal/d. EXERCISE CALORIES: = 340–380 kcal/session avg. SOMATIC SXS: h/o blood in vomit from throat cuts; occ. diarrhea, bloatedness, occ. excessive perspiration, recent hair loss, "strange" sleep patterns, excessive gland swelling, fluctuation in energy level.

Assessment. Pt has complicated, severe hx of bulimia w/frequent hospitalizations to stabilize medical condition only. No permanent, successful relationship w/therapist who specialized in eating disorders. Somatic sxs indicative of protein/calorie malnutrition and frequency of purging sxs. Recent 13# wt loss of 2 mo correlates w/recent excessive hair loss, energy fluctuations. Began education on metabolism, role of nutrients in the body and physiological consequences of binge/purge cycles. Discussed importance of normalizing physiological triggers to binge/purge due to inadequate energy intake over time and imbalance of calorie distribution throughout the day. Obtained contract to contact PhD. in order to normalize psychological triggers. Able to establish good rapport w/pt and initial trust foundation developed. Using current intake, obtained contract for selecting more appropriate food choices and improved caloric distribution in order to improve blood sugar fluctuations to help prevent binge triggers. Pt also agreed to complete safe food list prior to F/U. Discussed dangerous consequences of substituting alcohol for food binges; pt aware.

Plan.
1. Provided list of therapists to interview and encouraged initiating therapy as soon as possible.
2. Substituted whole grain crackers and fresh fruit @ bkft.
3. Contract for second alternative for bkft; Ovaltine, fresh fruit w/wheat germ.
4. Contract for consistent 'lunch' or afternoon snack 4–5 h after bkft; whole grain crackers, protein, fresh fruit
5. Dinner as is for now
6. Pt will complete safe foodlist, expectations handout, and food beliefs worksheet prior to F/U.
7. F/U in 1 week.

Courtesy of Tammy Beasley, RD, LD, CEDS.

EATING DISORDERS NOT OTHERWISE SPECIFIED

Disorders of eating that do not quite fit the full clinical picture for any specific disorder fall under the "not otherwise specified" diagnosis. Several examples are given in the DSM-IV, such as continuation of menses in an otherwise too thin person or recurrent episodes of binge eating in the absence of other symptoms of bulimia nervosa. People with problematic eating patterns that do not include the core features of anorexia nervosa or bulimia nervosa present a challenge to the MNT. However, individuals in this category or even those presenting with less acute symptoms may be better candidates for effective change than people who meet the clinical criteria for the other specific eating disorders. Difficulties arise in the diagnosis and treatment of individuals who may develop a clinical eating disorder because of a professional's hesitancy to label them as such. At the same time, third-party payment is usually not possible without this label. It is also interesting to note that over the years, the weight at which clients are diagnosed or hospitalized has become lower and lower. This correlates with the attitudes toward body image held by the population in general (Brumberg, 1988). These social factors may result in a failure to properly treat individuals who show signs of eating disorders soon enough to prevent anorexia nervosa or bulimia nervosa from developing.

A summary of the criteria for eating disorders not otherwise specified in the DSM-IV is listed in Box 9–3 (APA, 1994; p. 551).

BINGE EATING DISORDER

Although binge eating disorder was not included as a full criteria set in the DSM-IV, it was added to the appendix as a disorder worthy of further study. It is also included as an example of an eating disorder not otherwise specified. This delin-

---

Box 9–3

Diagnostic Criteria for Eating Disorders Not Otherwise Specified

DSM-IV 307.50 Eating Disorder Not Otherwise Specified
This category is for disorders of eating that do not meet the criteria for any specific eating disorder. Examples include:

1. All of the criteria for anorexia nervosa are met except the individual has regular menses.
2. All of the criteria for anorexia nervosa are met except that despite substantial weight loss, the individual's current weight is in the normal range.
3. All of the criteria for bulimia nervosa are met except binges occur at a frequency of less than twice a week or for a duration of less than 3 months.
4. An individual of normal body weight who regularly engages in inappropriate compensatory behavior after eating small amounts of food (eg, self-induced vomiting after the consumption of two cookies).
5. An individual who repeatedly chews and spits out, but does not swallow large amounts of food.
6. Binge eating disorder, recurrent episodes of binge eating in the absence of the regular use of inappropriate compensatory behaviors characteristic of bulimia nervosa.

Reprinted with permission from the *Diagnostic and Statistical Model of Mental Disorders*. 4th ed. Copyright 1994 American Psychiatric Association.

Diagnostic Criteria for Binge Eating Disorder

DSM-IV Binge Eating Disorder

A. Recurrent episodes of binge eating. An episode of binge eating is characterized by both of the following:

1. Eating, in a discrete period of time (eg, within any 2-hour period), an amount of food that is definitely larger than most people would eat during a similar period of time and under similar circumstances, and
2. A sense of lack of control over eating during the episode (eg, a feeling that one cannot stop eating or control what or how much one is eating).

B. The binge eating episodes are associated with at least three of the following:

1. Eating much more rapidly than normal.
2. Eating until feeling uncomfortably full.
3. Eating large amounts of food when not feeling physically hungry.
4. Eating alone because of being embarrassed by how much one is eating.
5. Feeling disgusted with oneself, depressed, or feeling very guilty after overeating.

C. Marked distress regarding binge eating.

D. The binge eating occurs, on average, at least 2 days a week for 6 months.

E. The binge eating is not associated with the regular use of inappropriate compensatory behaviors (eg, purging, fasting, excessive exercise) and does not occur exclusively during the course of anorexia nervosa or bulimia nervosa.

Reprinted with permission from the *Diagnostic and Statistical Model of Mental Disorders*. 4th ed. Copyright 1994 American Psychiatric Association.

eation is an interesting development in the field of obesity and has come to the forefront recently. Prevalence, comorbidity, and food intake studies are currently being documented. A summary of diagnostic criteria for binge eating disorder is presented in Box 9–4 (APA, 1994; appendix).

Profiles of People with Binge Eating Disorder

Binge eating disorder has been established as a distinct eating pattern among obese people. Binges are described as being similar to a "food orgy" followed by the person feeling severely uncomfortable and self-condemning. Because binging is not followed by purging, people with binge eating disorder tend to be obese. The excess weight contributes to low self-esteem, depression, and isolation (Gershoff, 1997). Comorbidities with certain forms of psychopathologies have been found. Food intake is similar to that observed in normal-weight bulimics (Mitchell & Mussell, 1996).

The onset of binge eating disorder usually occurs in late adolescence or in the early 20s. People affected are more likely to have been overweight as children and usually have a history of dieting (Bruce & Wilfley, 1996).

Treatment Strategies

This is a relatively new area and studies are still limited. It has been found that cognitive behavioral therapy and interpersonal psychotherapy lead to significant improvement in eating behavior and a decrease in binge eating in clients with this disorder. Agras and coauthors (1995), Zerbe (1995), and Bruce and Wilfley (1996) target areas of concentration of these treatments.

Cognitive behavior therapy emphasizes

▮ Establishment of a regular, balanced, heart-healthy eating pattern
▮ Decreased avoidance of specific foods
▮ Identification of alternative responses to triggers that evoke a binge

Interpersonal therapy focuses on

▮ Improving interpersonal problem areas
▮ Improving social functioning
▮ Enhancing self-esteem
▮ Decreasing negative mood

Fairburn (1995) suggests a three-stage approach in the cognitive-behavioral treatment of binge eating disorder. Stage 1 includes self-monitoring, nutrition education, use of alternative behaviors, and establishment of a regular eating pattern. Stage 2 emphasizes elimination of restrained eating, skill development in dealing with binge-triggering situations, challenge of distorted thinking, and consideration of the family and of social factors. Stage 3 considers plans for the future, such as expectations and recurrence prevention.

Medications are also being used experimentally. Desipramine and fluoxetine (antidepressants) have suppressed some binge eating.

MNTs treating patients for weight-related conditions should screen those patients suspected of binge eating. Dieting is associated with the onset of binge eating, but it has not been established what type of dieting may be predisposing to this eating disorder (Wilson, 1993). According to the dietary restraint theory, hunger induced by dieting produces a set of conditions that encourage binge eating. One study identified breaking rules of abstinence as one of the important precipitants to binging among obese patients. Box 9–5 lists suggested screening questions to aid in the detection of binge eating disorder (Zerbe, 1995).

Closed-ended questions often require follow-up to obtain additional information that is needed.

Box 9–5

Screening Questions to Aid in the Detection of Binge Eating Disorder

1. Are there times during the day when you could not have stopped eating, even if you had wanted to?
2. Do you ever find yourself eating unusually large amounts of food in a short period of time?
3. Do you ever feel extremely guilty or depressed afterward?
4. Do you ever feel even more determined to diet or to eat healthier after the eating episode?

From Bruce B, Wilfley D: Binge eating among the overweight population. Copyright the American Dietetic Association. Reprinted by permission from *Journal of the American Dietetic Association* 1996; 96:1.

CASE EXAMPLE ·

MNT: "Do you ever find yourself eating large amounts of food in a short time?"

CLIENT: "Yes."

MNT: "Give me an example."

· ·

Chart notes need to reflect clearly what happened during a medical nutrition therapy session. A sample of an MNT's chart note, using SOAP format (discussed in Chap. 11), and a follow-up note for an actual client with binge eating disorder are illustrated in Forms 9–7 and 9–8.

EATING DISORDERS AND MALES

It is estimated that males make up 5 to 10% of the population with anorexia nervosa and about 4% of the population with bulimia nervosa (Steiger, 1989). Current estimates of the age of onset in males range from 15 to 20 years. Onset of bulimia nervosa is around age 20. Socioeconomic status seems to be similar to that of the female population for both disorders. Although many individuals come from upper socioeconomic groups, there is a drift of both disorders into lower socioeconomic classes (Steiger, 1989).

Both males and females with eating disorders show similar family histories of weight disturbances and substance abuse disorders. Cultural pressures toward slimness are active in both genders. Psychological predisposing factors such as obsessive-compulsive behavior put both genders at risk.

Given that no marked differences are noted in terms of etiology (Steiger, 1989; Margo, 1987), there is no indication that special treatment techniques are needed for male clients. The likely biopsychosocial determinants (Garfinkel & Garner, 1982) of eating disorders in both genders suggest that "multimodel treatments, implicating biological therapies (nutritional rehabilitation and, where indicated, medications), psychotherapy aimed at eating and characterological disturbances, and often social reintegration and skills development, will be required in different measures. Identity problems seem particularly central in males and may need particular attention" (Steiger, 1989; p. 423).

Siever (1994) studied sexual orientation and gender as factors in socioculturally acquired vulnerability to body dissatisfaction and eating disorders. He found that gay men and heterosexual women, in particular, were dissatisfied with their bodies. This caused them to be vulnerable to eating disorders because of a shared emphasis on physical attractiveness and thinness that is based on a desire to attract and please men (sexual objectification). However, lesbians and heterosexual men were found to be less concerned with their own physical attractiveness, therefore less dissatisfied with their bodies, and consequently less vulnerable to eating disorders.

Chart Note for a Client with Binge Eating Disorder

CLIENT PROFILE REPORT

Initial Nutrition Consultation

DATE:
PATIENT:
DIAGNOSIS: Binge Eating Disorder (aka compulsive overeating)
PHYSICIAN:
THERAPIST:
DIETITIAN:

Subjective. Patient reports approximately 18 years of yo-yo dieting. Diets have included Weight Watchers, low-fat diets, to "every new fad diet on the market." States that she did have much success with Weight Watchers; however, something in her life triggered her to compulsively eat. Reports that she is presently at her highest weight.

Objective. yo female seen for medical nutrition therapy regarding binge eating disorder. Medical history includes mitral valve prolapse and high blood pressure. MEDS: include Calan, Coumadin, Zestril. HT: 5'8"; WT:; IBW approximately 170 lbs. (adjusted LARGE frame, diet history). Patient is 182% of IBW. LOWEST BW: 120 lbs (early 20s). HIGHEST BW: 310 lbs. (present body weight). Weight gain has been gradual and steady at 275 lbs approximately 5 years ago. Recently reports an increase in weight over the past years. BEE = 1474 calories $\times$ 1.25 ACTIVITY FACTOR = 1840 calories/day (ideal body weight used). Present caloric INTAKE ranges between 2000 and 3500 kcal/day. (Secretively eats, between 10 PM and midnight, foods that are high in fat and calorically dense. However, reports she is not a big sweets eater.) EXERCISE: Recently bought NordicTrack, reports that she has never been an exerciser in the past.

Assessment:. Very pleasant, open woman presents here with an interest in gaining control of her present eating habits. Admits that making the appointment with me was very difficult. Long discussion on her history, her goals, and her failures with diets in the past. One problem identified: fear of failure with regard to weight loss and exercise. Discussed my role as a nutrition therapist in a non-restrictive, non-diet approach to weight loss. The patient does not feel that she could face another diet secondary to her failures with them in the past.

A fasting program was discussed, and I provided basic information on the program. I personally do not feel that this program is warranted, at this time, due to her present fears, her dislikes for liquid meals, and her need to learn about her compulsion to eat. She does appear interested in medications: phen-fen for appetite control. Her MD presently does not want her to take this route for weight control and appetite control secondary to her history of irregular heartbeat and high blood pressure.

Education provided on binge eating disorder and basic metabolism. Discussed binge eating disorder, food triggers, and guilty eating and probed client's thoughts regarding these. Facilitated client development of strategies for meals and how to identify her triggers with regard to food and eating and appropriate substitute thought patterns. Stressed that our approach would be one of learning about herself and her issues that surround her eating activity level. She admits that she secretively eats, which was discussed at great detail. I reinforced the fact that she did restrict somewhat during the day which tends to set people up for physiological hunger in the evening. We discussed the importance of making peace with her eating and minimizing the labeling of good food versus bad food. The patient was extremely receptive.

Plan:. 1. Nutrition education packet provided on binge eating disorder.
    2. Safe food, unsafe food list provided and to be completed.
    3. Beliefs about hunger, food, and weight questionnaire to be completed.
    4. Meal journal to be completed.
    5. Contracts made for coping with difficult situations.

Thank you very much for this referral.

Courtesy of Tammy Beasley, RD, LD, CEDS

Follow-Up Note for a Client with Binge Eating Disorder

FOLLOW-UP REPORT

DATE OF REPORT:
TO:
FROM:
REGARDING: Follow-up nutrition consultation

Your patient, _____ continues to meet with me for medical nutrition therapy. This is a follow-up memorandum to discuss her continued progress in medical nutrition therapy.
     The sessions are summarized as follows:

Current Eating Patterns and Weight-Related Issues. Current weight is 239 pounds. Weight change over the past three months is 39 pounds. Total weight loss since starting nutrition therapy is 71 pounds (since January 1996).

Exercise Patterns. Exercises five to six times per week, ranging 20 minutes to an hour.

Assessment of Progress. Continues to do very well with nutrition therapy and the non-diet approach to weight loss. She continues to attend weekly medical nutrition therapy session. On a daily basis, she documents her meals, her exercise, and her moods as they relate to food. She has had problems with food over the past 3 months with regard to the resurfacing of guilty eating, and restrictive-like behaviors. We have spent much of our therapy sessions discussing guilt with eating and the importance of not being too restrictive with her calories, stressing thoughts and feelings that are detrimental. She has also been challenged over the recent months with regard to potentially exercising excessively. She is very receptive and has made several contracts for change, which she has kept. Her commitment is apparent. She is not aware of her weight loss with regard to the number of pounds that she has lost. She wishes to continue to not know her weight loss and her weight, for she feels this approach has worked very well. We will continue to weigh backward and continue to deal with her emotional issues as they relate to eating. Wishes to continue medical nutrition therapy on a weekly basis and to have her meals, exercise, and weight monitored.
     I will continue to keep you informed of her progress and/or any issues that may surface in nutrition therapy. I continue to enjoy working with her and look forward to her continued success with this approach. If you should have any questions, please do not hesitate to contact me.

Courtesy of Tammy Beasley, RD, LD, CEDS

SUBSTANCE-RELATED DISORDERS

There is a high rate of dual diagnosis of eating disorders and substance-related disorders (drugs and/or alcohol). Prevalence data show substance-related disorders in 9 to 55% of patients with bulimia nervosa, up to 19% of patients with anorexia nervosa, and from 10 to 44% of obese binge eaters (Varner, 1995). Disordered eating usually occurred before the onset of drug or alcohol problems.

In the past, substance-related problems received treatment first; but recently, support has been growing for concurrent treatment. Some people may substitute one problem for another if both problems are not addressed at the same time (Varner, 1995). The MNT needs to work closely with other members of a multidisciplinary health-care team to meet treatment goals for the individual. Also, the dietetic practitioner.needs to become proficient in nutrition management of both conditions.

EATING DISORDERS AND ATHLETES

Athletes are at increased risk of developing eating disorders and other pathogenic weight control techniques because sports often place significant emphasis on weight and body fat composition. Athletes may be asked or encouraged to lose weight quickly. Most will do this through restrictive dieting, which can be a precursor to eating disorders. Like some people with eating disorders, athletes may be perfectionists, have a strong desire to please others, and base their self-assessment on achievement and performance. They are willing to tolerate pain and to sacrifice themselves to meet their goals. Those sports that most emphasize weight control, thinness, and appearance include gymnastics, cheerleading, dancing, figure skating, diving, swimming, crew, track, wrestling, and equestrian sports. There have been some notable examples of athletes with eating disorders. Carling Bassett, 28 years old, suffered from bulimia nervosa while on the pro tennis tour. Cathy Rigby, 43 years old, a former Olympic gymnast, had bulimia nervosa for 12 years from the time she was 16. Christy Henrich, age 22, former gymnast, died of multiple-organ failure stemming from anorexia nervosa; at her death she weighed 47 pounds.

Athletes will go to great lengths to do what is necessary to improve performance. Often this involves reducing their body fat stores through pathogenic weight-control behaviors (Rosen et al, 1986; Clark, 1994). Fat reduction may in fact increase performance, as in gymnastics. However, in a survey of female runners, Clark and coauthors (1988) found that there was no relationship between fastest race times and thinner body weight or body mass index. This refutes the popular notion that the thinnest runner is the fastest. These investigators also found that, among runners, nutrition education needs included the following:

- How to balance fun foods with nutrient-dense foods
- How to prevent craving sweets
- How to get nutrients from wholesome foods
- How to select an iron-rich diet
- How to determine an appropriate body weight and then maintain it in a healthy manner

In November 1994, the American Anorexia/Bulimia Association and Eating Disorders Awareness and Prevention, Inc, issued a position paper regarding athletics as a risk factor in the development of eating disorders (Maine, 1994). The position it adopted follows:

Eating disorders seriously endanger the health and well-being of student athletes. All personnel involved in the teaching, coaching, training, and support of sports, dance and other physical activities should be aware of the risk factors and the pivotal role they can have in the prevention of eating disorders.

Risk Reduction

Some strategies that have been recommended to reduce risk of disorders among athletes include the following (Thompson, Sherman, 1993):

- Education for coaches and sports personnel in
  - eating disorders

- menstrual functioning
- consciousness-raising of male coaches (especially for female athletes)
- De-emphasizing weight
- Eliminating group weigh-ins
- Treating each athlete individually
- Establishing guidelines for appropriate weight loss
- Controlling the contagion effect of athletes mirroring unhealthy practices of other athletes

Box 9–6 presents a memory jogger that can be used as an aid to help screen for and prevent eating disorders among female athletes. It is just as well suited for male athletes.

The Female Athlete Triad

Young female athletes are at risk of developing a potentially fatal triad of disorders that are distinct yet inter-related. They are disordered eating, amenorrhea (cessation of menses), and osteoporosis. Eating disorders often lead to menstrual dysfunction and subsequent premature osteoporosis. Not only can amenorrheic clients develop osteoporosis in their teens and 20s, they may never regain their previous bone densities. The presence of one disorder of the triad in a young female client should prompt evaluation for the other two, according to Dr. Nattiv (1994) at UCLA. He suggests some screening questions for this triad:

- Do you use or have you ever used laxatives? Diet pills? Diuretics?
- Have you ever made yourself vomit to lose weight or get rid of a big meal?
- Do you skip meals or avoid certain foods?
- What have you eaten in the last 24 hours?

Other helpful questions include:

- Have you lost weight recently? What weight loss method did you use?
- What is the most and least you have weighed in the last year?
- What is your ideal weight?

MNTs also need to be attuned to the connection between menstrual status and nutritional status. In taking a menstrual history, the questions to be asked include:

- When did you start having your period?
- How regular has it been?
- Have you ever missed any periods? How many months in a row? How many cycles per year?

Female athletes who have irregular periods require further assessment, including questioning about nutrition, disordered eating habits, training, intensity, and life stressors. Additional questions include:

- How many hours per day and per week do you exercise?
- Do you take calcium supplements? How much dietary calcium do you get? (Ask about specific foods or food groups.)

Box 9-6

Memory Jogger: How to Identify Pathogenic Weight-Control Behaviors

Female athletes have gone to extraordinary lengths to lower their body fat stores in an effort to improve performance. A pattern of eating disorders has emerged from this desperate, health-threatening situation. The following protocol was developed to advise the athletic training staff how to identify symptoms in athletes who suffer from one or more features of pathogenic weight-control behavior. Many of the items do not by themselves prove the presence of an eating disorder, but identification of one or more may justify further attention to the possible presence of a problem.

Reports or observation of the following signs or behaviors should arouse concern:

1. Repeatedly expressed concerns by an athlete about being or feeling fat even when weight is below average.
2. Expressions of fear of being or becoming obese that do not diminish as weight loss continues.
3. Refusal to maintain even a minimal normal weight consistent with the athlete's sport, age, and height.
4. Consumption of huge amounts of food not consistent with the athlete's weight.
5. Clandestine eating or stealing of food (eg, many candy wrappers, food containers, etc., found in the athlete's locker, around her room); repeated disappearance of food from the training table.
6. A pattern of eating substantial amounts of food followed promptly by trips to the bathroom and resumption of eating shortly thereafter.
7. Bloodshot eyes, especially after trips to the bathroom.
8. Vomitus or odor of vomit in the toilet, sink, shower, or wastebasket.
9. Wide fluctuations in weight over short time spans.
10. Complaints of light-headedness or disequilibrium not accounted for by other medical causes.
11. Evidence of use of diet pills (eg, irritability fluctuating with lethargy over short periods of time).
12. Complaints or evidence of bloating or water retention that cannot be attributed to other medical causes (eg, premenstrual edema).
13. Excess laxative use or laxative packages seen in the athlete's area, locker, wastebasket, etc.
14. Periods of severe calorie restriction or repeated days of fasting.
15. Evidence of purposeless, excessive physical activity (especially in a thin athlete) that is not part of the training regimen.
16. Depressed mood and self-deprecating expression of thoughts following eating.
17. Avoiding situations in which the athlete may be observed while eating (eg, refusing to eat with teammates on road trips, making excuses such as having to eat before or after the team meal).
18. Appearing preoccupied with the eating behavior of other people such as friends, relatives, or teammates.
19. Certain changes in the athlete's physical appearance (eg, rounding or pouch-like dilation at or just under the angle of the jaw, ulcerations or scores at the corners of the mouth or on the tongue, thinning or loss of hair).
20. Known or reported family history of eating disorders or family dysfunction.

If an athlete who seems to have an eating disorder is practicing one or more pathogenic weight-control techniques, the following recommendations are in order:

1. The coaching or training staff person who has the best rapport with the athlete should arrange a private meeting with her.
2. The tone of the meeting should be entirely supportive. Express concern for the best interests of the individual and make it clear that this concern transcends the issue of the individual as an athlete.

Box 9-6

Memory Jogger: How to Identify Pathogenic Weight-Control Behaviors
(Continued)

3. In as nonpunitive a manner as possible, indicate to the athlete what specific observations were made that aroused your concern. Let the individual respond.
4. Affirm and reaffirm that the athlete's role on the team will not be jeopardized by an admission that an eating problem exists. Participation on a team should be curtailed only if evidence shows that the eating disorder has compromised the athlete's health in a way that could lead to injury should participation be continued.
5. Try to determine if the athlete feels that she is beyond the point of being able to voluntarily abstain from the problem behavior.
6. If the athlete refuses to admit that a problem exists in the face of compelling evidence, or if it seems that the problem either has been long-standing or cannot readily be corrected, consult a clinician with expertise in treating eating disorders. Remember, most individuals with this problem have tried repeatedly to correct it on their own and failed. Failure is especially demoralizing for athletes, who are constantly oriented toward success. Let the individual know that outside help is often required and that this need should not be regarded as a failure or lack of effort.
7. Arrange for regularly scheduled follow-up meetings apart from practice times, or, if the athlete is seeing a specialist, obtain advice as to how you may continue to help.
8. Be aware that most athletes resorting to pathogenic weight-control techniques have been told at various times that they had a weight problem. It is important to know what role, if any, past or present coaches or trainers may have played in the development of this problem. Let the athlete know that you realize that the demands of the sport may well have played a role in the development of this behavior.

What not to do:

1. Question teammates instead of talking directly to the athlete.
2. Immediately discipline the athlete if you find evidence that a problem exists.
3. Indicate to the athlete that you know what is going on, but tell nothing as to how or why you have become suspicious.
4. Tell the athlete to straighten up and that you will be checking back from time to time.
5. Conclude that if the athlete really wants to be okay, she will make it happen, and failure to improve shows a lack of effort.
6. Dissociate yourself and the demands of the sport from any aspect of the development of the problem.
7. Refuse to obtain outside assistance but rather "keep it in the family."

From Rosen LW, et al: Pathogenic weight-control behavior in female athletes. *Physician Sportsmed.* 1986; 14(1):89.

■ Have you ever used birth control pills?
■ Have you ever had a stress fracture or other fracture?

And, as with all eating disorders, the earlier the intervention, the better the outcome.

CASE EXAMPLE ·

The following is taken from the beginning of an initial interview. The client, a college student, was slim, but not underweight. The student was a walk-in at the student health clinic. She asked to see the dietitian.

M N T: "How can I help you today?"

C L I E N T: "Well, I just moved and my whole schedule has gone berserk, you know. I'm on the women's soccer team. I used to go to school in the daytime and work out nights. Now it's the opposite and that's my main problem. My eating pattern is all screwed up. I worry about getting enough vitamins. I know it's usually older women who get osteoporosis, but I worry about that. I'm all out of whack and I just want to get back into my old schedule." (Note that the client did not directly answer the MNT's questions, but did tell her in the last sentence what her goal was.)

M N T: (picking up on last sentence, also noting the "worry" about vitamins) "Tell me about your schedule."

C L I E N T: "Well, I usually would wake up about 8 AM and watch TV for an hour, then go the gym and work out. Oh, I would eat first. Then I'd be at the gym until 2 PM. I do free weights, then do the stairmaster, then run, then leg lifts. If there is an aerobics class scheduled when I'm there, I take it. When I was being good I would eat a yogurt and take one calcium. I used to eat breakfast, but I don't now. I used to be pretty tired by the time practice started, but nothing like now. Now, with night classes, I don't get up in time to eat breakfast."

M N T: (beginning to see that an eating disorder might be in the picture). "I am hearing you say that you work out about 5 hours a day and are no longer eating breakfast, is that correct?"

C L I E N T: "Yes."

M N T: "Have you been losing weight?"

C L I E N T: "Yes, but that's OK. I was too fat anyway and eating too much made me vomit a lot."

M N T: (realizing that the client was revealing clues to an eating disorder, began to pursue questions to clarify the problem) "Have you lost weight recently?"

C L I E N T: "Yes, about 10 pounds in a few months."

M N T: "Tell me what you've eaten the last 24 hours."

The remainder of the dialogue made it clear that although the student was not currently underweight, she was heading for trouble. The client was open and revealing and responded positively to a suggestion that she and the MNT ask a psychological counselor to help a better lifestyle.

• •

Anorexia Athletica

Anorexia athletica is a subclinical eating disorder. It is not yet part of DSM. It occurs when an athlete uses at least one unhealthy method to control weight, including fasting, vomiting, diet pills, laxatives, or diuretics. In a special Olympics '96 issue of *Eating Disorders Review,* such athletes are described as women with eating disorders who take up a sport and transpose the need for control from diet to performance. "Ironically, their persistence, perfectionism, concentration and ability to disregard hunger and fatigue all enable them to become outstanding athletes" (Yates, 1996; p. 100).

Body Builders

Weight cycling (the gain and loss of weight surrounding an athletic event) is a concern for athletes, especially males. Chronic dieting, preoccupation with food, and binge eating have been reported by men preparing for body building competitions. Also cited were troublesome psychological and behavioral changes. In one study, 81% of the men reported being preoccupied with food. As many as 10% binged during the week before a contest. The incidence of binge eating doubled immediately after an event. The body builders also reported having a wide range of negative feelings when preparing for a competition: 55% were irritable, 47% were angry, and 46% felt fatigued. About a third reported being anxious or depressed or feeling isolated (*Eating Disorders Review,* 1995).

Wrestlers

Wrestlers often participate in unhealthy practices to achieve a low body weight for competition. Most wrestlers agree that "making weight" is very important and that vomiting and laxative use are employed at times. In a 1994 study involving 197 adolescent wrestlers, the authors concluded that nutrition counseling needs to emphasize not only the risks involved in rapid weight loss but also motivation to adopt healthy weight-management strategies (Marquart & Sobel, 1994).

In Table 9–1, Clark (1994) outlines an overall nutrition treatment plan and goals for an athlete who has been diagnosed with anorexia nervosa.

TABLE 9–1

Overall Nutrition Treatment Plan and Goals for an Athlete with Anorexia	
Treatment Plan	**Goals**
Educate the athlete about the consequences of anorexia.	Establish a normal eating pattern. Optimize health.
Reduce preoccupation with food, weight, and body fat.	Attain peace with food and weight.
Gradually increase meals and snacks to an appropriate level.	Fuel body appropriately.
Rebuild the body to an appropriate weight.	Optimize strength and health. Maintain medically safe weights.
Establish regular menstrual periods.	Reduce risk of stress fractures. Optimize bone density.

From Clark N: Counseling the athlete with an eating disorder: A case study. Copyright the American Dietetic Association. Reprinted by permission from *Journal of the American Dietetic Association* 1994;94(6):656–658.

PREVENTION AND SCREENING

Primary prevention is aimed at reducing the incidence of eating disorders. This can be accomplished at the individual, family, and community levels (Shisslak & Crago, 1987). Prevention strategies can be outlined in the schools, starting in junior high school and through college, in the family, especially targeting parents, and in the community at spas, at grocery stores, and in public service announcements.

Individuals with eating disorders often seek medical treatment for secondary complaints. Physicians and dentists need to be educated to increase early recognition about these secondary consequences. Intervening in a client's development of risk factors for eating disorders can also serve as prevention by health-care professionals (White, 1992). Table 9–2 shows risk factors for women and eating disorders. This intervention can be emphasized by education and by guidance of parents and significant others.

One important function for the MNT is watchfulness for individuals who show a tendency toward an eating disorder. This will include some in-depth investigation of eating habits when some symptom or hunch suggests that a person is heading toward an eating disorder. Weight gain or loss for no apparent reason, for instance, would warrant further investigation (and careful listening to both verbal and nonverbal signs that suggest secretiveness). A screening questionnaire developed by the Renfrew Center can be used to help identify a person with an eating disorder (Box 9–7). These questions can be used with an individual who may not, at first, appear to have an eating disorder. When the answers are "yes," they need follow-up with open-ended questions to facilitate exploration.

There are times when clients might respond effectively to written questionnaires as opposed to oral questioning. For people attuned to computers, working with a computer may help them give open and revealing answers.

In children, there are variants in the criteria for eating disorders. To better identify and screen for eating disorders in children, the following features are suggested as criteria:

a disorder of childhood (defined here as below the age of 15) in which there is an excessive preoccupation with weight or shape, and/or food intake, and accompanied by grossly inadequate, irregular or chaotic food intake.

Bryant-Waugh & Lask, 1995; p. 191

TABLE 9 – 2

Women and Eating Disorders: Risk Factors		
Developmental	**Family**	**Biological**
Identity	Enrichment	Predisposition to obesity
Body Image	Cohesiveness	Predisposition to affective disorders
Autonomy	Overprotectiveness	
Separation-Individuation	Boundary rigidity	

Box 9–7

Questions That May Help Identify an Eating Disorder

1. Are you preoccupied with food and your next opportunity to eat?
2. Have you missed what someone was saying because you were thinking about food?
3. At parties, does the buffet or food supply feel like a magnet to you?
4. Have you made mistakes at work because you are thinking of food?
5. Does staying in touch with food make it hard for people to get in touch with you?
6. Is what to serve your first decision in planning a party?
7. Is eating out your chief form of entertainment?
8. Do you select and anticipate what you will be eating before you arrive home, at a party, or at a restaurant when you have eaten within 4 hours and are not genuinely hungry?
9. Do you wonder where your food went, because you do not remember finishing it?
10. Do you eat your food without tasting it very much? Do you find you've barely enjoyed your meal, snack, or binge?
11. Do you have some preference for eating alone?
12. Would you prefer not having others see what, how much, or how often you eat?
13. Do you snack behind the scenes while you are helping, visiting, or preparing food?
14. Do you eat in your car?
15. Do you seek food when you have a problem to solve?
16. Do you have specific foods or quantities of food which you use to help you handle uncomfortable emotions?
17. Do you eat to relieve tiredness or boredom or to keep yourself awake?
18. Do you eat when you are not hungry, because you might get hungry if you do not eat?
19. Do you feel strong emotions toward someone who tampers with your food supply?
20. Do you feel powerless over food?

From Renfrew Center: *Questions That May Help Identify an Eating Disorder,* 1991 The Renfrew Center, 7700 Renfrew Lane, Coconut Creek, FL 33073; 1-800-332-8415.

COLLABORATIVE PRACTICE

In the prevention, screening, and treatment of eating disorders, collaborative practices are vital. The position paper of The American Dietetic Association (1994) on nutrition intervention in the treatment of anorexia nervosa, bulimia nervosa, and binge eating gives models of collaboration (Box 9–8).

According to Beasley (1994), the nutritionist's main objectives as a member of the treatment team are to establish a trusting relationship and to aid the patient in feeling comfortable with food. She further states (p. 27) that "unlike the typical medical model of dietary counseling that offers short term intervention and a standardized plan of action with education as the primary goal, the nutritionist specializing in eating disorders must often set aside the traditional precepts of the profession."

Hospitalization and Residential Treatment

A hospital or residential setting can provide a safe, controlled environment for initiating medical, psychological, and nutritional rehabilitation. Criteria for admitting a person for inpatient treatment are as follows (Brownell & Foreyt, 1986):

1. Significant weight loss.
2. Metabolic abnormalities, especially hypokalemic alkalosis from bulimic conditions.

Box 9-8

Models of Collaboration Between the Dietitian and the Psychotherapist

Within the team context, a psychonutritional approach to the treatment of persons with eating disorders is recommended in which psychotherapy and medical nutrition therapy are considered very important throughout the entire recovery process. Of all the team members, the registered dietitian typically works most closely with the psychotherapist. Following are five possible models of collaboration between the dietitian and the psychotherapist member of the team.

The Continuous Contact Model. Both the dietitian and the psychotherapist work with the person with the eating disorder throughout the recovery process, although each focuses on a different aspect of treatment. This model requires the registered dietitian to have supervised training in counseling skills.

The Food Plan–Only Model. The registered dietitian does a one or two session consultation in which an individualized food plan is designed for the patient and specific questions are answered.

The Education-Only Model. The person with the eating disorder meets with the registered dietitian for a six- to ten-session consultation in which nutrition topics relevant to eating disorders are discussed.

The Education/Behavioral Change–Only Model. The therapist refers the person with the eating disorder to the registered dietitian (in this case, a dietitian with additional training and experience in the treatment of eating disorders is qualified to do the nutrition intervention) for education about nutrition concepts relevant to eating disorders early in treatment. The person then stops medical nutrition therapy to return at a later time when she or he is ready to work intensively on changing food- and weight-related behaviors.

The Intermittent Contact Model. The person with the eating disorder has intermittent contact with the registered dietitian (in this case, a dietitian with additional training and experience in the treatment of eating disorders is qualified to do the nutrition intervention) throughout her or his recovery as the patient and the psychotherapist deem it necessary.

The registered dietitian should present these five alternatives to team members, new referring professionals, patients, and their families as appropriate. The health-care team will select the model of collaboration to be used.

From American Dietetic Association: Position of The American Dietetic Association: nutrition intervention in the treatment of anorexia nervosa, bulimia nervosa, and binge eating. Copyright the American Dietetic Association. Reprinted by permission from the *Journal of the American Dietetic Association* 1994; 94(8):902–907.

3. Lowered mood or thoughts or intents of suicide.
4. Nonresponsiveness to outpatient treatment.
5. Demoralized, nonfunctioning family.
6. Lack of outpatient facilities.

Upon admission, a detailed nutrition history should be obtained in a supportive and nonjudgmental manner. Dietitians should then develop individualized care plans, specifying the parameters of nutrition rehabilitation. The care plan may include:

- Daily caloric intake
- Rate of weight gain
- Weight-range goal for discharge

■ Limitation of food choices
■ Necessity for meal supervision
■ Activity limitations

The inpatient setting also provides an opportunity for nutrition education groups such as cooking and structured eating experiences (Hornyak & Baker, 1989).

Arranging for outpatient follow-up is extremely important. The transition from a structured program to outpatient care can be difficult and frightening. An outpatient appointment with an MNT should be made before discharge so that progress can be sustained and continued without interruption (ADA, 1994).

Outpatient Settings

Outpatient settings may include individual therapy, group therapy, family therapy, or a combination of these. In any structure, a team approach is recommended. The American Dietetic Association (1994; p. 902) supports a multidisciplinary model of treatment for eating disorders:

> It is the position of The American Dietetic Association that nutrition intervention and education be integrated into the team treatment of patients with anorexia nervosa and bulimia nervosa during the assessment and treatment phases of outpatient and/or inpatient therapy.

Following are listed the advantages and disadvantages of an outpatient team approach (Beasley, 1995).

Advantages of an Outpatient Team Approach

1. Shared responsibility for the treatment of the patient.
2. The patient benefits from the pooling of knowledge: "two heads are better than one."
3. The team models a "family" that collaborates, solves problems together, makes decisions that meet the needs of all involved, and acknowledges that each person has strengths as well as limitations.
4. The patient has both male and female role models.
5. Increases the sense of security and confidence in the patient and her or his family.
6. Shared knowledge between the team members to use as a source of new ideas and approaches.
7. Enables the patient to better understand how food and weight-related behaviors interface with psychological, medical, psychiatric, and dental issues.

Disadvantages of an Outpatient Team Approach

1. Logistical problems due to different office locations.
2. Communication among team members can be difficult due to #1.
3. The patient may not like working with one of the team members.

4. Some professionals have difficulty in collaborating with others or are accustomed to making independent treatment decisions.
5. "Sharing a patient" may be perceived as threatening the stability of the professional's practice.
6. Insurance may cover some of the team members and not others, making it difficult for the patient to afford to see the recommended optional combination of team members.

Summary

Although eating disorders have received much attention recently, they have a long history. Understanding of them is beginning to develop, but remains rudimentary and tentative, as do treatments. Eating disorders among athletes seems to be a burgeoning problem. Medications and prevention are part of the approach to these disorders.

Of all areas in which nutrition counseling is being done today, the cadre of dietetic practitioners working with eating disorders has recognized the essential role of the dietetic practitioner as therapist, interacting effectively with the client. As time goes by, it is hoped that all dietetic practitioners who focus their practice on education and counseling will adopt similar attitudes and skills.

The suggested activities, additional references, and the forms provided throughout the chapter are all designed as guides to facilitate the reader's ability to counsel these interesting and complex clients.

Suggestions for Further Learning

1. Discuss situations in which eating disorders might have been a factor among your acquaintances.

2. Observe or participate with a dietitian or psychologist who specializes in counseling people with eating disorders. Identify the strategies used and evaluate the session with the professional.

3. Using the following client quotations, take these steps:

▌ Write your response.
▌ In groups, role-play the response.
▌ As a group, devise two responses that you believe would be productive.
▌ Have each group report to the full class.

Client 1: "I gained a pound since the last time. My stomach is bulging and I look disgusting!"
Client 2: "I put 2 tablespoons of dressing on my salad. I'm so depressed. I've lost total control of my diet plan."
Client 3: "I am terrified to do even one less than 100 push-ups because then I'll gain weight."

4. With a partner, role-play the following counseling scenario:

Client: You are a 34-year-old female. You have two very active children. They make you anxious and nervous. When you sit at the table with your family, you cannot eat. Often you eat alone, which is better for you. However, you sometimes vomit what you eat. You went to the doctor because of your fatigue. The physician notices that you have lost 20 pounds. She has referred you to the MNT in the out-patient clinic. You are a sweet person who tries to please others, but you do not want anyone telling you what to do. You may ad lib other things about yourself. After the dialogue begins, allow your feelings to direct your responses to the MNT.

MNT: You are a dietitian in a hospital outpatient clinic. This client was referred to the clinic by one of the staff physicians. Her chart has not yet arrived, although you know her diagnosis is anorexia nervosa. Your goal is to create a trusting environment and encourage the client to commit herself to appropriate nutritional change.

CITED REFERENCES

Agras WS, Telch CF, Arnow B, et al: Does interpersonal therapy help patients with binge eating disorder who fail to respond to cognitive-behavioral therapy? *J Consult Clin Psych.* 1995;63:356.

American Dietetic Association: Position of The American Dietetic Association: Nutrition intervention in the treatment of anorexia nervosa, bulimia nervosa, and binge eating. *J Am Diet Assoc.* 1994;94(8):902–907.

American Psychiatric Association: *Diagnostic and Statistical Manual of Mental Disorders.* 4th ed. Washington, DC: American Psychiatric Association; 1994, p.544, 549, 551.

Anonymous: Body Builders: Weight cycling can be a concern. *Eating Disorders Rev.* 1995, 6(6):4.

Arnow B, Kenardy J, Agras WS: Binge eating among the obese: A descriptive study. *J Behav Med.* 1992;15(2):155–170.

Bauer BG, Anderson WP: Bulimic beliefs: Food for thought. *J Counsel Dev.* 1989;67:416–419.

Beasley T: Inpatient vs outpatient approaches. Handout for lecture, Miami, FL, 1995.

Beasley T: The role of the nutritionist in the treatment of eating disorders. *Miami Medicine.* 1994;Sept:27–28.

Brownell KD, Foreyt JP (eds): *Handbook of Eating Disorders. Physiology, Psychology and Treatment of Obesity, Anorexia, and Bulimia.* New York: Basic Books, 1986.

Bruce B, Wilfley D: Binge eating among the overweight population: A serious and prevalent problem. *J Am Diet Assoc.* 1996;96(1):58–61.

Brumberg JJ: *Fasting Girls: The Emergence of Anorexia Nervosa as a Modern Disease.* Cambridge, MA: Harvard University Press, 1988.

Bryant-Waugh R, Lask B: Annotation: Eating disorders in children. *J Child Psychol Psychiat.* 1995;36(2):191–202.

Clark N, Nelson M, Evans W: Female runners. *Physician Sportsmed.* 1988;16:124–134.

Clark N: Counseling the athlete with an eating disorder: A case study. *J Am Diet Assoc.* 1994;94(6):656–658.

Crockett SJ, Littrell JM: Comparison of eating patterns between dietetic and other college majors. *Nutr Educ.* 1985;17:47–50.

Davis WN: The psychology of women and residential treatment for eating disorders. *Renfrew Perspe.* 1992;Fall:1, 5.

Drake MA: Symptoms of anorexia nervosa in female university dietetic majors. *J Am Diet Assoc.* 1989;89:97–98.

Eades MD: *Freeing Someone You Love from Eating Disorders.* New York: Putnam Publishing, 1990.

Engel GL: The clinical application of the biopsychosocial model. *Am J Psych.* 1980;137(5):535–543.

Fairburn CG: *Overcoming Binge Eating.* New York: Guilford Publications, 1995.

Garfinkel PE, Garner DM: *Anorexia Nervosa: A Multidimensional Perspective.* New York: Brammer/Mazel, 1982.

Gershoff SN (ed): Binge eating disorder comes out of the closet. *Tufts Univ Diet Nutrit Lett.* 1997;14(11):4–5.

Gilliland BE, James RK, Bowan JT: *Theories and Strategies in Counseling and Psychotherapy.* 2nd ed. Englewood Cliffs, NJ: Prentice-Hall, 1989.

Hornyak LM, Baker EK: *Experiential Therapies for Eating Disorders.* New York: The Guilford Press, 1989.

Howat PM, Beplay S, Wozniak P: Comparison of bulimic behavior incidence by profession: Dietitian, nurse, teacher. *J Nutr Educ.* 1993;25:67–69.

Hsu CK: Experiential aspects of bulimia nervosa: Implications for cognitive behavioral therapy. *Behav Modif.* 1990;14(1):50–65.

Jablow MM: *A Parent's Guide to Eating Disorders.* New York: Bantam Doubleday, 1992.

Johnston CS, Christopher FS: Anorexic-like behaviors in dietetic majors and other student populations. *J Nutr Ed.* 1991;23:148–153.

Kim SW: Drug reduces binge/purge frequency. *Eating Disorders Rev.* 1996;7(4):1–2.

Lawrence K: *Dietitian's Patient Education Manual.* Gaithersburg, MD: Aspen Publishers, 1993.

Leitenberg H, Rosen JC, Gross J, et al: Exposure plus response: Prevention treatment of bulimia nervosa. *J Consult Clin Psych.* 1988;56(4):535–540.

Levine P: Connections in primary prevention. *Renfrew Perspec.* 1995;1(3):4–5.

Maine M: *Father Hunger: Fathers, Daughters & Food.* Carlsbad, CA: Gurze Books, 1991.

Maine M: *Position of Eating Disorder Awareness and Prevention, Inc. and the American Anorexia/Bulimia Association: Athletics as a Risk Factor in the Development of Eating Disorders.* New York, EDAP and AA/BA, 1994.

Margo JL: Anorexia nervosa in males: A comparison with female patients. *Br J Psych.* 1987;151:80–83.

Marquart LF, Sobal J: Weight loss beliefs, practices and support systems for high school wrestlers. *J Adol Health.* 1994;15(5):410–415.

Maxmen JS: *Essential Psychopathology.* New York: WW Norton and Company, 1986.

McArthur LH, Ross JK: Attitudes of registered dietitians toward personal overweight and overweight clients. *J Am Diet Assoc.* 1997;97(1):63–66.

Mitchell JE, Mussell MP: Binge eating disorder: An update. *Eating Disorders Rev.* 1996;7(1):1–5.

Nash M: Conference on adolescent nutritional disorders: prevention and treatment. *Nutr Today.* 1996;31(2):68–72.

Nattiv A: The female athlete triad: Managing an acute risk to long-term health. *Physician Sportsmed.* 1994;22(1):60–68.

Pies RW: *Clinical Manual of Psychiatric Diagnosis and Treatment: A Biopsychosocial Approach.* Washington, DC: American Psychiatric Press, 1994.

Polivy J, Herman C: Dieting and bingeing, a causal analysis. *Am Psychologist.* 1985;40(2):193–201.

Polivy J, Herman CP: Diagnosis and treatment of normal eating. *J Consult Clin Psych.* 1987;55(5):635–643.

Rauch R: Comprehensive Review of Eating Disorders. Unpublished paper. Miami, FL, 1993.

Reiff DW, Lampson-Reiff KK: *Eating Disorders: Nutrition Therapy in the Recovery Process.* Gaithersburg, MD: Aspen Publishers, 1992.

Renfrew Center. *Questions That May Help Identify an Eating Disorder.* Coconut Creek, FL: Renfrew Center, 1991.

Rosen LW, McKeag DB, Hough DO, Curley V: Pathogenic weight-control behavior in female athletes. *Physician Sportsmed.* 1986;14(1):79–86.

Satter E: *How to Get Your Kid to Eat . . . but Not Too Much.* Menlo Park, CA: Bull Publishing, 1987.

Shisslak CM, Crago M: Primary prevention of eating disorders. *J Consult Clin Psych.* 1987;55(5):660–667.

Shure J: Sexual abuse linked to eating disorders. *Diet Dev Psych Disorder Newslett.* 1990;8(2):1.

Siever MD: Sexual orientation and gender as factors in socioculturally acquired vulnerability to body dissatisfaction and eating disorders. *J Consult Clin Psych.* 1994;62(2):257–260.

Snetselaar LG: *Nutrition Counseling Skills: Assessment, Treatment, and Evaluation.* 2nd ed. Rockville, MD: Aspen Publishers, 1989.

Spitzer RL: In DSM-IV: A Reply to Fairburn et al. The Classification of Recurrent Overeating: The Binge Eating Disorder Proposal. *Int J Eating Disorders.* 1993;13:162–168.

Steiger H: Anorexia nervosa and bulimia in males: Lessons from a low-risk population. *Can J Psychiatr.* 1989;34(5):419–424.

Thompson RA, Sherman RT: Reducing the risk of eating disorders in athletics. *Eating Disorders.* 1993;1(1):65–78.

Varner LM: Dual diagnosis: Patients with eating and substance-related disorders. *J Amer Diet Assoc.* 1995;95(2):224–225.

White JH: Women and eating disorders, part II: Developmental, familial and biological risk factors. *Healthy Women Int.* 1992;13:363–373.

Wilson GT: Cognitive behavioral and pharmacological therapies for bulimia. *In* Brownell KD, Foreyt JP (eds): *Handbook of Eating Disorders.* New York: Basic Books, 1986.

Wilson GT: Relation of dieting and voluntary weight loss to psychological functioning and binge eating. *Ann Intern Med.* 1993;119(7):727–730.

Yates A: Eating disorders in women athletes. *Eating Disorders Review.* 1996;7(4):1–4.

Zerbe KJ: *The Body Betrayed: A Deeper Understanding of Women, Eating Disorders and Treatments.* Carlsbad, CA: Gurze Books, 1995.

ADDITIONAL REFERENCES

American Dietetic Association: Nutrition Counseling Module. Self Assessment Series. Chicago, IL: Commission on Dietetic Registration, 1994.

Andersen AE: *Males with Eating Disorders.* New York: Brunner/Mazel, 1990.

Andersen AE: Eating disorders in males. *In* Brownell KD, Fairburn CG (eds): *Eating Disorders And Obesity: A Comprehensive Handbook.* New York: The Guilford Press, 1995.

Bryant-Wangh R: Anorexia nervosa in boys. *In* Dolan B, Gitzinger I (eds): *Why Women? Gender Issues and Eating Disorders.* London: Athlone Press, 1994; p. 124–133.

Davis C, et al: The role of physical activity in the development and maintenance of eating disorders. *Psychol Med.* 1994;24:957.

Drenowski A., Yee DK: Men and body image: Are males satisfied with their body weight? *Psychosomat Med.* 1987;49:626–634.

Eating Disorders Review, P.M. Inc. PO 2468, Van Nuys, CA 91404. 1-800/365-2468.

International Journal of Eating Disorders. John Wiley & Sons, New York, NY 10158.

Mitchell JE, Goff G: Bulimia in male patients. *Psychosomatics.* 1984;25:909–913.

Raynor H, Zemel P: Binge eating disorder and the dietitian's role. *J Am Diet Assoc* 1996;96:9.

Scott DW: Anorexia nervosa in the male: A review of clinical, epidemiological and biological findings. *Int J Eating Disorders.* 1986;5:799–817.

Stoutjesdyk D, Jevine R: Eating disorders among high performance athletes. *J Youth Adolescence.* 1993;22:271.

Sundgot-Borgen J: Risk and trigger factors for the development of eating disorders in female elite athletes. *Med Sci Sport Exercise.* 1994;26:414.

Weight Control Information Network (WIN): Win Way, Bethesda, MD 20892-3665, phone 201/951-1120, or online WINNIDDK@AOL.COM.

Yates A: Athletics, eating disorders and the overtraining syndrome. *In* Epling WF, Pierce WD (eds): *Activity Anorexia: Theory, Research, and Treatment.* Hillsdale, NJ: Lawrence Erlbaum Associates, 1996.

CHAPTER 10

Ethics

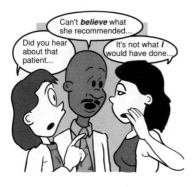

GOALS

The major goals of this chapter are (1) to increase the reader's understanding of ethical codes and principles, (2) to delineate issues in bioethics, counseling ethics, and business ethics, and (3) to stimulate analysis of personal thoughts, beliefs, and attitudes so as to enhance the reader's moral development.

Learning Objectives

At the end of this chapter the reader will be able to:

1. Define *ethics* and *bioethics.*

2. Describe the American Dietetic Association's code of ethics.

3. Elaborate on the five ethical principles discussed.

4. Give examples of ethical, legal, medical, and financial considerations in bioethics.

5. Describe advance directives.

6. Discuss issues that relate to counseling ethics.

7. Identify business ethics issues of honesty, integrity, and fairness.

Key Terms

▶ Moral Development: an ability to integrate ethical guidelines with personal and professional values. "In most cognitive developmental models, lower level thought characteristically tends toward dualism, rigidity, oversimplification, stereotyping, self-protectiveness, and authoritarianism. Whereas higher level of thought is more flexible, complex, contextually sensitive, and allocentric" (Neukrug et al, 1996).

▶ Informed Consent: consent voluntarily given by a person after an explanation and disclosure of a procedure has been given that is sufficient to enable that person to have a general understanding of the procedure and medically acceptable alternatives and to make a knowing health-care decision without coercion or undue influence.

You are driving in a truck on a narrow mountain road. There is a car driving toward you from the opposite direction. There is also a

Box 10-1

The American Dietetic Association Professional Code of Ethics

PREAMBLE

The American Dietetic Association and its credentialing agency, the Commission on Dietetic Registration, believe it is in the best interests of the profession and the public they serve that a Code of Ethics provide guidance to dietetic practitioners in their professional practice and conduct. Dietetic practitioners have voluntarily developed a Code of Ethics to reflect the ethical principles guiding the dietetic profession and to outline commitments and obligations of the dietetic practitioner to self, client, society, and the profession.

The purpose of the Commission on Dietetic Registration is to assist in protecting the nutritional health, safety, and welfare of the public by establishing and enforcing qualifications for dietetic registration and for issuing voluntary credentials to individuals who have attained those qualifications. The Commission has adopted this Code to apply to individuals who hold these credentials.

The Ethics Code applies in its entirety to members of the American Dietetic Association who are Registered Dietitians (RDs) or Dietetic Technicians, Registered (DTRs). Except for sections solely dealing with the credential, the Code applies to all American Dietetic Association members who are not RDs or DTRs. Except for aspects solely dealing with membership, the Code applies to all RDs and DTRs who are not ADA members. All of the aforementioned are referred to in the Code as "dietetic practitioners."

PRINCIPLES

1. The dietetic practitioner provides professional services with objectivity and with respect for the unique needs and values of individuals.
2. The dietetic practitioner avoids discrimination against other individuals on the basis of race, creed, religion, sex, age, and national origin.
3. The dietetic practitioner fulfills professional commitments in good faith.
4. The dietetic practitioner conducts him/herself with honesty, integrity, and fairness.
5. The dietetic practitioner remains free of conflict of interest while fulfilling the objectives and maintaining the integrity of the dietetic profession.
6. The dietetic practitioner maintains confidentiality of information.
7. The dietetic practitioner practices dietetics based on scientific principles and current information.
8. The dietetic practitioner assumes responsibility and accountability for personal competence in practice.
9. The dietetic practitioner recognizes and exercises professional judgment within the limits of his/her qualifications and seeks counsel or makes referrals as appropriate.
10. The dietetic practitioner provides sufficient information to enable clients to make their own informed decisions.
11. The dietetic practitioner who wishes to inform the public and colleagues of his/her services does so by using actual information. The dietetic practitioner does not advertise in false or misleading manners.
12. The dietetic practitioner promotes or endorses products in a manner that is neither false nor misleading.
13. The dietetic practitioner permits use of his/her name for the purpose of certifying that dietetic services have been rendered only if he/she has provided or supervised the provision of those services.
14. The dietetic practitioner accurately presents professional qualifications and credentials.
    a. The dietetic practitioner uses "RD" or "registered dietitian" and "DTR" or "dietetic technician, registered" only when registration is current and authorized by the Commission on Dietetic Registration.
    b. The dietetic practitioner provides accurate information and complies with all requirements of the Commission on Dietetic Registration program in which

Box 10-1

The American Dietetic Association Professional Code of Ethics (*Continued*)

he/she is seeking initial or continued credentials from the Commission on Dietetic Registration.

c. The dietetic practitioner is subject to disciplinary action for aiding another person in violating any Commission on Dietetic Registration requirements or aiding another person in representing himself/herself as a RD or DTR when he/she is not.

15. The dietetic practitioner presents substantiated information and interprets controversial information without personal bias, recognizing the legitimate differences of opinion exist.

16. The dietetic practitioner makes all reasonable effort to avoid bias in any kind of professional evaluation. The dietetic practitioner provides objective evaluation of candidates for professional association memberships, awards, scholarships, or job advancements.

17. The dietetic practitioner voluntarily withdraws from professional practice under the following circumstances:

a. The dietetic practitioner has engaged in any substance abuse that could affect his/her practice;

b. The dietetic practitioner has been adjudged by a court to be mentally incompetent;

c. The dietetic practitioner has an emotional or mental disability that affects his/her practice in a manner that could harm the client.

18. The dietetic practitioner complies with all applicable laws and regulations concerning the profession. The dietetic practitioner is subject to disciplinary action under the following circumstances:

a. The dietetic practitioner has been convicted of a crime under the laws of the United States which is a felony or a misdemeanor, an essential element of which is dishonesty and which is related to the practice of the profession.

b. The dietetic practitioner has been disciplined by a state and at least one of the grounds for the discipline is the same or substantially equivalent to these principles.

c. The dietetic practitioner has committed an act of misfeasance or malfeasance which is directly related to the practice of the profession as determined by a court of competent jurisdiction, a licensing board, or a governmental body.

19. The dietetic practitioner accepts the obligation to protect society and the profession by upholding the Code of Ethics for the Profession of Dietetics and by reporting alleged violations of the Code through the defined review process of The American Dietetic Association and its credentialing agency, the Commission on Dietetic Registration.

From the American Dietetic Association. Code of ethics for the profession of dietetics. Copyright the American Dietetic Association. Reprinted by permission from the *Journal of the American Dietetic Association* 1988; 88 (12):1592–1596.

biker on the side of the road. You have three choices. If you swerve to one side to avoid the car, you will hit and kill the biker. If you swerve to the other side, you will smash into the mountain and kill yourself. If you drive straight ahead, you will crash into the oncoming car and kill the occupant. What do you choose? What is the right thing to do? This modified scenario from Socrates' teachings illustrates a basic ethical dilemma that the study of ethics works to explore, what is the "right" thing to do when there is no clear-cut right and wrong.

Ethical principles are statements, usually developed by philosophers, that are intended to assist in coming to decisions when human dilemmas arise. Ethical principles are not used in "black or white" situations, but rather in those gray areas of right versus wrong, good versus bad. Often, but not always, laws reflect ethical principles. Something that is legal is not always ethical and some action may be deemed ethical but not legal. Ethical dilemmas are most often based on conflict with one's own sense of right and wrong.

Ethics is derived from philosophy and religion and is the general field of study that addresses issues of morality in human relationships. Although there is a set of ethical behaviors that is generally accepted by all human beings as a guide to our interactions, they differ somewhat from culture to culture (Curry-Bartley, 1987). What is ethically right in one culture may not be in another. For example, in some cultures it is deemed unethical for a person to take his or her own life, and in others, especially among the old, self-determined death is highly respected.

PROFESSIONAL ETHICS

Ethical Codes

All societies formally or informally establish codes of ethics. These pertain to the rational processes for determining the most desirable course of action in the face of conflicting value choices. They include standards of moral conduct that determine behavior. *Ethical standards* are systematized outlooks that have grown out of human experiences. They are guidelines to use when following rules does not suffice. These standards change according to the social milieu of the time. For example the "me generation" of the 1960s was a time when it was ethically right to do, generally, whatever you wanted; to be selfish was OK. Currently, there appears to be a movement toward an outlook that it is ethical to restrain oneself somewhat for the good of others. Such a standard is not written, but is apparent in the behavior of a society.

Formalized *ethical codes* are statements of certain ways of behaving that have stood the test of time for a given social group. The Ten Commandments is a good example of a formalized ethical code. Governmental constitutions are other examples of attempts to set forth statements of how people should behave.

A code of ethics is also one of the important documents that is produced by a group that wishes to distinguish itself as a profession. There are codes of ethics for lawyers, doctors, nurses, teachers, businesspeople, psychologists, and others who consider themselves professionals. The American Dietetic Association (1988) sets forth its ethical requirements in the *Standards of Professional Responsibility of the American Dietetic Association* (ADA's Code of Ethics). It is shown in Box 10–1.

The American Dietetic Association believes it is in the best interests of the profession and the public it serves that a code of ethics provide guidance to dietetic practitioners in their professional practice and conduct. Dietetic practitioners have voluntarily developed this code to reflect ethical principles guiding the dietetic profession. Also, the code serves to outline commitments and obligations of the dietetic practitioner to society, client, self, and the profession.

Some specific purposes of this code are to:

∎ Provide a position on standards of practice to assess each member of the profession in deciding what she or he should do when situations of conflict arise in his or her work. Examples of areas of possible conflict include: accepting perquisites (perks) from sales representatives, when to refuse to counsel a client, when to make referrals to other professionals, avoidance of discrimination, and personal bias.

■ Clarify the counselor's responsibilities to the client and protect the client from the counselor's violation of, or failure to fulfill, these responsibilities. For instance, a dietetic practitioner needs to provide sufficient information for the client to make his or her own decisions.

■ Give the profession some assurance that the practice of members will not be detrimental to its general functions and purposes. For instance, registered dietitians are expected to refrain from doing colonic irrigations, hair analysis, or iridology (study of the eye for the purpose of diagnosing diseases and identifying weakness in other body parts). These practices may be regulated on a state (legislative) level if licensure is in place.

■ Offer the counselor some grounds for safeguarding his or her own privacy and integrity. The dietetic practitioner does not reveal to others what he or she or the client says during counseling sessions. Also, he or she does not have to answer client's questions regarding his or her personal life.

Sometimes the code of ethics alone is not adequate for every decision or action with which the dietitian may be confronted. Other ethical principles must play a part in the decision-making process. This decision-making process should be a means of determining what is better or best in a particular situation under given circumstances, not what is right or wrong. What is considered ethical in one situation may not be considered ethical in a similar situation but under different circumstances.

Ethical Principles

According to Falvo (1994), ethical principles include autonomy, beneficence, non-maleficence, justice, and confidentiality.

Autonomy. Autonomy is the degree to which an individual is allowed to make his or her own choices and choose his or her own destiny. Individuals must be allowed to make decisions without coercion or undue influence. This is based on the assumption that the person is competent and understands the information given and the consequences of his or her decisions.

Beneficence. Beneficence is action taken by the professional to further enhance the client's welfare or well-being, providing more benefit than harm. An example of beneficence is using the client's food preferences and lifestyle in planning a nutrition plan.

Nonmaleficence. Nonmaleficence can be defined simply as "do no harm." Most dietitians would not deliberately give clients information that would cause harm. Yet, there are temptations, especially in weight control, to recommend unhealthy regimens. Dietitians need to recognize that most diets are still not completely "proven" and refrain from becoming dogmatic about any dietary regimen. Giving information is at times taken for granted as an innocuous activity that has little potential for causing harm. It must be kept in mind that there is no way of knowing all the potential risks or side effects that can occur if recommendations are followed.

Justice. Justice is a principle that implies fairness and consistency. It deals with issues that arise when there are too few resources to serve all of the people who need to be served. An example of application of this principle in dietetic practice can be cited in programs such as the WIC program in which criteria are set to limit who can receive care. If the decision were made based on the ethnic or religious background of the clients, the principle of justice would be violated.

Confidentiality. Confidentiality has to do with privacy rights. Most dietetic practitioners understand that client information is considered private and is not to be shared with others without the client's consent. However, as more dietitians go into private practice they are likely to be told things that present a conflict between the client's right to privacy and action that would be in the best interest of the client. For instance, if a teenaged client tells you that she has AIDS you might believe that this information should be passed on to prolong the person's life. A dilemma is present, and an ethical solution must be thought out.

Model of Ethical Decision-Making

The classic theory on moral development was proposed by Kohlberg. A study using Kohlberg's six stages of moral development found that dietetics students who had a sufficient duration of exposure to experiences promoting moral growth (clinical rotations with patients, ethical issues discussions with peers, access to ethics-trained instructors) demonstrated a higher level of moral development (Edelstein, 1992).

Table 10–1, six stages of moral development according to Kohlberg, outlines this classic theory (Kohlberg, 1969).

Models of ethical decision-making have been devised when ethical codes do not suffice. For example, Corey and coauthors (1993) developed a problem-solving model. It consists of seven steps that address ethical-moral and practical concerns.

1. Identify the problem.
2. Identify the potential issues.
3. Review the pertinent ethical guidelines.
4. Obtain consultation.
5. Consider possible/probable courses of action.
6. Determine the consequences of decisions.
7. Decide on the best possible course of action.

The counselor's general skill at making ethical decisions tends to increase over time and with experience (Neukrug et al, 1996). This moral development usually changes as the person matures. A higher level of ethical thought is attainable wherein ethical codes are used only as tools in soul-searching, culturally sensitive decision-making processes.

BIOETHICS

For the purpose of this book, *bioethics* is defined as ethical issues found in areas of nutrition treatment. Although not directly counseling ethics, bioethics, especially

Six Stages of Moral Development According to Kohlberg	
Stage	**What Is Considered to Be Right**
Level One: Preconventional	
Stage One: Obedience and punishment orientation	Sticking to rules to avoid physical punishment. Obedience for its own sake.
Stage Two: Instrumental purpose and exchange	Following rules only when it is in one's immediate interest. Right is an equal exchange, a fair deal.
Level Two: Conventional	
Stage Three: Interpersonal accord, conformity, mutual expectations	Stereotypical "good" behavior. Living up to what is expected by people close to you.
Stage Four: Social accord and system maintenance	Fulfilling duties and obligations to which you have agreed. Upholding laws except in extreme cases where they conflict with fixed social duties. Contributing to society, group.
Level Three: Principled	
Stage Five: Social contract and individual rights	Being aware that people hold a variety of values; that rules are relative to the group. Upholding rules because they are the social contract. Upholding nonrelative values and rights regardless of majority opinion.
Stage Six: Universal ethical principles	Following self-chosen ethical principles. When laws violate these principles, act in accord with principles.

From Kohlberg L: Moral stages and moralization: The cognitive development approach. *In* Lickoner T (ed): *Moral Development and Behavior: Theory, Research and Social Issues.* Orlando, FL: Holt, Rinehart & Winston, 1969, pp 34–35.

in institutional settings, often interplays with the ethical considerations in interpersonal relationships. For the dietitian, this usually refers to situations in which decisions to feed or not feed patients occur. The need for such decisions can occur for patients of any age. Among members of the medical community, as well as the population of this country, there is significant conflict regarding what is ethical behavior in treating the terminally ill. The American Dietetic Association has addressed this issue and published a position paper regarding terminally ill adults.

It is the position of the American Dietetic Association (King & O'Sullivan-Maillet, 1992; p. 996) that "the dietitian take an active role in developing criteria for feeding the terminally ill adult within the practice setting and collaborate with the health-care team in making recommendations on each case. The dietitian, like other health-care professionals, has an inherent ethical responsibility to respect the sanctity of life and the dignity and rights of all persons and to provide relief from suffering."

The most important ethical principle to consider in the argument to feed or not to feed is the patient's right of self-determination, or autonomy. Each patient considers death, quality of life, pain and suffering, and feeding differently, according to his or her own religion, philosophy, values, culture, morals, and so on. The dietitian's responsibility is to provide both emotional and nutrition support so that each patient can reach his or her goals. Even if the patient elects not to have nutrition support, the dietitian still needs to support the dying patient emotionally. These patients most frequently fear physical and emotional abandonment. Also, the rejection of food should not be interpreted as a sign of professional inadequacy or failure. It is important for all dietetic practitioners, and especially MNTs, to be cognizant of their own values and personal attitudes toward the dying patient, issues in feeding, and professional responsibility (King & O'Sullivan-Maillet, 1992).

Legal Considerations

- What is the legal duty of health-care facilities in providing nutrition support for the terminally ill?
- Is nutrition an integral part of mandatory palliative care or an optional medical treatment?
- Is iatrogenic (hospital-induced) malnutrition or dehydration grounds for a professional negligence lawsuit? (Butterworth and Blackburn [1975] discuss this issue in the classic article "Hospital malnutrition.") MNTs are not exempt from professional negligence malpractice suits.
- Does a mentally competent adult have the right to refuse nutrition support? Legally, patients have the right to refuse treatment. This includes their constitutional right to privacy—not to be invaded or treated against their will (eg, feeding tubes). This is part of a patient's informed consent.

The Patient Self-Determination Act, which took effect in December 1991, requires that all Medicare/Medicaid health-care providers inform patients of their right to prepare advance directives and to refuse treatment (La Puma et al, 1991). The ethical responsibility is to ensure that the patient, not the family, institution, or others, make his or her own health-care decisions.

Legal counsel can provide information on patient's rights and professional obligations. In the past 10 years, there have been numerous landmark judicial decisions addressing the issue of when nutrition support can be withdrawn or foregone.

Landmark Judicial Decisions

The Conroy case was a landmark decision by the New Jersey Supreme Court in 1985. It ruled that there was no distinction between a feeding tube and a respirator in determining whether to withdraw life-sustaining care for a patient with a limited life expectancy, "provided that is what the patient wants or would want."

The Nancy Cruzan case is probably the most famous. Following is a description of the events of the case as reported by King and O'Sullivan-Maillet (1992).

On January 11, 1983, Nancy Cruzan, then age 25, lost control of her automobile and lost consciousness when she was thrown into a ditch. Cardiopulmonary resuscitation was performed for approximately 12 to 14 minutes at the site of the accident. She was transferred to a hospital and diagnosed as having a lacerated liver and coma secondary to anoxia. She did not respond to rehabilitative programs and remained in a persistent vegetative state (PVS). She was not brain dead and therefore didn't require a respirator to breathe. A gastrostomy tube had been surgically inserted approximately 1 month after her accident.

For 5 years Cruzan's parents drove 90 miles a week to visit her. Then, after agonizing deliberation and with the counseling of religious, medical, and legal experts, they requested that the hospital remove the feeding tube. They strongly believed that their daughter would not want to live indefinitely in a "locked up" existence as a human "vegetable." When the request was refused by hospital medical administration, they petitioned the court on March 9, 1988, to seek judicial sanction for their request.

The trial court, the lowest court in Missouri, concluded from the testimony presented by Cruzan's parents, sister, and a close friend that her conversations shortly before the accident strongly suggested that she would not want to indefinitely exist in a persistent vegetative state. Permission was granted to remove the feeding tube. This judicial decision was consistent with the prevailing national trend of other court cases involving PVS patients on feeding tubes who had not left written directives but had discussed their preferences not to be sustained as a human vegetable.

The lower court's decision was immediately appealed and action was suspended to remove the feeding tube. The Missouri Supreme Court reversed the lower court's decision and denied permission to remove the feeding tube from an incompetent patient who had not left a written expression of her wishes to discontinue all treatment, including artificial feeding. The court disregarded the testimony given by the family, as well as the recommendation of the court-appointed guardian, who said it was in Cruzan's best interest to discontinue tube feeding. The court held that this was not "clear and convincing evidence" because it was inherently unreliable. The Missouri Supreme Court said that the state's interest was not in the "quality" of life but in the preservation of life, no matter how severely diminished the quality of life.

The US Supreme Court granted certiorari (permission) to hear the Cruzan case as the first case regarding right to refuse life-sustaining treatment. The question was whether Missouri had violated Nancy Cruzan's constitutional rights by not requiring the hospital to withdraw life-sustaining treatment, the feeding tube, under the specific circumstances. On June 25, 1990, in a close vote of 5 to 4, the US Supreme Court affirmed the state of Missouri's discretion to impose a very strict standard for "clear and convincing" evidence. Each state may set its own standard on what "clear and convincing" means. In November, 1990, the state of Missouri withdrew from the case which meant that now no one objected to removal of the feeding tube. The tube was removed on December 14, 1990.

Twelve days later she died.
Courts have decided that:

▪ Capable adults have the right to refuse treatment, including artificial feeding.
▪ For incompetent adults, caretakers and family need to try to ascertain the patient's wishes. What is "clear and convincing evidence" of the patient's desired wishes is often unclear.
▪ The use of advance directives (living wills) and patient-appointed surrogates will help in the decision-making process.
▪ If those wishes can be determined, they should be followed. If not, a decision must be made in accordance with the patient's "best interests."

Advance Directives

Advance directives (living wills) are witnessed, written documents or oral statements in which instructions are given by a principal or in which the principal's desires are expressed concerning any aspect of the principal's health care, including, but not limited to, the designation of a health-care surrogate, a living will, or orders not to resuscitate issued pursuant to §. 401.45. In other words, advance directives allow people to specify that they do not want their life artificially prolonged should they become terminally ill and unable to express their wishes. They can provide medical instructions. Some doctors, hospitals, and nursing and funeral homes give out living will forms, as do various patients' rights organizations. Forty-seven states have laws acknowledging living wills. Massachusetts, Michigan, and New York do not. However, a New York–based nonprofit patients' rights group, Choices in Dying, will send a state-specific living will and instruction booklet on request. The first one is free. After that, each set costs $2.50. The telephone number is 1-800-989-WILL.

A Miami Herald article, written by John Barry, appearing Sunday, June 6, 1994, discussed the issue of facing our mortality. "When Richard Nixon and Jacqueline Onassis each set the terms for their own passing through living wills, they became symbols of the new way of approaching death. Taking personal control of medical decisions." Assisted suicides, brought to the forefront by Dr. Jack Kevorkian, raise serious and complicated ethical questions.

A recent study showed that a surprisingly high number of seriously ill patients, their families, and their doctors are deciding not to resuscitate (DNR, do not resuscitate). The study followed 4301 seriously ill patients admitted to five hospitals. Of the 1150 patients who died, doctors tried to revive only one of eight who went into cardiac arrest (Barry, 1994). Many think that hospice has contributed to these changed attitudes. Hospice is a program of choice enabling terminally ill patients to live comfortable until they die. Services provided usually include trained volunteers, nurses, doctors, spiritual support, bereavement counseling, and emotional support groups. They focus on pain control and symptom management rather than fighting an inevitable end. Patients remain at home or at home-like hospital settings if necessary. Many doctors admit that death is no longer the enemy; unnecessary suffering is.

Cost/Benefit Issues

Another ethical issue is related to cost. The question of whether cost should be a factor in clinical ethical decision making is coming to the forefront as resources become more scarce (O'Sullivan-Maillet, 1995). The need to ensure a just and fair allocation of resources continues to be a moral dilemma. Managed care brings with it limitations of access to treatment and the resulting ethical problems.

Ethical issues raised by managed care will be receiving much attention in the immediate future. Already laws have been passed, such as one that requires insurance coverage for at least 48 hours of hospital stay for women giving birth. The percentage of national health dollars spent at the end of life—as high as 30% in the final months, by some estimates—has been one trigger for rethinking the do-everything approach (Barry, 1994).

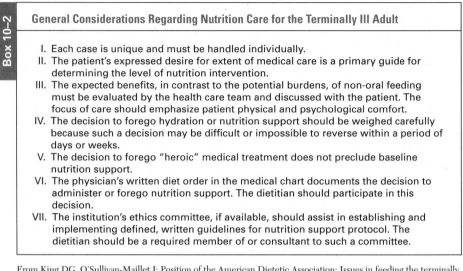

Box 10–2 presents a set of considerations regarding nutrition care for the terminally ill adult.

Medical Issues

Medical issues focus on decisions such as aggressive versus palliative care for the terminally ill. The focus of palliative care for terminally ill patients is to lessen the pain, psychological distress, and other symptoms without actually attempting to cure. Common objectives include reduction of nausea, vomiting, insomnia, and anxiety. Emotional comfort and support should be continuously provided by the health-care staff to both patient and family.

Food and drink both have psychological and physical roles to play in the care of the terminally ill. For patients able to eat and enjoy food orally, previous dietary restrictions can be minimized or eliminated depending on potential consequences. Many terminally ill patients cannot take in food orally. Sometimes the risks (eg, infection, aspiration pneumonia), burdens of pain (eg, deteriorated veins), and discomfort (eg, diarrhea) of providing nutrition support substantially outweigh the benefits.

Box 10–3 describes some considerations for examining the efficacy of providing aggressive nutrition support.

Dietitians need to consider both objective and subjective criteria for making nutrition care plans and the kind of counseling that would be most appropriate for terminally ill patients. A team approach to decision-making usually yields the best results (patient, family, doctor, nurse, social worker, therapists, dietitian, ethicist, attorney). If the facility has an ethics committee, the dietitian is well advised to become a full-time or a consulting member.

Box 10–3

Considerations for Examining the Efficacy of Providing Aggressive Nutritional Support

I. Will nutrient support, either oral or mechanical, improve the patient's quality of life during the final stages of morbidity by increasing physical strength or resistance to infections?

II. Will nutrient support, either oral or mechanical, provide the following to the patient: emotional comfort, decreased anxiety about disease cachexia, improved self-esteem with cosmetic benefits, improved interpersonal relationships, or relief from the fear of abandonment?

III. Oral feedings are the preferred choice. Tube feeding is generally the next logical step. Parenteral nutrition should be considered only when other routes are impossible or inadequate to meet the comfort needs of the patient.

IV. Oral intake
   a. Oral feeding should be advocated whenever possible. Food and control of food intake may give comfort and pleasure. The most important priority is to provide food according to the patient's individual wishes.
   b. Efforts should be made to enhance the patient's physical and emotional enjoyment of food by encouraging staff and family assistance in feeding the debilitated patient.
   c. Nutrition supplements, including commercial products and other alternatives, should be used to encourage intake and ameliorate symptoms associated with hunger, thirst, or malnutrition.
   d. The therapeutic rationale of previous diet prescriptions for an individual patient should be reevaluated. Many dietary restrictions can be liberalized. Coordination of medication or medication schedules with the diet should be discussed with the physician, with the objective of maximizing food choice and intake by the patient.
   e. The patient's right to self-determination must be considered in determining whether to allow the patient to consume foods that are not generally permitted within the diet prescription.

V. Tube feeding or parenteral feeding
   a. Palliative care is the usual realistic goal. However, a palliative care plan does not automatically preclude aggressive nutrition support.
   b. Facilities should provide and distribute written protocols for the provision of and termination of tube feedings and parenteral feedings. The protocols should be reviewed periodically, and revised if necessary, by the health-care team. Legal and ethical counsel should be routinely sought during the development and interpretation of the guidelines.
   c. The patient's informed preference for the level of nutrition intervention is paramount. The patient or guardian should be advised on how to accomplish feeding if the patient wants maximal nutrition care.
   d. Feeding may not be desirable if death is expected within hours or a few days and the effects of partial dehydration or the withdrawal of nutrition support will not adversely alter patient comfort.
   e. Potential benefits vs. burdens of tube feeding or parenteral feeding should be weighed on the basis of specific facts concerning the patient's medical and mental status, as well as on facility options and limitations.

From King DG, O'Sullivan-Maillet J: Position of the American Dietetic Association: Issues in feeding the terminally ill adult. Copyright the American Dietetic Association. Reprinted by permission from *Journal of the American Dietetic Association* 1992; 92(8):996–1005.

COUNSELING ETHICS

Ethical considerations begin as soon as nutrition interventions start at the student level. Even simulated counseling sessions must be based on ethical standards. The ethical codes that set these standards include the American Dietetic Association Code of Ethics and ethical codes of counseling professions. The following standards have been drawn from several statements.

- **A counselor should complete his or her training before practicing.** Student dietitians often provide counseling in various supervised practice settings. It should always be supervised by a registered dietitian or other qualified person. Supervision can be done by observation of the student, review of taped sessions, or reports presented by the student. There is a vast difference between the actual counseling of clients and other interviews to determine food likes and dislikes, conduct nutrition assessment, or gather other data. Such interviews do not demand the same close supervision that counseling sessions do.
- **A counselor should restrict his or her practice to the areas encompassed by his or her training.** For instance, a dietitian should not include in his or her practice physical therapy, nursing, or psychotherapy, unless qualified. A dietitian who has not had adequate counseling education and experience should attend training sessions to learn proper counseling interventions before counseling. Dietitians who do not interact well or who do not use appropriate intervention and effective communication techniques with clients can become part of the problems rather than facilitators for finding solutions. Referrals to other professionals should be made when necessary.
- **The counseling interviews and the counselor's records should be confidential.** It is acceptable to discuss clients with colleagues or other health-care professionals as long as it is in privacy and is for information gathering or professional sharing purposes. It should not be done in a public place (like the hospital cafeteria where visitors frequent). Discussing a patient's case for educational purposes (eg, lecture, in-service, documentation of activities) is also acceptable as long as the client's identity remains anonymous; refer to patient as Mr. G, Mrs. H, or patient XY.
- **A counselor's responsibility is to the client, not himself or herself.** For example, you do not counsel a client for the purpose of boosting your own ego or to meet your need for control or power. You would not counsel to fulfill your need to be nurturing and helpful. Although this may seem noble, the focus of attention is on you and your needs instead of the client's needs. It is also not ethical to counsel with missionary zeal to change others in the direction toward your own values. For example, you are a vegetarian, and you really want to change all your clients to vegetarianism because you fervently believe it is the best way to eat. This kind of missionary zeal is not appropriate in nutrition counseling.
- **A counselor's responsibility is to his or her client, not society.** This means that, even though our society in general feels that thin is better, you need to support your female client who wants only to get down to 200 pounds.

Another example is not asking a client to eliminate his favorite foods, no matter what his medical nutrition therapy dictates, unless it is life-threatening.

■ **Confidentiality may lapse when the common welfare demands revelation.** For example, when the client shares that he or she is contemplating suicide, this information may need to be shared with the client's family and the client referred to a psychologist or psychiatrist. Other issues that might arise include: "Do you tell a teenager's family when she shares that she is pregnant?" When a client is aggressive or abusive toward you, other than some normal displacement of anger, you need to talk with your supervisor or with the police.

Ethical Cross-Cultural Counseling

Ethical implications in cross-cultural counseling include (1) the MNT's world view and how it affects client welfare, (2) self-determination and cultural autonomy, and (3) ethical issues in counselor preparation. Although it is not realistic for MNTs to become intimate with many different cultures, it is possible to instill a foundation of appreciation and consideration of the unique cultural circumstances that influence client behaviors (Burn, 1992). Listening closely to clients usually reveals the cultural norms of the client.

> If counselors fail to integrate an appreciation for a client's own belief systems, the ethical principle of beneficence is violated. Beneficence, defined as "doing good" by preventing harm to the patient and, furthermore, acting in such a way as to benefit the patient, is a principle that governs the counselor-client relationship.
>
> *Cayleff, 1986, pp. 345–346*

A more in-depth discussion to enhance a strong ethical foundation in cross-cultural counseling is found in Chapter 7.

The self-inventory of attitudes relating to ethical issues, shown in Box 10–4, was developed by Gerald Corey for psychology students at California State University (Corey, 1991). Most of his questions can be effectively extrapolated to counseling as an MNT for the purpose of self-examination and analysis of possible ethical dilemmas. Some suggestions for using this self-inventory are made in Suggestions for Further Learning at the end of this chapter.

BUSINESS ETHICS

In business, codes of ethics have not been quite as formalized as those established for professional groups. However, there are some general concepts concerning a moral sense of responsibility within the business community. Broom and Longenecker (1975) discuss ethics in *Small Business Management* and recognize some basic ethical practices. They suggest that consistency of honesty is important. Failure to be honest about small things can jeopardize trust placed in an individual even if he or she is honest in big matters; insincerity and lack of integrity are soon recognized and trust is lost. In addition, small hypocrisies soon begin to distort the individual's perceptions of honest behavior.

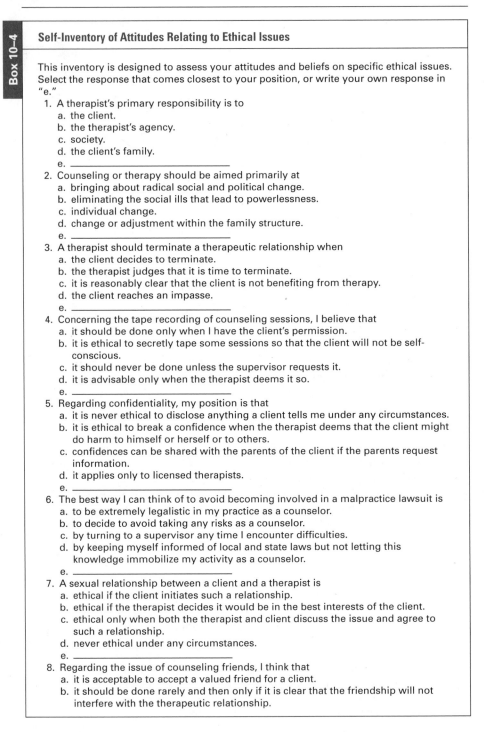

Box 10–4

Self-Inventory of Attitudes Relating to Ethical Issues

This inventory is designed to assess your attitudes and beliefs on specific ethical issues. Select the response that comes closest to your position, or write your own response in "e."

1. A therapist's primary responsibility is to
   a. the client.
   b. the therapist's agency.
   c. society.
   d. the client's family.
   e. _____

2. Counseling or therapy should be aimed primarily at
   a. bringing about radical social and political change.
   b. eliminating the social ills that lead to powerlessness.
   c. individual change.
   d. change or adjustment within the family structure.
   e. _____

3. A therapist should terminate a therapeutic relationship when
   a. the client decides to terminate.
   b. the therapist judges that it is time to terminate.
   c. it is reasonably clear that the client is not benefiting from therapy.
   d. the client reaches an impasse.
   e. _____

4. Concerning the tape recording of counseling sessions, I believe that
   a. it should be done only when I have the client's permission.
   b. it is ethical to secretly tape some sessions so that the client will not be self-conscious.
   c. it should never be done unless the supervisor requests it.
   d. it is advisable only when the therapist deems it so.
   e. _____

5. Regarding confidentiality, my position is that
   a. it is never ethical to disclose anything a client tells me under any circumstances.
   b. it is ethical to break a confidence when the therapist deems that the client might do harm to himself or herself or to others.
   c. confidences can be shared with the parents of the client if the parents request information.
   d. it applies only to licensed therapists.
   e. _____

6. The best way I can think of to avoid becoming involved in a malpractice lawsuit is
   a. to be extremely legalistic in my practice as a counselor.
   b. to decide to avoid taking any risks as a counselor.
   c. by turning to a supervisor any time I encounter difficulties.
   d. by keeping myself informed of local and state laws but not letting this knowledge immobilize my activity as a counselor.
   e. _____

7. A sexual relationship between a client and a therapist is
   a. ethical if the client initiates such a relationship.
   b. ethical if the therapist decides it would be in the best interests of the client.
   c. ethical only when both the therapist and client discuss the issue and agree to such a relationship.
   d. never ethical under any circumstances.
   e. _____

8. Regarding the issue of counseling friends, I think that
   a. it is acceptable to accept a valued friend for a client.
   b. it should be done rarely and then only if it is clear that the friendship will not interfere with the therapeutic relationship.

Box 10–4

Self-Inventory of Attitudes Relating to Ethical Issues (*Continued*)

   c. friendship and therapy should not be mixed.
   d. a friend could be accepted as a client only when the friend asks to be.
   e. _____

9. Concerning the issue of physically touching clients, my position is that
   a. touching is an important part of the therapeutic process.
   b. touching a client is not wise, because it can be misinterpreted by the client.
   c. touching a client is ethical when the client requests physical closeness with the therapist.
   d. it should be done only when the therapist feels like doing so.
   e. _____

10. The way I can best determine my level of competence in working with a given type of client is
    a. by having training, supervision, and experience in the areas in which I am practicing.
    b. by asking my clients whether they feel they are being helped.
    c. by possessing an advanced degree and a license.
    d. by relying on reactions and judgments from colleagues who are familiar with my work.
    e. _____

11. If I thought that my supervision as a counselor intern was inadequate, I would
    a. take the initiative and talk to my supervisor about it.
    b. seek supervision elsewhere, even if I had to pay for it.
    c. continue to work without complaining.
    d. attempt to compensate for lack of supervision by doing extensive reading, attending conferences and workshops, and talking with fellow interns about my work.
    e. _____

12. Continuing education for those who counsel others
    a. should be mandated by professional organizations.
    b. should be left to the discretion of the practitioner.
    c. should be a requirement for relicensure of mental-health professionals.
    d. is appropriate primarily for professionals who are open to new learning, because requiring it will simply lead to complying with the letter of the law.
    e. _____

13. I would tend to refer a client to another professional
    a. if it were clear that the client was not benefiting in the relationship with me.
    b. if I felt a strong sexual attraction to the person.
    c. if the client continually stirred up painful feelings in me (reminded me of my mother, father, ex-spouse, and so on).
    d. if I had a hard time caring for or being interested in the client.
    e. _____

14. Regarding the ethics of social and personal relationships with clients, it is my position that
    a. it is never wise to see or to get involved with clients on a social basis.
    b. it is an acceptable practice to strike up a social relationship once the therapy has ended if both want to do so.
    c. with some clients a personal and social relationship might well enhance the therapeutic relationship by building trust.
    d. it is ethical to combine a social and therapeutic relationship if both parties agree.
    e. _____

15. One of the best ways that I can think of to help me determine on what occasions and under what circumstances I would break confidentiality with a client is
    a. to confer with a supervisor or a consultant.
    b. to check out my perceptions with several colleagues.

Box 10–4

Self-Inventory of Attitudes Relating to Ethical Issues *(Continued)*

   c. to follow my own intuitions and trust my own judgment.

   d. to discuss the matter with my client and solicit his or her opinion.

   e. _____

16. If I were an intern and became convinced that my supervisor was encouraging trainees to participate in unethical behavior in an agency setting, I would
   a. encourage those trainees involved to report the situation to the director.
   b. report the supervisor to the director of the agency myself.
   c. ignore the situation, because there is really not much I would do about it.
   d. look the other way of fear of making the situation even worse.
   e. _____

17. I believe that the real reason for professional licensing and certification is
   a. to protect the public by setting minimum standards of competent practice.
   b. to protect licensed people from competition from unlicensed people and to preserve a "union shop."
   c. to increase the stature of the profession.
   d. to give the consumer a sense of confidence in the counseling profession.
   e. _____

18. My view of supervision is that it is
   a. a threat to my status as an independent professional.
   b. essential whenever I feel that I am at an impasse with a client.
   c. something that I could use on a continuing basis.
   d. a way that I can keep growing both personally and professionally.
   e. _____

19. If I thought that a client was at high risk for committing suicide, my course of action would be to tell my client that
   a. I would offer support for whatever decision she made.
   b. it would help to look at all the positive things to live for.
   c. I had certain legal and ethical responsibilities to take action to prevent her suicide.
   d. I intended to seek consultation with another professional because of my concern in this case.
   e. _____

20. In terms of appreciating and understanding the value of clients who are culturally different from me,
   a. I see it as my responsibility to learn about their values and not impose mine on them.
   b. I would encourage them to accept the values of the dominant culture for survival purposes.
   c. I would attempt to modify my counseling procedures to fit their cultural values.
   d. it is imperative that I learn about the specific cultural values my clients hold.
   e. _____

21. In working with clients from different ethnic groups, I think it is most important to
   a. be aware of the sociopolitical forces that have affected these clients.
   b. understand how language can act as a barrier to effective cross-cultural counseling.
   c. refer these clients to some professional who shares their ethnic and cultural background.
   d. help these clients modify their views so that they will be accepted and not have to suffer rejection.
   e. _____

22. To be effective in counseling clients from a different culture, a counselor must
   a. possess specific knowledge about the particular group he or she is counseling.
   b. be able to accurately "read" nonverbal messages.

Box 10–4

Self-Inventory of Attitudes Relating to Ethical Issues *(Continued)*

    c. have had direct contact with this group.
    d. treat these clients no differently from clients from his or her own cultural background.
    e. _____

23. If my philosophy were in conflict with that of the institution I worked for, I would
    a. seriously consider whether I could ethically remain in that position.
    b. attempt to change the policies of the institution.
    c. agree to whatever was expected of me in that system.
    d. quietly do what I wanted to do, even if I had to be devious about it.
    e. _____

24. Of the following, I consider the most unethical form of counselor behavior to be
    a. using the client to satisfy my personal needs.
    b. promoting a dependent relationship.
    c. continuing therapy with a client when it seems clear that the client is not benefiting from it.
    d. practicing beyond my level of competence.
    e. _____

25. My definition of an ethical therapist is one who
    a. knows the right thing to do in each problem situation in counseling.
    b. follow all of the ethical codes of the profession.
    c. continually devotes time to self-examination on issues.
    d. does not take advantage of the client.
    e. _____

Manual for Theory and Practice of Counseling and Psychotherapy by Gerald Corey. Copyright © 1995, 1990, 1985, 1981. Brooks/Cole Publishing Company, Pacific Grove, CA 93950, a division of Thomson Publishing, Inc. By permission of the publisher.

Honesty, Integrity, Fairness

Business ethics generally address issues of honesty, integrity, and fairness. Examples of honesty in the business setting include:

▌ Being honest with your clients, especially telling them when you do not know the answer to something.
▌ Being honest when you have made a mistake to take responsibility for it, not blaming others or trying to cover up.
▌ Filing claims under correct codes for insurance payments.

Examples of integrity include:

▌ Competing honestly and cooperatively.
▌ Not accepting perks from salespeople.

Examples of fairness include:

▌ Reporting infractions of other dietitians or other health-care professionals.
▌ Keeping charges competitive and adequate for your service while not being prohibitive for your clients.

Ethical Conduct

Advertising must be done in such a manner as to accurately and professionally inform the public about services, expertise, profession, and techniques of counseling. Clarity and accuracy are stressed in the American Association for Counseling and Development (AACD) 1981 Ethical Standards. A related ethical warning is the misuse of an institutional affiliation to recruit clients for a private practice (DePauw, 1986).

The Better Business Bureau (BBB) has been established to promote ethical conduct in the business world. This agency is responsive to the public and to businesses that may have complaints, as well as seeking out and stopping unethical practices when they occur. It is supported by local business firms.

In addition to articulating the principles by which a profession governs its professional conduct, the BBB serves as a vehicle for educating prospective members and the public as to the ideals of the profession and the manner in which the business community protects the public against those who would use credentials for immoral or illegal purposes.

Box 10–5

Timeline of Ethical Considerations

1. Initiation Phase Issues
   a. Precounseling considerations
      i. Advertising
      ii. Avoiding misuse of institutional affiliations
      iii. Financial arrangements
      iv. Donated services
   b. Service provision issues
      i. Adequacy of counselor skills, experience, and training
      ii. Better service option for the client
      iii. Concurrent therapist involvement
      iv. Conflicting dual relationship
   c. Informed consent issues
      i. Structures to educate regarding purposes, goals, and techniques
      ii. Explanation of rules of procedure and limitations
      iii. Supervision and consultation release concerns
      iv. Experimental methods of treatment
2. Ongoing Counseling Issues
   a. Confidentiality
   b. Special issues of confidentiality with minors
   c. Consultation
   d. Record keeping
3. Dangerousness and Crisis Concerns
   a. Threat to self
   b. Threat to others
   c. Child abuse
   d. Gray areas
4. Termination Phase Considerations
   a. Referral if unable to assist
   b. Professional evaluation

From DePauw ME: Avoiding ethical violations: A timeline perspective for individual counseling. *J Counsel Dev.* 1986; 64:303–305. © ACA. Reprinted with permission.

Box 10–5 depicts a timeline of ethical considerations for individual counseling (DePauw, 1986). It includes both business and counseling ethical issues.

Summary

Issues of morality in human relationships (ethical issues) have received attention since ancient times. Ethics portray the conscience of the professional and the profession. Implementation of the ethical component of practice demands an awareness and understanding of persons' needs and rights and a respect for justice (Kreigh & Perko, 1983).

Ethical issues faced by MNTs are diverse. In medical and clinical settings, patients' rights, confidentiality, and the provision of food and water are the primary issues that are faced (Payne-Palacio & Canter, 1996). In management settings, ethical issues revolve around honesty, integrity, and fairness in money management, personnel, materials, and time. A reiteration of the patient's right to self-determination in ethical treatment is worthy, as is the caveat for the MNT not to inflict his or her own personal values on patients and clients.

The integrity and continuing development of a profession depends in part on a willingness to examine the ethical implications of activities, to establish and update standards, and to implement strategies to foster ethical behavior (Gibson & Pope, 1993).

Suggestions for Further Learning

1. In small groups, discuss the following case study and report your recommendations to the class. Assume that the MNT is on the treatment team.

CASE EXAMPLE ·

Mrs. T is a 70-year-old woman who was admitted to the geropsychiatric unit of Middle South Psychiatric Institute (MSPI) for treatment of depression. Approximately 6 months ago, her husband died following a stroke. After a brief period of mourning, Mrs. T seemed to adjust and became interested in redecorating her small house and participating in her church's surrogate grandmother program.

When Mrs. T's son and daughter-in-law visited recently, they found that although she was still cooking meals for herself and walking out to the mailbox, she had not read her mail or washed her dishes for some days. She told them that she could not seem to get interested in anything and "just felt sad." Upset by her changed emotional state, her son suggested that Mrs. T be admitted to MSPI. She agreed to go and said that she "wanted to feel better because there were things that [she] wanted to do, but just couldn't right now."

The MSPI treatment team agreed that Mrs. T should be treated for her depression both pharmacologically and with therapy for her grief. At mealtimes, the nursing staff noted that Mrs. T ate with moderate enthusiasm, but frequently retained portions of previous mouthfuls in "pouches" of her mouth and occasionally had difficulty swallowing. MSPI policy dictates that all geriatric patients observed to have difficulty swallowing normally must be evaluated to determine their risk of aspiration. This aspiration risk policy was instituted after a patient in the geropsychiatric unit died while eating; although choking was determined not to be the cause of death, this policy was drafted to address concerns about patient welfare and MSPI's liability exposure.

Mrs. T was evaluated by an aspiration team, who determined that she was suffering from oral stage dysphasia. The team recommended pureed food and spoon-feeding in a location with few distractions. A speech pathologist was asked to train Mrs. T to swallow so as to minimize the aspiration risk.

Mrs. T was first angered and subsequently disheartened by the "diagnosis that [she] couldn't even eat right anymore." She has become combative during spoon-feeding attempts and has not had adequate nutrition for 5 days. Although she cooperates with the speech pathologist, no progress has been made in reducing her aspiration risk. The speech pathologist is concerned that Mrs. T's swallowing ability will deteriorate if she refuses to eat while being spoon-fed. The nursing staff is concerned about Mrs. T's nutritional state, the effect of her feelings of failure at eating upon her overall psychological state, and the effect of her disruptive, combative behavior on nursing staff morale and unit atmosphere. Several nurses have expressed their intention not to report future patients' swallowing difficulties. Although they are concerned about her nutritional and psychological conditions, Mrs. T's resident and attending physician are adamant that she not be allowed to feed herself because of both the risk to her life or health (eg, pneumonia) from aspiration and the hospital's liability. They are considering placing a feeding tube if Mrs. T refuses to be spoon-fed.

How should these conflicts be resolved? (Reproduced by permission © the Hastings Center, 1994.)

· ·

2. Some suggestions for using the self-inventory by Corey (1991; p. 27) are the following:

■ On completing the inventory, circle several items that have stimulated your thinking the most. Bring them to class to discuss.
■ Work in pairs on certain questions. Compare and contrast your positions.
■ Divide the class in small groups for discussions. Good material for debates are generated with divergent viewpoints.

CITED REFERENCES

American Dietetic Association: Code of ethics for the profession of dietetics. *J Am Diet Assoc.* 1988;88(12):1592–1596.

Anonymous. Case study: A hard policy to swallow. Hastings Center Report, July-August 1994; p. 23.

Broom HN, Longenecker J: *Small Business Management.* Cincinnati: Southwestern Publishing Company, 1975.

Butterworth CW, Blackburn GL: Hospital malnutrition. *Nutr Today.* 1975;10:18.

Cayleff SE: Ethical issues in counseling gender, race, and culturally distinct groups. *J Counsel Dev.* 1986;64:345–347.

Corey G: *Manual for Theory and Practice of Counseling and Psychotherapy.* 4th ed. Pacific Grove, CA: Brooks/Cole Publishing Company, 1991.

Corey G, Corey M, Callahan P: *Issues and Ethics in the Helping Professions.* Pacific Grove, CA: Brooks/Cole Publishing Company, 1993.

Curry-Bartley K: *Dietetic Practitioner Skills: Nutrition Education, Counseling, and Business Management.* New York: Macmillan Publishing Company, 1987.

DePauw ME: Avoiding ethical violations: A timeline perspective for individual counseling. *J Counsel Dev.* 1986;64:303–305.

Edelstein SF: Development of moral judgment and its relationship to the education and training of dietitians. *J Am Diet Assoc.* 1992;92(8):938–941.

Falvo DR: *Effective Patient Education. A Guide to Increased Compliance.* 2nd ed. Gaithersburg, MD: Aspen Publishing, 1994.

Gibson WT, Pope KS: The ethics of counseling: A national survey of certified counselors. *J Counsel Dev.* 1993;71:330–336.

King DG, O'Sullivan-Maillet J: Position of the American Dietetic Association: Issues in feeding the terminally ill adult. *J Am Diet Assoc.* 1992;92(8):996–1005.

Kohlberg L: Moral stages and moralization: The cognitive developmental approach. *In* Lickoner T (ed): *Moral Development and Behavior: Theory, Research and Social Issues.* Orlando, FL: Holt, Rinehart & Winston, 1969; pp 34–35.

Kreigh HZ, Perko JE: *Psychiatric and Mental Health Nursing: A Commitment to Care and Concern.* 2nd ed. Reston, VA: Reston Publishing Company, 1983.

LaPuma J, Orentilicher D, Moss RJ: Advanced directives on admission: Clinical implications and analysis of the Patient Self-Determination Act of 1990. *JAMA.* 1991;266:402–405.

Neukrug E, Lovell C, Parker R: Employing ethical codes and decision-making models: A developmental process. *Counsel Values.* 1996;40:103.

O'Sullivan-Maillet J: Position of the American Dietetic Association: Legal and ethical issues in feeding permanently unconscious patients. *J Am Diet Assoc.* 1995;95(2):231–234.

Payne-Palacio J, Canter DD: *The Profession of Dietetics: A Team Approach.* Englewood, NJ: Prentice-Hall, 1996.

ADDITIONAL RESOURCES

Anderson GR, Glesnes-Anderson VA: *Health Care Ethics: A Guide for Decision Makers.* Rockville, MD: Aspen Publishing, 1987.

Bowie NE: *Making Ethical Decisions.* New York: McGraw-Hill, 1985.

Dalton S: What are the sources and standards of ethical judgment in dietetics? *J Am Diet Assoc.* 1991;91(5):545–546.

Edelstein S, Anderson S: Bioethics and dietetics: Education and attitudes. *J Am Diet Assoc.* 1991;91(5):546–548.

Heaney RP, Dougherty CJ: *Research for Health Professionals: Design, Analysis, Ethics.* Ames, IA: Iowa State University Press, 1988.

Oxendind B: Are you ethical? Why ethics are important in your career. *Florida Leader.* 1992;7.

Russell CA: Role of dietitians in enteral feeding. *Gut.* 1986;27(S1):58–60.

Strein W, Hershenson DB: Confidentiality in nondyadic counseling situations. *J Counsel Dev.* 1991;69:312–315.

Wall MG, Wellman NS, Curry KR, Johnson PM: Feeding the terminally ill: Dietitian's attitudes and beliefs. *J Am Diet Assoc.* 1991;91(5):549.

Zeatch RM: *Medical Ethics.* Boston: Jones & Bartlett Publishers, 1989.

CHAPTER 11

Professional Considerations

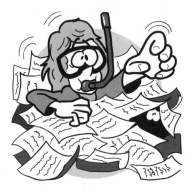

GOALS

The goals of this chapter are (1) to discuss various aspects of professional communications, both verbal and written, (2) to summarize the professional environments in which dietetic practitioners counsel, and (3) to review marketing strategies.

Learning Objectives

At the end of this chapter the reader will be able to:

1. Recognize and begin to practice effective verbal and written communications.

2. Give examples of assertive, aggressive, and passive behaviors.

3. Describe various settings that are conducive to counseling clients.

4. Identify business procedures, including the importance of third-party reimbursement and managed care.

5. Describe marketing strategies employed in inpatient and outpatient settings.

6. Develop a view toward the future of medical nutrition therapy and nutrition counseling.

Key Terms

▶ **Assertiveness:** characterized by behavior that gives empathic honest expression to thoughts, feelings, and creativity.

▶ **Clinical Pathways:** a tool to improve managed-care outcomes. Also called practice guidelines, patient care protocols, care maps, and multidisciplinary action plans (MAPs). Data from large numbers of patients are pooled to create these pathways.

▶ **Licensure:** formal permission from state and/or local government to practice nutrition counseling.

▶ **Managed Care:** prepaid health plans that offer a mechanism for cost-effective health care. HMOs, PPOs, and IPAs are examples. Managed care applies standard business practices to the medical industry.

▶ **Marketing:** the process of promoting services and/or business in a competitive environment.

▶ Medicaid: a state and federal program of hospitalization and medical insurance for people of all ages within certain income limits.

▶ Medicare: a federal program of hospitalization and medical insurance for persons aged 65 years and over.

▶ Negotiate: to arrange for or to bring about by discussion and settlement of terms, a process of give and take.

▶ Nonassertiveness: encompasses characteristics and behaviors that discount the needs and wants of self and/or others. It can take the form of aggression or passivity.

▶ Profession: a self-regulated occupational group that has a unique function in society, usually requiring extensive training.

▶ Third-Party Payment: the process by which various types of insurance plans pay for medical and health coverage.

The unique and central purpose of dietetic and nutrition professionals is to translate nutrition knowledge into nutrition lifestyle. Burgeoning beliefs in wellness and prevention of disease have created many opportunities for dietetic practitioners. The way in which the opinions of dietetic practitioners will be received by other professionals and the public will depend on their communication skills. For the MNT, success in meeting this challenge requires three general qualities: nutrition knowledge, communication skills, and a professional demeanor.

The rest of this book has focused on counseling and interpersonal communication. This chapter discusses interprofessional communication, both verbal and written, in groups and individually, and the professional environment in which medical nutrition therapy occurs. The focus here is more on outpatient departments, clinical settings, and private practice arenas for professional considerations. As emphasized throughout the text, effective medical nutrition therapy is unlikely to occur in a single session with a client; however, this is what usually occurs in acute-care settings. Since many practicing professionals do work in hospitals and perform inpatient care, some acute care issues are addressed. It is hoped that inpatient dietitians exert a good degree of time and energy during their one session in directing patients to continued care of nutrition therapy after discharge (King-Helm & Klawitter, 1995). Fiscal procedures, including third-party payment, managed care, and health-care reform, are reviewed. The need for marketing is detailed in step-wise fashion, and future trends are explored. To some extent, this chapter is a discussion of how the MNT sells himself or herself and presents ideas so that individuals and policies are influenced.

PROFESSIONAL ENVIRONMENT

In much the same way that body language tells the client more about the MNT than spoken words, the environment in which MNTs work communicates to the client many things about the MNT. The client gains clues as to the counselor's self-concept and power from the work surroundings.

Picture a health clinic. What is noticed? Is it crowded? Empty and bleak? Quiet? Noisy? Cluttered? Neat? How does it smell? Is it clean? Dirty? Antiseptic? Bright with light? Too bright? What expectations are there in the environment just created? What status could be attributed to the people who work in such an environment and how much confidence would be placed in them?

Now shift thoughts to the private office of a physician, lawyer, or psychological counselor. How does the environment contrast with that in the first example? What does the environment in the second situation bring to mind as far as expectations about the people who will provide service and the expected outcomes?

Each person may draw significantly different conclusions from this exercise, yet some general conclusions can be reached: (1) some people will be comfortable and some uncomfortable in each environment; (2) the more control an MNT has (as does the person in a private office) over the environment in which she or he works, the better able she or he will be to surround himself or herself with the desired message to communicate to the client; (3) by recognizing the different reactions people have to different environments, the chances of success can be increased wherever the practice may be. The environment should be suited to the clientele whom you expect to serve.

Certain aspects of any environment are more conducive to success no matter where the MNT works. A neat, but not stark, work space certainly helps set the tone for clear thinking and comfortable feelings. In addition, a clean smell is important. These two things are a minimum for environmental control. It is true that a dynamic person can overcome almost any environment, but most professionals need to pay attention to establishing a workplace that helps create a desirable environment, one that is consistent with the practitioner's goals and purposes.

Dietetic practitioners work in a variety of environments. A quick eye and a creative mind can be of service in arranging the physical environment in any situation. In many cases, assertiveness and a refusal to accept an undesirable environment are essential. There are many ways to develop an environment in which effective nutrition counseling can take place.

Hospitals

In hospitals, it is sometimes necessary for nutrition care and counseling to take place at the bedside. However, whenever possible, this practice should be discontinued. The very fact that the client is in bed reduces his or her capacity as a decision-maker and problem-solver. At the very least, have the patient seated in a chair. Turn off the television, close the door, and request that the phone not be answered. If the patient is ambulatory, bring him or her to an office or to a conference room that is comfortable. Some dietitians now have offices on the patient floors for just this reason. Select chairs that will be comfortable yet allow each person to assume a posture suitable for problem-solving. Be sure the room is tidy, the light comfortable, and the noise level acceptable. Place the chairs so that the light does not interfere with communication. Decide whether or not a table is needed. If needed, place the chairs at the table so that there is no barrier between the nutrition counselor and the patient. If there is a physical object in between, the patient may interpret that as an indication of your discomfort with interpersonal contact. If the temperature can be controlled, make sure that it is within the comfort zone for your patient, realizing that in some types of illnesses the patient may respond to temperature erratically. Then relax, realizing that you have done all you can, and refuse to let the patient use any discomfort he or she may experience (unless it is significant enough that it should be dealt with) as a method of avoiding the issue at hand.

If a hospital does not already have a private area for counseling, one should be established. In this situation, influence needs to be exerted to create a favorable environment for the counseling and instruction of clients. An ideal situation would include an area in which there is sufficient space for the storage of audiovisual equipment and supplies and other educational material, a teaching center, and a counseling center appropriate for individual or group counseling. The minimum space that can accommodate these basic needs is a room at least 10 by 14 feet. The walls should be painted or papered and have a flat surface, and there should be highlights of color in the room to indicate calmness, yet lightness.

A room that can serve for individual counseling, group counseling, or small group instruction will need the following basic furniture: a desk, a desk chair, two side chairs, a table lamp or a floor lamp in addition to the installed lighting, a bookcase, a storage cabinet for audiovisual materials, six to 10 classroom-style chairs, one folding table approximately 30 by 72 inches, one comfortable chair, a chalkboard, a bulletin board, and a plant or two, which may add warmth.

Outpatient Clinics and Community Facilities

In an outpatient clinic, group instruction space can and should be an area that can be used by various professionals. In such situations, the dietetic practitioner has the responsibility for exerting influence on the development of this space and for creating the private area needed for one-on-one counseling sessions. If at all possible, an office with a door is preferable. Minimal furniture includes a desk, desk chair, two side chairs, a cabinet for audiovisual equipment, and a bookcase. If the room is small, neatness will be of the utmost importance. Other personnel, such as secretaries or clerks, should not share this space.

Schools

Dietetic practitioners often have a central office and are only part-time in schools. Every effort must be made to adapt to a wide variety of environments. At the same time, assertive attempts to change undesirable environments should be made. A special classroom for nutrition education can help create the environment needed to help children recognize the vital nature of good nutrition, although this is rare. Sometimes a cafeteria may provide a good setting. Exciting, attention-getting audiovisual aids on bulletin boards and as part of a movable educational system can also be highly effective in school systems.

Corporate Settings

In settings in which the dietetic practitioner is working as part of a corporate structure, insistence on an appropriate environment is essential if the credibility of the dietetic practitioner is to be established and maintained. It is a professional responsibility to become familiar with what is possible in each situation and to include negotiation for space in initial employment agreements. Unless there is an overwhelming reason for another arrangement, a private office should be expected. Space in a wellness center may be shared with others and can also be negotiated.

Space can be shared with other professionals efficiently if cooperation is obtained in meeting the various needs of the different individuals and their clients. Some of the environmental requirements for nutrition counseling are similar to those for occupational therapists, psychologists, and others.

Individual Office Space

Initial planning of office space should consist of imagining the ideal situation, without regard to restrictions. After outlining the first plan, priorities can be established and the plan modified to fit economic constraints. The goals of nutrition counseling must guide the development of an environment that will foster success in reaching them. The essential environmental consideration is to make the physical surroundings as free of distractions as possible so that attention can be focused on the task at hand (Berne, 1966).

In the beginning, think of as many variables as possible that will make the setting ideal for nutrition counseling. Make a list of the time needed, the amount of space required, and the supplies and equipment necessary to conduct counseling and nutrition classes. From this list, evaluate the relative value of different ideas and determine the costs incurred in creating an ideal setting. An office that meets these criteria will be comfortable in regard to size, color, temperature, and furnishings and be free of objects that would distract clients from the business at hand. Decor should be warm, light, calm and non-distracting. Wall hangings should be unobtrusive. Credentials can be placed on the walls, but such items as family pictures and nutrition education posters tend to distract clients. A waiting room is desirable and is the appropriate place for nutrition education materials and perhaps aesthetic educational posters. What type of space fits this ideal depends on each individual's own goals, plans, and dreams, and may be quite different for each professional.

ORAL COMMUNICATION

Communication and getting along with others often makes the difference between success and failure in persuading people that you are knowledgeable. Poor communication with colleagues and supervisors can get even the most competent person fired. It is just common sense to know that communication is an essential ingredient for professional success. It is also an essential ingredient in establishing the role of the medical nutrition therapist in patient care. We know that nutrition is important, yet we all too often forget that we must persuade others to accept our role, appreciate our expertise, and recognize our competence, as well as the benefits of a healthy nutrition lifestyle. Assertiveness plays a major role in effective communication. It is explored here in detail to promote a solid professional communication foundation.

Assertiveness

Assertiveness is a form of interpersonal communication that gives empathic, honest expression to one's thoughts, feelings, and creativity. Assertiveness assumes equality between communicators. It is a characteristic found among successful counselors. Assertive counselors exhibit an authentic style that shows respect for clients and themselves (Meadors & Rogers, 1984).

Descriptions of Assertiveness

The assertive person is able to ask for what he or she wants, refuse requests without undue stress, and accept that other people also have the right to be assertive. Assertiveness requires willingness to accept responsibility for one's own thoughts, feelings, and behaviors (Alberti & Emmons, 1986). Behaviors are confident yet considerate, as opposed to tentative behaviors (passive), or overwhelming behaviors (aggressive). People who are highly assertive have been shown to be more internally controlled than less assertive people (Williams & Stout, 1985).

Foundations of Assertiveness

The basic building block of assertiveness is the belief that you have the right to assert yourself. For the fortunate, this belief is established in early childhood. Among developmental psychologists there is wide acceptance of the idea that consistent, firm control combined with parental warmth promotes the development of high self-esteem and assertiveness in children. Children need outside control to serve as a model for inner control. Inner control provides a sense of autonomy. Autonomy, an integral part of assertiveness, implies self-control, relinquishing control of others. Children who grow up in environments of overcontrol or undercontrol struggle with self-esteem and tend to develop nonassertive behavior patterns (Bronstein, 1994).

Emotional autonomy has been defined as the ability to define oneself, rather than to be defined by others, and freedom from pressing needs for approval and reassurance. Instrumental autonomy is the ability to act, cope with problems, and meet one's needs. Autonomy includes relinquishing attempts to control others and accepting that others have the same rights as you and can act in their own best interests.

Women are sometimes thought of as passive, submissive, dependent, and helpless. Submissiveness in women is sometimes more appreciated than assertiveness. It has been pointed out that women find themselves in a double bind when they strive for assertiveness. Often women who act assertively are seen as aggressive, yet those who are submissive are viewed as compliant and overdependent and are considered ineffective (Josefowitz, 1984). Whatever behavior is exhibited, women may encounter accusations of being incompetent and sometimes of being irrational even when exhibiting behavior that is accepted as assertiveness in men (Chenevert, 1994). The field of health, under the medical model of patient care, has been no exception. Women often choose health professions because of a need to nurture and a tendency to define themselves by their success in relationships.

Protecting or providing for these "others" may inhibit assertive behavior because of concern that assertiveness is a threat to others (Phelps & Austin, 1987). Women in the medical field frequently face the dilemma of being expected to perform professionally and autonomously while remaining traditionally feminine and passive (Slater, 1990).

Professional Rights and Responsibilities

Professional rights and the responsibilities that accompany them have been outlined for health-care professionals. Emphasis generally has been on the rights of women because of the overwhelming number of female health-care professionals. Sincere belief in one's rights underlies assertiveness. Listed here are some essential aspects of an assertive belief system.

1. Assertiveness is appropriate.
2. Expertise brings with it rights to decision-making and responsibility for decisions made.
3. It is OK to be independent of the good will of others, ie, "I am still OK even if others are mad at me."
4. Mistakes are inevitable, and it is appropriate to take responsibility for them.
5. It is OK to change your mind, to not care, and to be illogical at times.

Need for Assertiveness

Assertiveness is a desirable characteristic for MNTs in every aspect of dietetics and nutrition practice. Opportunities to be effective MNTs and nutrition care managers often depend upon other professionals' and the public's recognizing the value of dietetic and nutrition services. Increased assertiveness is needed in at least three ways: (1) delivery of competent nutrition care, (2) documentation of the effectiveness of medical nutrition therapy and other nutrition services, and (3) pursuit of leadership and decision-making positions in the health-care arena.

Perceptions of Assertiveness

Although the overall description of assertiveness is generally accepted among professionals, the lay public does not always have a clear understanding of assertiveness (Boisvert et al, 1985). Men and women do not always perceive assertiveness quite the same way. A study has shown that both men and women perceive assertiveness as:

forceful
dominating
pushy
influencing
knowing what you want
self-confidence

However, men were more likely to perceive assertiveness as aggressiveness, goal-driven, and getting what you want, whereas women more likely perceived assertiveness as direct expression of feelings, respecting one's self and others, and not feeling guilty when saying "no." Women in the study also perceived consideration of others as a part of assertiveness, whereas the men did not.

It is clear from this that the women in the study were more internally focused than the men. Distinctions between assertiveness and aggressiveness seem fuzzy among both men and women. No one mistook passive behaviors for assertiveness (Wilson & Gallois, 1993).

Responses to Assertiveness

Assertiveness is not always well received. Change in a person's behavior is frequently unsettling to those close to the person, because predictability is lowered. In addition, the exhibition of assertiveness in a person who was previously passive changes the balance of power in relationships and usually causes friction. For these reasons, efforts to become assertive should be undertaken slowly and in limited areas, gradually developing into overall assertiveness. There are indications that even though assertiveness among women is sometimes regarded as aggressive (and undesirable), women's self-esteem rises as they become more assertive (Delamater & McNamara, 1986).

Styles of Assertiveness

Styles of assertiveness vary from situation to situation, and from person to person. Consistent efforts are required to build medical nutrition therapy programs. "They won't let me" must become a sentence no longer heard among MNTs. In interprofessional communication, one presents oneself with confidence to express ideas and feelings, and to pursue these in the face of rejection. The MNT often must be an advocate in assisting individual clients make use of the health-care system, as well as advocating for effective service.

In the counseling situation, the MNT presents herself or himself with sufficient self-confidence to withhold self-expression when it is in the best interest of the client. Withholding ideas is frequently a challenge, especially for a novice counselor. A client may attempt a "yes, but" game, asking the MNT for help when the client really knows the acceptable answer to a question. The nonassertive MNT may fall into the trap. The following case example illustrates this.

CASE EXAMPLE ·

CLIENT: "What do you think I should say to my wife when she goes ahead and makes ham for the family, and I know I should not eat salty foods?"

MNT: " 'No, thank you,' is probably the easiest thing to say."

CLIENT: "She'll just go right ahead and ask me again, putting the pressure on."

MNT: "Explain the reasons why you don't want to eat the ham."

CLIENT: "That will just start a fight."

To stop this game, the MNT could assertively answer the very first question with a question herself.

M N T: "What do you think is the thing to say?"

C L I E N T: "Well, I could take some and just leave it on my plate."

The client may answer, "I don't know." In this case the MNT might answer, "Make a guess." In most cases, the client will provide an answer that he or she is willing to use. This interchange could be followed up with practice of the selected responses.

• •

Assertive Communication

Even though each situation is unique, there are systematic ways of communicating assertively. Following are examples of assertive communication.

1. Straightforward requests. "I expect you to be at work on time."
2. Consistent, calm, but not nagging, repetition of what is wanted when it is not granted upon first request and is still desirable; for example, contacting insurance companies several times with requests for payment or extended counseling sessions. "I am calling again to see if we can work out payment for medical nutrition therapy."
3. Negotiation when several people have different needs; for example, when two people want off from work on the same day: "Let's see how we can work this out."
4. Responses to criticism that may not be true or is manipulative that are calm and acknowledge the possibility that the criticism might be partially correct. "I am not sure I agree with your assessment, but I will take note of it and use the information."
5. Acknowledgment, with no excuses, when criticism is true. "Yes, I see I made an error. It is a good thing you noticed. I'll correct it."
6. Expression of unsolicited feelings in a noncritical (of self or others) manner. "I was concerned when you didn't arrive for your appointment last week."
7. Keeping the conversation on the topic rather than on personalities in the face of personal attacks. "Boy, you really are aggressive." "Whether I am aggressive or not is not the issue, the issue is . . ."
8. Accepting compliments without excuses or self-deprecating comments. "Thank you for the compliment."
9. Silence can be assertive when appropriately used.
10. Aggression is sometimes necessary. "You **will** listen to me."

Regardless of the situation, keep the following in mind: (1) when dealing with issues use words to address the issues, not personalities involved; (2) body language consistent with verbalization—firm voice, steady (but not staring) eye contact, erect yet relaxed body, and direct communication; (3) show empathy for others.

Effective use of the word "I" deserves special attention. Assertive expressions of the self: "I feel angry," "I think you did a fine job" indicate that you are responsible for your own thoughts and behaviors, and indicate confidence in yourself. By contrast, "You make me mad" or "That was a fine job" distance the feeling and thought and suggest that a person feels uncomfortable with self-responsibility.

A Communication Model. Butler (1976) in *Self-Assertion for Women* presented some concepts of assertive communication. She addressed the ability to express both positive and negative feelings, the ability to set limits and initiate the assertion of need. Some examples of assertiveness in these areas are:

Positive Feelings

Counselor to client, "I am proud of your accomplishment."
Counselor to colleague, "Thank you for sending me clients."

Negative Feelings

Counselor to client, "I am upset by your repeated tardiness for your appointment."
Counselor to physician, "I am frustrated when my calls aren't returned."

Setting Limits

Counselor to client, "My fee is $75.00 per session."
Counselor to supervisor, "It usually takes at least an hour to conduct an effective initial interview."

Self-Initiation of Expression of a Need

Counselor to supervisor, "I need to take care of some unexpected business tomorrow and will need to have the day off. I will arrange for my absence."
Counselor to colleague, "I really need some professional shop talk. Let's have lunch tomorrow and split the check."

These statements are all direct, to the point, and nonmanipulative. They are assertive.

Descriptions of Nonassertiveness

Nonassertiveness, a form of communication that discounts the needs and wants of individuals, assumes inequality between communicators. It is essentially dishonest and manipulative. Solutions to problems that are satisfactory to those involved are usually avoided. In transactional analysis terms, the transactions are ulterior and a basis for game playing, blaming others for difficulties.

Nonassertiveness serves to prevent close relationships, hinder creativity, and foster overly competitive win-lose relationships, professionally as well as interpersonally. The result is poor problem-solving. Nonassertiveness can be expressed by passivity or aggression. Passivity can be seen in the overcompliant individual. Aggressiveness is seen in people who seem to be "driven." Few people can sustain passive or aggressive behavior over a long period of time, but most people vacillate between the two, being passive for a period of time, then becoming aggressive. Often indirect aggression is exhibited, a behavior commonly thought of as passive-aggressive.

Types of Nonassertiveness

Aggression. Aggressive behavior is manipulative and controlling in an overt and intimidating manner. A win-lose situation generally results, in which aggressors come out on top but never seem satisfied or secure in winning. Aggressors are compelled to try to prove themselves again and again. They may be ruthless, willing to do anything to get what they want. Interpersonal relationships are strained, and much energy is diverted from creative activities because that energy is consumed in controlling merely for the sake of controlling. Conversations are intimidating, insulting, or sarcastic. Threatening remarks are used, and voice tones as well as words are "other-blaming" and accusatory. Aggression may serve the purpose to hide a low self-concept. It usually comes from a belief that life is very competitive, and that winning is essential to be successful in life (Dainow, 1986).

Passivity and Overcompliance. Passive, overcompliant behavior, on the other hand, is self-blaming, conciliatory, and at first can be perceived as "mature," especially in women. However, overcompliance is also non-problem-solving and calculated to prevent close relationships and maintain low self-esteem. Hurts are turned inward, resulting in feelings of guilt and depression. People who are overcompliant may follow directions, always trying to be good, and often manifest physical symptoms of distress. The energy level in overcompliant individuals is very low. They may work hard, but they frequently have little ability to do anything without being told what to do. They have little initiative, and often just do not get things done. They have little influence on others because their energy is turned inward, keeping them under control. Overcompliant people spend their time trying to smooth things over and often become victims of aggressive individuals.

Passive-Aggressive Behaviors. Most people exhibit patterns of behavior that are sometimes passive and sometimes aggressive. People are compliant for a while until energy is built up to the point where hostile feelings are at a sufficient tension level to precipitate aggressiveness and an outburst of emotion. During the compliant stage (passive), behaviors are manipulative and controlling in indirect ways. This hidden aggression is often perceived by others as confused and unclear communications or as a "mixed message." Teasing, sarcasm, and inconsistencies between verbal and nonverbal messages are common examples of such indirectly aggressive behavior (Dainow, 1986). Individuals attempt to hide hostile feelings, yet hostility is apparent in teasing and sarcasm. During the overtly hostile stage (aggressive), the outsider often perceives that the aggressor is "over-reacting." Within a short time, the energy will be expelled, guilt over the outburst will emerge, and a retreat to a resentful passivity will occur. A common reason people have difficulty moving out of the passive aggressive cycle is the retention of unresolved anger.

Distinguishing Among Behaviors. There is often difficulty in distinguishing between assertive and aggressive behaviors. Tactics used to assert one's rights can be labeled both assertive and aggressive. In addition, assertiveness in women and minorities is often labeled as aggressive (Wilson & Gallois, 1993). Empathy in the delivery of assertive messages seems to be a key factor in the perception of assertive behaviors, especially assertiveness in environments of conflict. Passivity is rarely confused with assertiveness or aggression.

Following are descriptions to help distinguish between assertive and nonassertive thoughts, feelings, and behaviors.

Situation. You have a client who has not paid you for one session and is now telling you that she cannot pay you for the session you have just completed.

Passivity and Overcompliance

Thoughts: I should consider how difficult it is for people to pay for nutrition counseling. If I confront the client she probably won't come back and I'll lose a client. Maybe she will even discourage other clients. I can't afford to lose clients.

Feelings: Resentment and hidden anger.

Behavior: Smiles, "Well, I guess that will be OK, but I hope you will pay next time."

Aggressiveness

Thoughts: "Boy, I don't have to take this. After all the energy I put into this lady how can she not pay? I better take care of myself. She's just no good."

Feelings: Obvious anger and impatience.

Behavior: "You don't need to come back until you have paid your bill in full."

Assertiveness

Thinking: "I wonder what might be happening in her life that has brought this about."

Feelings: Neutral

Behavior: "You seem to be having some financial problems. We need to discuss a method of payment that will be satisfactory to both of us. Let's take a moment to do that right now."

CASE EXAMPLE ·

Assertive

MNT on the phone to an insurance company:

"Hello, this is Janet Walker, medical nutrition therapist with Health Care Systems, I would like to obtain permission to see Mrs. Smith, whom you insure, for medical nutrition therapy over a period of at least 3 weeks. She can improve her condition quite dramatically, I believe, with appropriate nutrition counseling. There are a number of advantages . . ."

Nonassertive

"Hello, uh, this is Janet Walker, I, uh, wonder if you would, uh, give permission, for me to see Mrs. Smith, for a few times, she, uh, doesn't know her diet very well, you know". (nonassertive, passive).

"Hello, this is Janet Walker, medical nutrition therapist. Your company really doesn't provide adequate coverage for medical nutrition therapy. You are going to have a lot of trouble with Mrs. Smith if she doesn't learn her diet better. I can't do the right kind of job if I don't get permission to see her for several weeks." (nonassertive, aggressive).

• •

Distinctions between assertiveness and nonassertiveness are evident in a number of behavior categories. Table 11–1 presents a comparison of assertive, aggressive, and passive aggressive behaviors (Curry-Bartley, 1987).

Barriers to Assertiveness

From birth, it is more likely for boys than for girls to be taught assertiveness in many societies. Girls are more often taught to be compliant, putting others' needs before their own. Consequently, girls are less likely to develop high self-esteem or beliefs that they have rights of assertiveness. It appears that particular pressure to be feminine begins to take place around the age of 8 years (Sheehy, 1995). Consequently, feelings of conflict are common among women as to their adult role. The anxiety model in Chapter 8 depicts such conflicts effectively.

Irrational thoughts and negative feelings underlie unassertiveness. Studies have shown that less assertive people have more irrational thoughts (Delamater &

TABLE 11–1

Comparison of Assertive, Aggressive, and Passive Aggressive Behaviors			
	Assertive	**Aggressive**	**Passive Aggressive**
Time Orientation	Usually on time	Early, pacing	Late
Helpfulness	Allows independence *or* Gives help when needed	Unhelpful	Overly helpful
Criticism	Gives objectively	Intimidates	Takes blame
Problem-Solving	Negotiates Gets problem solved	Demands control Scolds Problems remain	Too agreeable *or* Stubborn and sneaky Sarcastic Problems remain
Responsibility	Objectively determined	Blames others	Blames self

From Curry-Bartley KR: *Dietetic Practitioner Skills: Nutrition Education, Counseling and Business Management.* New York: MacMillan, 1987.

McNamara, 1986). A series of irrational thoughts becomes a system of irrational beliefs that contribute to the retention of unassertive behaviors. People talk themselves out of assertiveness, so to speak. Some underlying irrational beliefs that support nonassertivenss are summarized here:

Beliefs that Support Passivity

- I am responsible for other people's feelings and I must be careful not to hurt them.
- I will be unloved if I stand up for myself.
- People will think I am not nice.
- Nothing works for me so I might as well not try.

Beliefs that Support Aggressiveness

- I am not responsible for anybody, and they can look out for themselves.
- I have a right to say anything I want.
- Winning is all that counts. If I don't win, I have to lose, and that is unacceptable.

Feelings

Feelings are a major inhibitor of assertiveness. Anxiety was described earlier in this text. Anger and fear are also inhibiting when they are intense and interfere with thinking in a problem-solving situation. Attempts to suppress feelings are usually counterproductive. When the difference between having feelings and acting out feelings is recognized, a person is able to use energy to solve problems rather than suppress feelings.

Anxiety regarding the outcomes of being assertive may inhibit assertiveness. Changes in behavior make it more difficult for others to predict the outcome of your behavior. The first result of new assertive behaviors may be negative (Wilson & Gallois, 1993). Family, friends, and colleagues will put on pressure to get you to change back to behavior patterns to which they are accustomed. It is only after new behaviors have become routine that people will begin to respond differently to you, and positive effects will occur. It is often best to exhibit behavior changes with people who are less important to you first and when you have increased confidence begin to be more assertive with people closer to you. When you believe that assertiveness training may be useful to a client, be sure that she or he also understands that immediate results can be negative.

Steps to Assertiveness

The way to gain assertive skills is to analyze situations in which there is difficulty being assertive and compare them to situations in which it is easy to be assertive. Examine thoughts, beliefs, feelings, and behaviors in each situation. Plan and practice changes, beginning with behaviors that create minor stress before moving on to situations in which you are more vulnerable. Josefowitz (1984) suggests that one begin steps to assertiveness with the honest expression of feelings. When that becomes comfortable, move on to request, demand, insist, confront, and then to refuse, reject, criticize, or dismiss.

Other authors suggest starting the process of becoming assertive by saying "no" (Weiss, 1982). People may even need to be aggressive in refusal in the early stages because of an intense emotional state. Continued practice will reduce tension and the calmer, empathic assertiveness will emerge.

When assertiveness has been established as a lifestyle, people behave much more spontaneously, judging each situation more realistically, and making judgments as to whether assertiveness, passivity, or aggression will be the most appropriate behavior.

PROFESSIONAL COMMUNICATION IN GROUPS

Some professionals have responsibilities for serving on committees in professional settings. The more you become aware of group dynamics and your own role in the group, the better you will be able to influence the groups to your own ideas—and that is what communication is all about. Aristotle told us thousands of years ago, the purpose of all communication is to persuade others to your way of thinking.

Facilitative and Obstructive Communication

A person's behavior is shaped by his or her own attitudes and beliefs about how she or he fits into a particular group, which can vary from group to group. Types of groups to which MNTs belong include inter- and intradepartment committees, multidisciplinary teams, and educational groups.

In the group setting, generally there are two types of communicators, those who facilitate and those who obstruct. Although individuals who obstruct may be sometimes seen as powerful, their power is poorly used and they prevent problem-solving. Facilitators focus on problem-solving and creativity. The behaviors can also be recognized as valid descriptions of assertiveness (facilitating) versus passive-aggressiveness (obstructive). Table 11–2 outlines the characteristics of both.

The behaviors exhibited in group meetings can indicate how much of what you want you will get out of the group. This includes not only the things that are acknowledged as part of your official membership in the group, but also the influences you want to exert because of your own psychological needs. These needs are often referred to as the "hidden agenda." Everyone brings some degree of a hidden agenda to meetings. Hidden agendas regulate the social interactions and also the ideas that are endorsed by the group. Generally, whether one is a facilitator or an obstructer is part of the hidden agenda.

Negotiating

Resolving all the different ideas that are brought up by committee members requires negotiating. Usually work progresses best when goals are negotiated and agreed on first. This approach may seem time-consuming at the moment, but it saves time later because group members become goal-oriented.

Central to negotiating is the ability to disagree with others without being disagreeable. It is important to recognize that when you are negotiating, you are al-

 Characteristics of Facilitative and Obstructive Communication	
Facilitative Communication	**Obstructive Communication**
Referring to others by name	Using big words to show off
Asking for clarification when you do not understand something	Asking questions to attract attention
	Interrupting others
Keeping your mind open to the ideas of others	Changing the subject to attract attention
Building on the ideas of others	Talking too much
Speaking in a logical, organized manner	Repeating the same thing over and over
Using simple, straightforward language	Saying things to discount what others have said
Complimenting others freely	
Using a pleasant tone of voice	Using foul language
Speaking clearly, and loudly enough to be easily heard by all	Shouting unnecessarily, arguing
	Talking too fast or too slowly
Looking people in the eye without staring	Looking bored or angry; fidgeting
Sitting as though interested, leaning forward	Shaking your head no while someone is trying to make a point
Making nonverbal signs of receipt of the message, to encourage others to speak	Rolling eyes while others are talking
Wearing clothes that tell others that you care enough about the group to dress appropriately	Exhibiting inconsistencies between verbal and nonverbal behavior

TABLE 11 – 2

ways at odds with the others in the group. Each person attempts to persuade every other person to share limited resources or accept his or her goals as group goals. Negotiation always entails communication to express goals, exchange ideas, debate the issues, and reach a compromise. When it is done well almost everyone comes away feeling as if they have won.

Good negotiators have similar characteristics and most of them can be learned. However, the characteristics are attitudinal, and learning them requires more commitment than learning intellectual concepts does. Table 11–3 describes characteristics of a good negotiator. A good negotiator is an assertive negotiator. The assertive negotiator is willing to compromise and recognizes the she or he will sometimes give up more and sometimes get more than the others.

WRITTEN COMMUNICATIONS
Inpatient Settings
Hospital Charts

Written communication with other professionals through the medium of patient charts is one of the most vital of all communications. Both the substance and the method of charting have a strong influence on the attitude that other professionals have toward the dietetic practitioner and his or her power to affect patient care.

TABLE 11 – 3

Characteristics of a Good Negotiator	
Well organized	Exhibits patience and perseverance
Ability to think under stress	Open-minded
High tolerance for ambiguity and uncertainty	Able to perceive and exploit power
Plenty of common sense	Observant
Good listener	Respects opponent and opponent's position
Good talker	Possesses power of concentration
Does "homework" before coming to negotiate	Does not get sidetracked by obstructive communicators
Possesses integrity and honesty	Quick to shift mental gears as the situation changes
Courageous, takes cautious risks	Willing to make reasonable compromises

Others will recognize this individual as an assertive, thoughtful professional, an inept dietitian, or something in between. It is the responsibility of the dietitian to develop a style of reporting that communicates to others a good degree of professionalism.

The problem-oriented medical record is the most common form currently used in health-care institutions and is an effective communication vehicle. As with oral communication, good communicating through the medical records occurs only when the purpose is clear. The problem-oriented medical record provides a vehicle for directing patient care and for recording the patient's status and response to interventions. To be effective, gather data from the chart, other health-care professionals, and the patient and come up with a viable assessment and plan. When there is a need for change, make suggestions for treatment based on your own findings. Charting will include notes suggesting alterations in treatment.

The documentation process is necessary to review and evaluate the function of total quality management. Continuous quality improvement is the process of continual information feedback evaluation and improvement of services to the patient. Institutions differ in documentation formats, but since the Joint Commission on Accreditation of Healthcare Organizations (JCAHO) standards have been shifting toward outcome evaluation, changes may occur in the way some institutions chart. See Additional References for in-depth information on JCAHO standards. Variance charting is defined under the Clinical Pathway section. More and more facilities are using electronic charting, whereby all documentation is done on computer. Some charting formats include FOCUS, SOAP, and SOAPIER (see the examples following). PIE (problem, intervention, evaluation) charting is currently more of a nursing process (King-Helm & Klawitter, 1995).

Focus Charting. Focus: Altered knowledge: diabetic diet

D (data). "I don't understand my diet. It's much too complicated for me. My wife will have to take care of it." 32-year-old male admit with newly diagnosed diabetes, to receive oral hypoglycemic agent coupled with diet for control of blood glucose. Admission labs: glucose 255, cholesterol 245. Height: 72″ Weight: 215#. Order received for instruction on 1800-calorie, low-fat, low-cholesterol diet for discharge. Diet history reveals erratic meal patterns, frequent soda and alcohol intake (had four beers night before admission). Eats out frequently, usually fast foods or convenience store items. Wife working and not available for counseling before discharge. Strong family history of heart disease and diabetes.

A (action). Assist client in identifying diet changes he can make. Suggest use of diet soda and provide suggestions for lower-fat, lower-cholesterol options when eating out. Monitor menu selections and intake while hospitalized. Provided qualitative diabetic guidelines and started counseling on lifestyle changes (diet and activity) that client can consider. Instructed on use of exchanges for menu completion. Continue with counseling inpatient with follow-up as outpatient (including wife) recommended.

R (response). Client expresses willingness to make some changes, eg, drink diet soda and decrease alcohol intake. Client able to state importance of controlling blood sugars and cholesterol levels. Able to complete menu with assistance using exchanges.

Soap Charting

S (subjective data). "I don't understand my diet. It's much too complicated for me. My wife will have to take care of it."

O (objective data). 32-year-old male admit with newly diagnosed diabetes, to receive oral hypoglycemic agent coupled with diet for control of blood glucose. Admission labs: glucose 255, cholesterol 245. Height: 72″ Weight: 215#. Order received for instruction on 1800-calorie, low-fat, low-cholesterol diet for discharge. Diet history reveals erratic meal patterns. Wife working and not available for counseling before discharge. Strong family history of heart disease and diabetes.

A (assessment). Lack of knowledge regarding diabetic and low-fat, low-cholesterol diet principles. Client appears resistant to participating in counseling.

P (plan). Assist client in identifying diet changes he can make. Suggest use of diet soda and provide suggestions for lower-fat, lower-cholesterol options when eating out. Monitor menu selections and intake while hospitalized. Will refer patient to diabetic clinic for follow-up post discharge, to include wife if possible.

Soapier Charting

S (subjective data). "I don't understand my diet. It's much too complicated for me. My wife will have to take care of it."

O (objective data). 32-year-old male admit with newly diagnosed diabetes, to receive oral hypoglycemic agent coupled with diet for control of blood glucose. Admission labs: glucose 255, cholesterol 245. Height: 72″ Weight: 215#. Order received for instruction on 1800-calorie, low-fat, low-cholesterol diet for discharge. Diet history reveals erratic meal patterns. Wife working and not available for counseling before discharge. Strong family history of heart disease and diabetes.

A (analysis/assessment). Lack of knowledge regarding diabetic and low-fat, low-cholesterol diet principles. Client appears resistant to participating in diet counseling.

P (plan).   Assist client in identifying diet changes he can make. Suggest use of diet soda and provide suggestions for lower-fat, lower-cholesterol options when eating out. Monitor menu selections and intake while hospitalized.

I (interventions).   Provided qualitative diabetic guidelines and started counseling on lifestyle changes (diet and activity) that client can consider. Instructed on use of exchanges for menu completion.

E (evaluation).   Client expresses willingness to make some changes. Client able to state importance of controlling blood sugars and cholesterol levels.

R (revisions).   Maintain current diet as ordered and monitor menu completion. Continue with counseling inpatient with follow-up as outpatient (including wife) recommended.

Good chart notes serve to increase the visibility of nutrition as a vital part of patient care when you represent yourself as an evaluator, a decision-maker, and an implementer of effective patient care.

Clinical Pathways

"Clinical pathways are interdisciplinary plans of care that outline the optimal sequencing and timing of interventions for patients with a particular diagnosis, procedure or symptom" (Ignatavicius & Hausman, 1995; p. 10). They are tools used to identify patient outcomes, which in turn are used to determine reimbursement parameters. Patients on clinical pathways typically have a case manager or coordinator. She or he oversees, coordinates care, and documents variances or deviations from the pathway.

Table 11–4 discusses the benefits of clinical pathways (Ignatavicius & Hausman, 1995).

Potential dilemmas include using clinical pathways as evidence for malpractice claims. Variances made from pathways could imply that an error was made. Also, physicians may not actually use them, and there may not be adequate data to demonstrate the value of pathways.

The four general features of a clinical pathway are:

- Patient outcomes
- Collaboration
- A time line
- Comprehensive aspects of care

Variance is the difference between what is expected and what actually happened. Variances may be positive or negative. For example, a positive variance occurs when a patient recovers more rapidly than expected, and is discharged earlier. A negative variance happens when pathway activities are not completed as expected and patient discharge is delayed. Some professionals chart by variance. For example, documentation occurs only when the care or the patient's response to care varies from what is on the clinical pathway. Many causes of variance exist and all variances should be monitored either concurrently or retrospectively. As a re-

Benefits of Clinical Pathways		
Patient	**Health-Care Team Members**	**Health-Care Agency**
Consumer involvement	Standardized, organized care	Supported by JCAHO
Patient education	Improved communication	Supported by third-party payors
Mutual goal setting	Reflection of current practice	Integration of quality improvement, utilization, management, and risk management
Increased patient satisfaction	Increased staff satisfaction	
	Educational tool for students and new graduates	Improved communication
		Better competitive position
		Decreased length of stay
		Decreased costs
		Availability of data for evaluating care

TABLE 11–4

From Ignatavicius DD, Hausman KA: *Clinical Pathways for Collaborative Practice.* Philadelphia: WB Saunders, 1995.

sult of this analysis, clinical pathways may be modified or changed, or the need for staff education may be exposed.

A clinical pathway may be a part of the official medical record or it may be a separate documentation vehicle that is discarded after the patient is discharged. An example of a clinical pathway involving nutrition intervention is given in Table 11–5.

Screening

Clinical dietetic practitioners often use comprehensive nutrition screening programs to identify patients at nutrition risk and therefore in comorbid nutritional conditions. Computer linking between departments facilitates this process. In some studies of diagnostically related groups, comorbid nutrition conditions have been found to contribute up to $312,000 in additional costs of care. (King-Helm & Klawitter, 1995) Screening is an inexpensive way to streamline clinical nutrition care.

Discharge Referrals

Inpatient nutrition counseling continues to decline as patients are discharged sooner and sicker. Although discharge planning should start at the time of the patient's admission to the hospital, rapid patient turnover and short preparation times limit the ability of the dietetic practitioner to provide counseling services. Many dietitians agree that it is most appropriate to counsel the patient on "need to know" information during hospitalization and to refer patients after discharge to outpatient settings for more comprehensive care.

T A B L E 1 1 – 5

Nutrition Component of Typical Cardiac Pathway

Goals: to improve patient outcomes, promote recovery, and promote healthy eating behaviors. Nutrition concerns are:

- Maintenance of lean body mass (LBM)
- Anorexia
- Meeting 50% of nutritional needs prior to discharge
- Infection
- Effects of drugs
- Anemia
- Protein-calorie malnutrition (PCM)
- Initiation of oral intake
- Fluid imbalance/hydration status

Nutrition Interventions:

Post Op Day #1 (POD #1)
- NPO (nothing by mouth)
- Nutritional assessment

POD #2
- Active bowel sounds in all four quadrants
- Tolerating solid food without nausea and/or vomiting
- 4 gm sodium, heart-healthy diet

POD #3
- Evaluate adequacy of oral intake via nutrient intake analysis
- Assess for constipation
- Supplements to supply additional kcal, if necessary
- Initiate tube feeding if patient is still intubated

POD #4
- Instruct on nutritional requirements for wound healing (first 6 weeks post op)
- Instruct patient/family on heart-healthy diet

POD #5
- Eating 50–75% of nutritional needs without nausea and/or vomiting
- Patient and family will describe the benefits of the heart-healthy diet and how they will meet the requirements
- If patient is assessed to have inadequate knowledge, a discharge summary/plan for continuum of care is initiated (refer to the outpatient clinic dietitian or referring health-care provider)

POD #6
- Patient is discharged

From DeHoog SJ: Re-engineering clinical nutrition processes. *In* WA Redmond (ed): Diagnostic Related Nutritional Care Plans. Seattle, WA: University of Washington Medical Center, 1995.

As has been mentioned repeatedly and is well-documented and theoretically supported (by the concept of process of change), little is accomplished in a 20-minute inpatient interview. For most patients, a referral to an outpatient setting or a rehabilitation inpatient or nursing home setting is desirable. In some hospitals, this is routine.

Outpatient Settings

Initial Interview

The initial interview is generally a time of gathering substantial amounts of data for use through the term of counseling. Included should be information regarding health status, dietary habits, and dietary needs pertinent to the problems presented. A diet history should be attached, along with referral forms, for easy access. In addition, summaries of counseling sessions and progress notes are helpful in reminding you of the progress you are making and noting overall trends that you may miss as you work on the details of specific problems. These summaries can be filled out in the presence of the client or recorded immediately after a session.

Documentation of the instructional materials used should appear in client records. Copies of nutrition plans, as well as the titles of pamphlets, computer programs, or other instructional media used should be included, along with a note as to their effect.

Consent for Treatment

A standard form consenting to treatment should be signed by each client on the first visit. It should explain that the service or educational materials you provide are for their use alone and cannot rightly be given to another person because the nutrition care plan has been individually developed for them and perhaps would not be appropriate for another person. A carbon copy of this form should be kept in your files, and the original given to the client. Figure 11–1 is a sample adapted from material from the Canadian Dietetic Association. Although this form for printed material permission is not widely used in the United States, it is a good standard practice.

I, _____ , understand that the nutrition information materials with which I have been provided are solely for my use, and that the Author is not liable for any nonauthorized transfer, sale, or reprinting of such information or the use of such information by others for whom it was not intended.

Date _____ Client signature _____

FIGURE 11–1. Sample printed material consent permission form.

Records Documentation

Accurate client records are also an aid to good counseling and provide protection in case of legal questions. They should contain documentation of all communication to or about a client. There are various opinions about the length of time records should be kept, but 5 years is probably sufficient. If documentation of sessions with clients takes place outside the arena of hospital charts, it is important to remember that records are confidential documents. Under no circumstances, except perhaps in response to a subpoena from a court of law, should this confidentiality be violated without the express consent of the client.

Report Writing

When a patient is referred to you by another professional or by an agency, a report to the referral source is expected. These reports are vital for the collaboration needed to enhance the care and management of the client. The purpose of reports is to keep other professionals apprised of what is occurring in the aspects of treatment for which you are responsible and to provide information pertinent to other aspects of the treatment of the patient. There are a number of ways to approach this task. A checklist can be used which you check appropriately and send in as a report; telephone conferences can occur (with notes made in your files); or short anecdotal notes describing the client's progress can be written. All these techniques may have their use, but it is important that all communication be very professional. Checklists used alone may seem so impersonal that the person receiving them may sense a lack of feeling toward the patient. On the other hand, notes that are too long and tedious are unimpressive and are often not read.

> Reports written by private practitioners should reflect a high degree of professionalism, high ethical standards, and legal responsibility. Inaccuracy, vagueness, ambiguity, wordiness, and meaningless professional jargon all reflect on the individual capabilities of the practitioner. For those in private practice, there is no large organization or institution to back up such errors in judgment. The private practitioner must communicate effectively through both oral and written language.
>
> *Knepflaar, 1978; p. 116*

Knepflaar goes on to list the essentials of writing reports: "They should be concise, complete, well organized, and labeled for ease in finding different types of information, honest and carefully worded for legal purposes."

Nutrition Education Materials

Many nutrition education materials are distributed free from governmental agencies. There are also many new and exciting materials available for purchase that are useful. In addition, materials that are unique or are improvements on items available on the market may be developed by each professional. All materials developed should be copyrighted. Further discussion of the appropriateness and level of nutrition education materials can be found in Chapter 7.

Client Referral

When a physician or other professional refers a client to an MNT, it should always be in writing. Requests can be made to those from whom you seek referrals to use their letterheads or prescription blanks. Medical nutrition therapy prescriptions should be specific, and any pertinent information that communicates progress toward physician-requested goals should be included. Relevant laboratory test results may also be included.

Client Scheduling

It is important to schedule clients in a systematic and efficient manner. Office hours should be established and kept. Time must be allowed for recording information at the end of each interview or counseling sessions as necessary, and time must be allotted for administrative activities such as report-writing and financial record-keeping. The length of a counseling session depends on two things: the complexity of nutrition education needed and the complexity of the client. Generally, the first interview will take about an hour, and in many cases follow-up visits can be scheduled for 1/2-hour time increments. However, if a client is having trouble meeting his or her goals, you may need 1-hour appointments with that person. When appointments are made, the client's telephone number should be indicated on the computer or manually so that she or he can be reached if the appointment needs to be changed in some way. If clients are scheduled 15 or 20 minutes apart, time will be available for record keeping and one client will not have to wait in a reception room while you finish with another. In addition, time for making telephone calls should be included in your scheduling plan. The management of clients includes not only a counseling relationship to facilitate nutrition lifestyle changes but also appropriate management of business relationships. The records normally needed for both include those listed in Table 11–6. All these records can be computer-generated. If financially feasible, the use of the computer is definitely the most efficient and professional.

TABLE 11–6	Counseling/Business Records Needed
	▎ A written diet prescription when appropriate
	▎ An appointment book/computer program in which client appointments are always recorded
	▎ Appointment cards
	▎ An initial interview sheet
	▎ Interview records
	▎ A diet history and food records
	▎ Copies of instructional materials
	▎ Itemized bills and receipts
	▎ A ledger for recording payments
	▎ Report forms for professional sources of referrals
	▎ All communication regarding the client
	▎ Referrals made to other professionals

FISCAL PROCEDURES

For each fiscal policy established, the procedure for enforcing the policy is important. This includes a system of billing and keeping financial records and the interpersonal system of communication developed to conduct business with clients, consultants, and sources of referrals.

Collecting Immediate Payment

There are assertive ways of collecting bills effectively. If you are alone in your office, you will have to handle everything yourself, but if you have secretarial assistance, she or he can help in this delicate task. The first step is to give the client a clear statement of your fees in writing, in addition to providing this information orally at the time she or he first requests an appointment. At the appropriate point in the first contact with the client, if fee information has not been requested, say, "Let me explain my fees and billing policy to you" and then do so. Tell the client how much you charge and when you expect payment and list the alternative methods of payment. If the client cannot comply with the form of payment expected, you will have to use professional judgment to decide if you are going to negotiate some other system.

For clients expected to pay on receipt of service, a simple and assertive way to request payment when they are hesitant about taking their responsibility is to say, "How would you like to pay today? Cash, check, or credit card?" If you have a receptionist, she or he can do this.

Collection for services rendered is as vital to the health and success of the counseling service as it is to the individual's financial well-being. It is especially important in interactions with manipulative clients who will be quick to recognize any discomfort regarding reimbursement of services. You do a disservice to your client as well as to yourself if you do not expect the same compliance with the fiduciary contract between you as you expect with the nutrition changes you help the client decide to make. When relationship is the essence of the treatment, and when that relationship is tainted by the realization of both parties that trust and respect were violated, the treatment gains are also jeopardized (Barker, 1982).

Payment Records

There are many computer systems for recording charges and payments. Manually, some are structured so that the receipt and the record can be completed with one entry on carbon-backed paper. If there is a policy of accepting third-party payment, everyone should utilize the same system that is set up for third-party reimbursement.

Collecting Bad Debts

The collection of bad debts is a difficult part of practice for most people and there are collection agencies that can assist in this process. The best way to deal with this problem is to enforce appropriate payment policies assertively so that the situation does not occur. If you have a number of clients with poor payment records, examine your own assertive behaviors and make changes to reduce or eliminate the problem.

In addition to payment policies, a policy should be established for missed appointments. There are two ways in which clients can avoid paying the counseling fee. One is to avoid paying for services, and the other is to fail to keep appointments. This is one of the most difficult areas of business with which to deal because it impinges on the crucial trust relationship between the counselor and the counselee as well as on business management. Making a clearly written statement of fees and appointment cancellation policies available to every client will help reduce difficulties in receiving payment. Professionals vary in their policies regarding missed appointments. Some think that nonpayment encourages clients to be careless about keeping appointments, and others believe that it is better for the relationship if payment for missed appointments is not required. Some MNTs require 24 to 48 hours notice if the client cannot keep the appointment. Otherwise, the client is charged for a missed appointment.

Third-Party Reimbursement

Nutrition services should be covered in the basic benefits package under Medicare, Medicaid, and other public, private, and corporate insurance programs, according to the American Dietetic Association as part of their legislative highlights in 1994 (ADA, 1994; Coulston & Rosen, 1994). An excellent summary of the economic benefits of nutrition services in acute care, outpatient care, home care, long-term care, and preventive care can be found in the ADA's health-care reform legislative platform (ADA, 1993).

Also, the ADA stated in its strategic framework for 1996–1999 (1996; p. 2) that the vision of the ADA will be to "obtain reimbursement for comprehensive nutrition services, including health promotion and disease prevention services, and medical nutrition therapy." The goal is to persuade policy-makers at federal, state, and community levels, as well as the insurance industry, to incorporate the value of nutrition services so that there can be an overall reduction in the cost of health care. It is becoming more common for MNTs to be reimbursed by third-party payment when nutrition care is clearly documented to be part of the medical treatment. Payment by a third party is most successful when one correctly and precisely completes its reimbursements forms, using the terminology the paying party expects as documentation of reimbursable services.

Currently, the primary third-party payee is the federal Medicare system. A system of payment based on diagnostically related disease groups (DRGs) has been established for payment of cost for Medicare patients. Retrospective data are collected, and future payments are based on average previous costs for treating disease groups. It is possible that other third-party reimbursement systems will follow its lead in payment policies. There are many ramifications of the use of diagnostically related groups as a basis for deferring payment for services.

According to Medicare guidelines, most dietetic professionals, like other non-physician health-care providers, do not have provider status and therefore cannot be directly reimbursed for services. However, it is possible to apply for provider status with managed-care companies. Otherwise, arrangements can be made with an accepted provider under certain situations to perform nutritional counseling activities under its supervision. Providers can receive third-party reimbursement for these services. The dilemma created by this situation concerns the problem of lack of appropriate recognition of the dietetic practitioner as the best qualified provider of nutritional counseling.

Claims submitted to Medicare must list standard services and fees. The *Nutrition Service Payment System,* published by ADA (1985), includes estimated times for many nutrition services in a number of settings. These guidelines, along with additional documentation of actual services and the time required, can be used to support the development of future regulations that will better recognize dietetic practitioners. The following options for a payment policy are suggested (ADA, 1984):

1. Payment at the time services are rendered. Patient/client submits insurance claim directly for reimbursement.
2. A percent of fee is paid at the time services are provided. Insurance is billed directly from the office, and the outstanding balance following insurance is billed to the patient/client.
3. No payment is requested at the time of service; insurance forms can be generated from the office and any balance owing billed to the patient.

One study was conducted on strategies for increasing reimbursement of outpatient services. The clinical dietitians instructed clients about how to file claims and provided them with form letters of medical necessity to submit with claims. The form letters increased the reimbursement rate but client instruction did not increase the submission of claims rate. Many clients said they did not have time to submit a claim. The study concluded that claims submitted by the professional or by the professional's office or clinic may increase the reimbursement rate (Bolonda et al, 1994).

Cost-Effectiveness

Dietitians are challenged to provide cost-effective care and to justify their interventions with positive treatment outcomes (Eiger et al, 1996). The JCAHO evaluates the dietitian's effect on patient health. Studies of positive outcomes are currently being published for a variety of dietetic settings. In a recent study of the National Cholesterol Education Program, it was found that intensive nutrition counseling enhanced outcomes and reduced the need for costly medication intervention (Rhodes et al, 1996). Self-report questionnaires are useful as outcome measures in total quality management projects.

Because of some chronic conditions and disease progression, clients may not exhibit physical improvements after nutrition counseling interventions. Influence on a patient's quality of life offers a different approach as outcome measures. Table 11–7 outlines the values of a nutrition education and counseling framework and definitions (Hauchecorne et al, 1994). An actual questionnaire instrument and guidelines for use are detailed in Hauchecorne et al, pp. 431–440.

It is important for dietetic practitioners to take the responsibility for documenting nutrition services and their effectiveness. The dietitian works in an environment in which the potential for success is great, and the entire profession will ben-

TABLE 11 – 7

Value of Nutrition Education Framework and Definitions

Improved Physical Well-Being	Fulfillment of Interpersonal Psychological Need	Reduction of Uncertainty	Control	Accessibility
Achievement of nutrition goal relieve symptoms *or*	Attention/ individual care Empathy/ understanding	Dietitian integrity/ competence/trust° Reassurance/ dietary change appropriate for condition¶	Interaction/ partnership† Achievable dietary change°°	Available for consultation‡
Restore function *or*	Support§	Goal perceived as possible#		
Improve nutrition assessment parameter	Emotional relief			

°Confidence in the dietitian as a credible source of information and advice.
†Agreement between the patient and dietitian in identifying nutrition needs and goals.
‡By telephone or at the clinic.
§Encouragement and assistance provided by the dietitian.
¶Dietary change(s) to be made are perceived as appropriate for the patient's condition/situation.
°°Positive experience at home in making dietary changes that correspond with nutrition goals.
Decreased anxiety, worry, or fear of eating (related to appropriateness of food choices for the condition or fear of symptom exacerbation brought on by consumption of inappropriate foods).
#Patient understands plan for nutrition care, dietary changes to be made, and his or her role in carrying out the plan; patient feels proposed changes are possible.
From Hauchecorne CM, Barr SI, Sork TJ: Evaluation of nutrition counseling in clinical settings: Do we make a difference? Copyright the American Dietetic Association. Reprinted by permission from *Journal of the American Dietetic Association* 1994;94(4):437–440.

efit by documentation of nutritional counseling services. The public also deserves this accountability.

Managed Care and Health-Care Reform

It is the position of The American Dietetic Association that health maintenance organizations and systems of managed care provide nutrition services as an essential component of preventive and therapeutic health care and that these services be provided by qualified nutrition professionals.

Neville, 1993; p. 1171

Increased nutrition education to the public and to other health-care professionals, along with research aimed at the development of new information, goes hand in hand with disease prevention and health-care reform (Kretchmer, 1994). President Clinton's Health Security Act (*J Am Diet Assoc,* 1994) addressed the issues of health-care reform. Nutrition has been recognized in the legislative language of this proposal. The grassroots lobbying efforts of all dietitians and nutrition therapists continue to be crucial in promoting inclusion of more therapies in the final legislation. A managed care glossary of terms is provided in Box 11–1 (Palumbo, 1995).

Box 11–1

Managed Care Glossary of Terms

Bundling. Inclusion of multiple services under a pre-established rate of reimbursement, either a per diem or capitated rate.

Capitation. Contracted providers provide and pay for covered services for a fixed per member per month payment.

Case Management. A collaborative process that assesses, plans, implements, coordinates, monitors, and evaluates services to meet an individual's needs through communication and available resources to promote quality, cost-effective outcomes.

Exclusions. Specific services or conditions that the policy will not cover or that are covered at a limited rate.

Fee Schedule. A list of predetermined payments for medical services

HMO (Health Maintenance Organization). An organization that provides comprehensive health services to its members in return for a fixed prepaid fee.

Independent Practice Association (IPA). An organization of independent physicians that contracts with managed care.

PPO (Preferred Provider Organization). A network of physicians and other providers who agree to provide services at a discounted rate.

Provider. The person in relation to the insurance program who provides covered services and supplies to the beneficiary.

Superbill. A multipart form that provides sufficient information so that patients may file their own insurance claim forms.

Unbundling. The process of breaking a single charge into multiple components to "game the system" for higher payment.

Utilization Review. The process of reviewing services provided to determine if those services were timely, medically necessary, and appropriate.

From Palumbo C. Managed care is here to stay. Copyright the American Dietetic Association. Reprinted by permission from *Ventures Newsletter of Nutrition Entrepreneurs of the American Dietetic Association.* 1995;XI(3):2–3.

LEGAL REGULATION OF PRACTITIONERS

Professional Credentials

The basic credential for dietetic practitioners is the designation of Registered Dietitian (RD). Several states have enacted entitlement or licensure laws limiting the practice of dietetics. Currently, individuals who pass the registration examination meet the criteria needed to practice in states with legislation; however, this may not continue to be the case as more states pass entitlement and licensure laws. State regulation of dietetic practitioners will no doubt make significant changes in the credentials under which RDs practice in the future.

There are specialty groups within the ADA concerned with the standards of practice for women and men claiming expertise in specialty fields such as oncology, nutrition support, and renal dietetics. They may pursue credentialing beyond initial registration or licensure. For example, a dietitian may use the initials CNSD after his or her name to signify Certified Nutrition Support Dietitian. At the same time, the growing number of dietetic practitioners working as private practitioners rather than being employed by institutions may change the way in which specialization works. In addition, concepts of appropriate standards of practice for dietetic practitioners are likely to change with the changing environment in which they work.

Licensure and Entitlement

Licensure of practitioners qualified to perform nutritional counseling and other related activities is particularly difficult for a number of reasons. Many individuals who have no affiliation with the ADA are involved in such activities. Many of them use the term "nutritionist" or "nutrition counselors" to identify themselves, as do many RDs. Non-registered nutritionists or nutrition counselors are unlikely to support licensure efforts unless they are included.

There are several ways in which dietetic practitioners can seek regulation under state licensure. The options include entitlement legislation, optional licensure, and mandatory licensure. Entitlement legislation entitles a professional group to participate in regulated professional activity. Optional licensure provides the opportunity for a profession to establish standards and let people who meet such standards obtain a license but does not require people to become licensed before they can practice. Mandatory licensure can be much stronger than the other two unless the description of the professional activities is so broad that it becomes meaningless. Florida is a state that has mandatory licensure. In 1995, from April to December, the state board of medicine issued disciplinary actions against six nutrition counselors for violating Florida licensure laws. All disciplinary actions are published in a quarterly newsletter. One such action is anonymously described:

> . . . found guilty of violating a board rule; attempting to obtain, obtaining or renewing a license to practice dietetics and nutrition by bribery or fraudulent misrepresentation. Action—License suspended until respondent documents completion of 15 hours CEU required for the 1993 license renewal; $250 fine due prior to reinstatement. Upon reinstatement, the Board may impose further discipline.
>
> *Florida Board of Medicine, 1996; p. 5*

The complexities of licensure will result in different regulations in different states. It is important to become familiar with the regulations in various states, especially in any state in which you intend to practice.

PROFESSIONAL GROWTH

Retention of professional status as a registered or licensed dietitian is a major impetus for continuing education. A number of avenues are available, and workshops, various self-teaching programs, professional meetings, and regular graduate class work will keep you up-to-date in the wide range of expertise you need in practice.

These represent only a portion of professional growth. You should expect to acquire a growing reputation as an authority in nutritional counseling and consultation. If you write, continue to do so. Be sure to copyright what you write, but share it. Do not hesitate to charge reasonably for the work that you produce. Workshops, professional achievement, and civic contributions should be publicized so that your reputation as a professional leader is maintained. You and your business will both grow if you use educational opportunities to develop innovative ways to deliver your services.

Because of the restrictions placed on continuing education criteria for the maintenance of registration, only a limited portion of your continued growth should involve self-study. Especially for the private practitioner, communication and sharing with colleagues are very important in keeping your information and techniques up-to-date and in keeping your mind open and excited about professional growth. The networking, more than the actual facts you learn, may be the vital force in your growth and development.

A form of continuing education that should become a part of the field of dietetic practice, as the counseling aspect of the profession grows, is a system of collegial supervision. This can be accomplished through peer review or arrangements with consultants appropriate for your situation. For instance, if you wish to increase your skill as a counselor rather than being merely an information giver, you may find that consultation and educational activities supervised by a psychological consultant will develop this ability even further. As time goes by, MNTs who have developed exceptional skill can become mentors and supervisors of new practitioners. Mentoring is advantageous to both sides, and it can occur at any time during a career. A mentor is usually described as a teacher, sponsor, role model, guide, or counselor (ADA Courier, 1996). Although this concept is a new one, it must soon be initiated if the quality of care is going to improve as the profession matures. Intraprofessional consultation and referral is in its infancy in dietetics, and its growth will be a sign of the growth of the profession.

In fact, emerging opportunities for referrals among dietitians include referrals from inpatient to outpatient clinics, home health agencies, private practice, or long-term-care facilities, and back again to inpatient if warranted.

The Need for Marketing

Dietetics and nutrition professionals, as well as students, know the benefits of good nutrition, but not everyone else does. Some may know about it but not be willing to do anything about it. Still others may know about appropriate nutrition lifestyles, but not be willing to pay for assistance in changing their food habits. If you expect to be paid for sharing your expertise, it is up to you to make people aware of their needs and to provide motivation that will bring them to your doorstep willing to pay for your services. There are a number of ways to market services. The Physician Nutrition Education Program, sponsored by the ADA, is designed to help market dietitians' services to physicians. The program is a training seminar for dietitians to learn how to teach physicians to incorporate nutrition personally and professionally (ADA Courier, 1996). ADA also has a consumer nutrition hotline. It has both an 800 number for general questions and a 900 number for consumers seeking customized answers to food and nutrition questions. Consumers and businesses can also find dietitians on ADA's home page on the World Wide Web. See Additional References for direct information.

If you are starting a private practice, you may not have ideal visibility if you are situated in a retail outlet. You must develop a way to make your potential clientele realize that you can provide a service. Even if you are well established with physicians before you open your own office, marketing strategies and procedures must be formulated and executed.

In the beginning, few people will know about you outside of some of your own colleagues. Be sure to include them in your marketing strategies. Marketing can help establish productive communication with colleagues, as well as with others. The methods you use at the beginning are not the ones you will use after your business has opened.

The First Step

The first step in the marketing process is to approach the potential market in an indirect method. As soon as you know your address and telephone number, get a letterhead, perhaps with a logo. Purchase stationery, business cards, appointment cards, and announcements and start to work by sending out mailings. The essential mailing should be to people from whom you wish to receive referrals. If you are in a large metropolitan area, send out about 1000 letters to physicians, osteopaths, local corporations, and organizations that might be interested. Dentists, mental health workers, nursing practitioners, and other professionals are all potential sources of client referrals. Other items such as announcements, postcard surveys, letter enclosures, and any creative ideas you have for a mailing are good advertising. If you intend to practice in a small town, set your market boundaries at a feasible distance for travel and still include enough referral sources. You may extend your mailings to include a wider segment of the population. Each letter should be personal, but to be efficient, a form letter with the basic information you wish to convey should be the foundation of your mailings.

The letters you write to potential sources of referrals should contain the following basic information: the announcement that you are in business at a specific location, a description of your services, a statement of your credentials and expertise, and a request for referrals. You need to express the attitude that your services will help them serve their clients better. The request for an appointment should reassure each recipient of your letter that you will need only a very small amount of time (10 to 12 minutes) to introduce yourself personally and to describe your expertise and services. Medical doctors are among the most valuable sources of clients. An example of a letter to a physician is given in Figure 11–2.

If you have not already made a list of potential referral sources as part of a market survey, such a list should be made at this time. In addition, establish a mailing list of friends, colleagues, professionals, and organizations with whom you will wish to communicate. Other mailings may include announcements of your opening, postcards sent to interested parties, and mailings to organizations, corporations, or anyone you think would be a good contact for you.

If you have a computer, you have a convenient tool for preparing this list and having it available for use or updating. A clerical employee or service is the other option for completing mailings.

Letters create awareness but will not motivate a specific physician or other professional to send a specific client to you. Referrals always result from a more per-

Title of Practice

Address, Telephone Number, and Date

Stephan Combs, M.D.
1283 Ramsey Blvd, Suite 330
Douglas, OH 34281

Dear Dr. Combs:

I am a registered dietitian in private practice where I provide medical nutrition therapy services for individuals with disease-related therapeutic needs such as cardiovascular disease, diabetes, eating disorders, and weight control.

I am interested in accepting referrals from you in the hope that these services will assist you and your patients.

May I have ten to twelve minutes of your time to introduce myself and further explain the services I provide? I will be contacting your office within the next few days to request an appointment to see you. I believe I can assist your practice in a cost-efficient manner.

Sincerely,

Sarah Martin, RD

FIGURE 11–2. Sample letter to a physician.

sonal contact with those from whom you expect to receive referrals or with people who have used your service and recommend it. The recipient of your letter does not know you and is not sure of your credentials. Other professionals cannot take a chance on sending people to someone about whom they know little or nothing and who is just starting a business. The assurance of your legitimate credentials and your personality are vital to them before they send you clients. It is important to follow up your letters with personal contacts.

The Second Step

Direct Approaches. Direct approaches to potential referral sources should be undertaken to follow up your introductory letters. Good work habits and effective management are important at every juncture, but they are crucial at this stage. Systematically, every person or organization who received a letter must be called on the telephone to request an appointment. Keep good records of your contacts and remember to call again after you have been turned down. Schedule a part of each day for this activity and be prepared for a high proportion of refusals in the beginning. One appointment as a result of 100 telephone calls is the average return at this stage. If you persist, the percentage of success will rise.

Even when you get appointments, this does not mean you will get referrals every time. Many people are afraid to send clients to beginners. Some may be beginning professionals themselves and cannot afford to take this risk. Keep your patience and your perseverance. You will begin to be recognized, and people will take notice that you are still around, that you are not a fly-by-night operation. Some will change their minds and can prove to be good resources for clients. Keep giving people the opportunity to know you.

The Interview. Be as well prepared as possible when you make personal calls and keep to your appointment time of 10 to 12 minutes. Describe your services in an attractive and meaningful way. Express your belief in yourself and what you are doing and be sure to present a one-page summary of your credentials.

Many of your first interviews will be with physicians. When you have presented your case, and you sense an opportunity, ask to see some of his or her difficult patients, and those who would benefit from the two of you working together. Mention, for instance, that you would be glad to see someone who needs very specific nutrition information or who has great difficulty in complying with a diet prescription and is at risk of serious complications because of it. Give the doctor a clear direction to pursue in thinking of patients who would be logical referrals.

Appointments with health-care professionals should center on making them aware that people who come to them for treatment of eating disorders will solve their problems even more satisfactorily when they have accurate nutrition facts as well as better problem-solving techniques. Your combined efforts can have a synergistic effect. These contacts may lead to client referrals, and they can help you locate a mental health professional to use as a consultant and to whom you may send referrals when you see the need.

The Third Step

The third step in marketing has two facets. One is to establish yourself as an authority in nutrition and dietetic counseling and consultation. The other is to make yourself known in the community as a civic-minded leader.

Establish Yourself as a Nutrition Authority. Letters to organizations need to be followed by telephone calls in which you offer yourself as a speaker. There are many topics of interest in nutrition. Offer guidelines about the topics you can speak on and be open to any special topic a group might request. Set a goal to book at least one speech every week, but do not be discouraged if at first you fail to meet this goal.

Prepare one general speech about a current popular nutrition topic, 20 minutes long, in which you include the best example of your professionalism that you have to offer. Memorize it and practice it until it is so much a part of you that is seems spontaneous. There are a variety of ways in which you can compose your speech, but there are two essential elements. First, your nutrition information must be up-to-date and well-documented; and second, you must tell your audience in an indirect way that you are in the practice of dietetics. Otherwise you will sound so erudite that they will think you are a college professor. Tell your audience through your personal anecdotes of success stories that you see clients privately for dietetics consultation and counseling. Although private practice is not too likely to be the option for a first job in dietetics, even students moving from their educational program straight into private practice will have some experience in counseling clients to share.

One such anecdote might sound like this: "I once had a client who had been on dozens of weight loss diets and could never keep the weight loss for more than 3 months. We worked together to develop a nutrition plan and support system to lose the weight and when that was accomplished, we developed a food intake plan and support system to keep the weight off. One way he found to keep the weight off was to. . ."

If you are asked for information about special nutrition topics, you can easily add pertinent comments to your standard speech. This will also serve as motivation for keeping it up-to-date.

The mass communication media are an excellent resource for gaining visibility and present an opportunity to establish your authority. Make contacts with people in the mass media. Talk on the telephone with health, food, and nutrition writers. Write letters to the editor about controversial nutrition subjects. Offer articles about nutrition and about the benefits of nutrition counseling. Get yourself on radio and television but stay away from situations where you have to debate nutrition concepts with those you think are engaged in unethical nutritional counseling.

Materials you produce for use with your own clients or for presentations should always have your name on them as author. If you find good materials produced by others, use them. You do not have to do everything yourself. Give appropriate credit to the people who have developed the materials you use, and you will gain allies in addition to providing effective service. Be sure to observe copyright laws in utilizing nutrition education materials.

Civic Leadership. In addition to making speeches and personal contacts with other professionals, it is important for you to become established as a civic-minded leader. Join civic groups such as The American Heart Association (AHA) in addition to the professional groups to which you belong. Investigate the options and become a member of those that share your interest. Become active and consider becoming an officer. This will provide you with visibility within the community. Your activities in these organizations will help establish your standing in the community and your reputation as a doer. It is also a good place to network.

It is important that you become active in organizations that you enjoy. The final criterion for these activities is the same as that mentioned in regard to the services you offer. You must like to do what you do if you are to be successful. Going through the motions will not produce the results you want.

All these activities will keep you busy for the first 2 years of your practice. You will be establishing the groundwork for your business, but do not expect quick income and profits. Your rewards will be in the pride of achievement and the self-motivation you will have developed along with the characteristics of careful preparation, enduring patience, and steady persistence. Furthermore, these activities will serve to reduce the feelings of depression that could arise if you sat in your office day after day waiting for clients who did not come (Curry-Bartley, 1987).

The marketing tactics you use after your business is established will not be the same as those you used in the beginning. You will maintain and increase your clientele based on the satisfaction of your clients and those who refer clients to you. As you become successful, you will have options to explore further, such as specialization and expansion.

FUTURE TRENDS IN DIETETICS

"Nontraditional" roles used to be defined as dietetic practitioners working outside the area of direct providers of health-care services. Dietitians are now successful in businesses of marketing, advertising, sales and sales support, journalism, sports nutrition, government policy making and lobbying, product development, manufacturing, distribution, and so on (Dowling, 1996).

Home Health Care

Home health care is emerging as a new worksite for dietitians who monitor nutrition support. As health care is shifting more services to outside the hospital, dietitians' services are shifting as well. The ADA has promoted dietetics in the home by endorsing coverage of in-home nutrition services by Medicare and Medicaid (Pantalos, 1993). Typically, the dietitian is employed by the home infusion therapy company. The service costs of the RD are often included in overhead charges. The role of the home health-care dietitian is similar in many ways to that of a dietitian in an acute care setting: assessment, nutrition care planning, monitoring, and screening. Also, the psychosocial concerns of the persons receiving home nutrition support are addressed by the dietitian. Allowance for expression of feelings of loss (independence, control, and inability to eat) and patient participation in the formulation of their plans of care are essential.

Documentation

Documentation in the home health-care setting usually includes the following:

- Objectives of treatment
- Care plan
- Specific feeding regimen
- Training activities
- Patient's response to care
- Complications
- Monitoring results
- Revisions in care plan

When intervention is complete, documentation includes a summary statement, complications, outcome, and follow-up care (Pantalos, 1993).

Reimbursement is subject to policies of public and private payors, which vary widely by carrier and policy. Dietitians' visits do not qualify for reimbursement per visit at this time. Documentation of outcomes and cost-effectiveness of nutrition intervention can help expand coverage. Standard documentation of home health-care services provided to third-party payors includes:

- Medical necessity for nutrition therapy
- Duration of treatment
- Dependence on artificial feeding
- Caloric requirements
- Need for specialized formulas

Hospital dietitians should become knowledgeable about which companies in their community employ home health-care dietitians for continuity of care.

Multiskilling

The dietetics profession has begun to discuss the issue of multiskilling and cross-training as pressures continue to reduce costs by eliminating redundancies and to increase department collaboration. For example, a home health dietitian could increase cost-effectiveness if she or he were also able to assess for edema and complete simple screens for functional status and hearing impairment while in the client's home. Alternatively, it might be beneficial to train a physical therapist making a home visit to complete a simple nutrition screen to determine the need for a dietitian's intervention. Many dietary managers possess skills to effectively manage other departments as well.

New Directions for the Dietetic Professional

The following are some major forces that will affect the profession of dietetics (Payne-Palacio & Canter, 1996):

1. Downsizing in hospitals
2. Emergence of mergers and coalitions
3. Emergence of managed care

4. Formation of integrated networks and cooperation between health-care facilities and services
5. Alterations in referral patterns (referrals from primary-care physicians)

Dietitians who see change as opportunity will be forerunners who take the dietetics profession into the 21st century. A willingness to seize opportunities to market themselves and their abilities is crucial for success in new arenas.

New arenas may include the development of new foods, new approaches to nutrition education and counseling, new computer software and applications, and new programs aimed at children, minorities, women, the elderly, and dual-career families.

Summary

This chapter focused on the elements necessary to support successful medical nutrition therapy and nutrition counseling. Professional environments wherein counseling takes place, such as hospitals, outpatient and community facilities, schools, and corporate settings, were described. Both verbal and written communication must be effective with clients, other professionals, and the lay public. Assertiveness was explored in depth as a useful tool in this endeavor of professional effectiveness and success.

Legal regulation of the profession continues to change and it would be wise for the reader to keep abreast of these and other pertinent legislative issues. Professional growth and continued marketing of dietetic practitioners and their services are paramount. Without marketing, the value of medical nutrition therapy will not be recognized.

It is exciting to experience the expansion of dietetic practitioner roles. Many practitioners have recognized opportunities and assertively developed them.

Suggestions for Further Learning

1. Review the monthly "President's Page" in the *Journal of the American Dietetic Association* in the last year to determine relevant issues currently facing the profession.
2. Write a chart note using both Focus and SOAPIER formats.
3. Describe an ideal medical nutrition therapy environment.
4. In groups of five, pick issues, take sides, and negotiate a solution for a specific problem. Have one person be the observer and document the group's processes.
5. Select uncomfortable situations. Determine what you want to change, use the empty chair technique or role-playing, and practice assertive behaviors. Then, try these techniques in real life.

CITED REFERENCES

Alberti RD, Emmons ML: *Your Perfect Right: A Guide to Assertive Behavior.* 4th ed. San Luis Obispo, CA: Impact Publishers, 1986.
American Dietetic Association: Platform: Health care reform legislative platform: Economic benefits of nutrition services. *J Am Diet Assoc.* 1993;93(6):686–690.

American Dietetic Association: *Courier.* 1996;35: 2, 4, 10.

American Dietetic Association. *Nutrition Service Payment System: Report of 1984 Study Commission on Dietetics.* Chicago: American Dietetics Association, 1985.

Barker R: *The Business of Psychotherapy: Private Practice Administration for Therapists, Counselors and Social Workers.* New York: Columbia University Press, 1982.

Berne E: *Principles of Group Treatment.* New York: Grove Press, 1966.

Boisvert JM, Beaudry M, Bittar J: Assertiveness training and human communication processes. *J Cont Psych.* 1985;15(1):58–73.

Bolonda KL, et al: Strategies for increasing third-party reimbursement for nutrition counseling. *J Am Diet Assoc.* 1994;94(4):390–393.

Bronstein P: Patterns of parent-child interaction in Mexican families: A cross-cultural perspective. *Int J Behav Dev.* 1994;17(3):423–446.

Butler: *Self-Assertion for Women: A Guide to Becoming Androgynous.* San Francisco: Canfield Press, 1976.

Chenevert M: STAT: *Special Techniques in Assertiveness Training for Women in the Health Professions.* 4th ed. St. Louis: Mosby-Year Book, 1994.

Coulston AM, Rosen C: American health care reform: Implications for medical nutrition therapy. *Am J Clin Nutr.* 1994;59:1275–1276.

Curry-Bartley KR: *Dietetic Practitioner Skills: Nutrition Education, Counseling and Business Management.* New York: MacMillan, 1987.

Dainow S: Assertiveness: Believe in yourself. *Int Nurs Rev.* 1986;33(6):171–173, 177.

Delamater ARJ, McNamara JR: The social impact of assertiveness: Research findings and clinical implications. *Behav Mod.* 1986;10(2):139–158.

Dowling R: Role expansion for dietetics professionals. *J Am Diet Assoc.* 1996;96(10):1001–1002.

Eiger MR, Christie BW, Sucher KP: Change in eating attitudes: An outcome measure of patients with eating disorders. *J Am Diet Assoc.* 1996;96(1):62–64.

Florida Board of Medicine Newsletter, Summer 1996, p. 5–6.

Hauchecorne CM, Barr SI, Sork TJ: Evaluation of nutrition counseling in clinical settings: Do we make a difference? *J Am Diet Assoc.* 1994;94(4):437–440.

Ignatavicius DD, Hausman KA: *Clinical Pathways for Collaborative Practice.* Philadelphia: WB Saunders, 1995.

Josefowitz N: *Paths to Power: A Working Woman's Guide from First Job to Top Executive.* Reading, MA: Addison-Wesley, 1984.

King-Helm K, Klawitter B: *Nutrition Therapy: Advanced Counseling Skills.* Lake Dallas, TX: Helm Seminars, 1995, p. 172.

Knepflaar KJ: *In* Battin RR, Fox DR (eds): *Private Practice in Audiology and Speech Pathology.* New York: Grune & Stratton, 1978, p. 116.

Kretchmer N: Nutrition is the keystone of prevention (editorial). *Am J Clin Nutr.* 1994;60:1.

Legislative Highlights: ADA's advocacy stresses access to nutrition in health care reform and children's feeding programs. *J Am Diet Assoc.* 1994;94(5):496.

Legislative Highlights: Clinton's Health Security Act recognized value of nutrition: An update in the legislative debate over health care reform. *J Am Diet Assoc.* 1994;94(1):25–26.

Meadors BD, Rogers CR: Person-Centered Therapy. *In* Corsini RJ (ed): *Current Psychotherapies.* 3rd ed. Itasca, IL: FE Peacock Publishers, 1984.

Neville JN: Position of the American Dietetic Association: Nutrition services in health maintenance organizations and other forms of managed care. *J Am Diet Assoc.* 1993;93(10):1171–1172.

Palumbo C: Managed care is here to stay. *Ventures Newsletter of NE of ADA.* 1995;XI(3):2–3.

Pantalos DC: Home healthcare: A new worksite for dietitians monitoring nutrition support. *J Am Diet Assoc.* 1993;93(10):1146–1151.

Payne-Palacio J, Canter DD: *The Profession of Dietetics: A Team Approach.* Englewood Cliffs, NJ: Prentice-Hall, 1996, p. 177.

Phelps S, Austin N: *The Assertive Woman: A New Look.* San Luis Obispo, CA: Impact Publishers, 1987.

Rhodes KS, et al: Intensive nutrition counseling enhances outcomes of National Cholesterol Education Program dietary therapy. *J Am Diet Assoc.* 1996;96(10):1003–1010.

Sheehy G. *New Passages.* New York: Random House, 1995.

Slater J: Effecting personal effectiveness: assertiveness training for nurses. *J Adv Nurs.* 1990;15:337–356.

The American Dietetic Association: *Creating the Future: 1996–1999 Strategic Framework.* Chicago, IL: 1996, p. 2.

Weiss L: Getting past "no". *Women Therapy.* 1982;1(4):9–14.

Williams JM, Stout JK: The effect of high and low assertiveness on locus of control and health problems. *J Psych.* 1985; 119(2):169–173.

Wilson, Gallois: *Assertion and Its Social Context.* Oxford, UK: The Pergamon Press, 1993.

ADDITIONAL REFERENCES

American Dietetic Association Website: http://www.eatright.org/

American Dietetic Association National Nutrition Network: 800/877–1600 ext 4848; 900/225–5267 ($1.95/first minute, $0.95/minute thereafter).

Dawson R. *The Secrets of Power Negotiating* (audiotape). Niles, IL: Nightingale-Conant Corp, 1995; 800/323–5552.

Hill L. Women's changing work roles: Implications for the progress of the dietetic profession. *J Am Diet Assoc.* 1991;91:25–27.

Lathrop JP. *Restructuring Health Care.* San Francisco, CA: Jossey-Bass, 1994.

Lodi KJ. *Tapping Potential: Achieving What You Want with the Abilities You Already Have.* Los Angeles, CA: Kenneth Lodi, 1995.

McKenzie L. Cross-functional teams in health care organizations. *Health Care Supervisor.* 1994;12(3):1–10.

Membership in ADA's DPG Nutrition Entrepreneurs (NE). 9212 Delphi Road SW, Olympia, Washington 98512.

Pritchett P. *New Work Habits for a Radically Changing World.* Dallas, TX: Pritchett and Associates, 1994.

Rinke WJ, Finn SC. Winning strategies to excel in dietetics. *J Am Diet Assoc.* 1990;90(7):935–938.

Smith PS, Rhoades PK, Tolman NM: The seven personal habits of highly effective dietitians. *J Am Diet Assoc.* 1994;94:377–378.

INDEX

Note: Page numbers in *italics* refer to illustrations; page numbers followed by t refer to tables.